Psychosocial Adaptation to Pregnancy

Regina Lederman • Karen Weis

Psychosocial Adaptation to Pregnancy

Seven Dimensions of Maternal Role Development

Third Edition

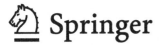 Springer

Regina Lederman
University of Texas
Galveston, TX
USA
rlederma@utmb.edu
reginalederman@yahoo.com

Karen Weis
United States Air Force
School of Aerospace
Medicine, Brooks-City Base
TX, USA
karen.weis@us.AF.MIL
afnurse87@yahoo.com

1st Ed., Prentice Hall - November 1984
2nd Ed., Churchill Livingstone (Springer Publishing) - 1 Mar 1996

ISBN 978-1-4419-0287-0 (hardcover)   e-ISBN 978-1-4419-0288-7
ISBN 978-1-4419-8175-2 (softcover)
DOI 10.1007/978-1-4419-0288-7
Springer Dordrecht Heidelberg London New York

Library of Congress Control Number: 2009933092

Printed on acid-free paper

Springer is part of Springer Science+Business Media (www.springer.com)

Preface

The subject of this book is the psychosocial development of gravid women, both primigravid and multigravid women. Seven personality dimensions, or developmental challenges, are discussed and intended to serve as a guide for understanding and assessing the gravidas' adaptation to pregnancy and expectant parenthood.

The book is an outgrowth of research projects[1] that investigated the relationship of maternal psychosocial adaptation in pregnancy to maternal anxiety and labor progress during childbirth, to prenatal and parturition obstetric complications, to newborn birthweight, and to maternal and infant postpartum adaptation. Verbatim statements made by the women who participated in the study are used throughout the text to provide examples of good and poor adaptation for each dimension. The excerpts from prenatal interviews illustrate specific conflicts and fears, as well as methods used to cope with them, which are also indicative of levels of adaptation. The chapters have been expanded to incorporate recent literature and research results in the analysis and interpretation of interview statements, with examples of good, moderate, and low maternal adaptation for each dimension.

The items on interview schedules and on a subsequently developed questionnaire were specifically designed to assess the universal aspects of each personality dimension. Questionnaire scales to assess the prenatal dimensions have consistently produced reliable and valid results over time in different cultures, socioeconomic classes, and family constellations.

Furthermore, there has been limited advancement in the development of theory or alternative theories to explicate maternal psychosocial development or adaptation during pregnancy. For these reasons, the original theoretical model and the results obtained with interview and questionnaire assessment remain current and significant to date, and are utilized in this third edition.

Research results over the past 30 years support the validity and significance of the personality dimensions. These results and an overview of each dimension are

[1] The research projects were supported by grant awards from: (1) the Division of Nursing, Bureau of Health Professions, Health Resources and Service Administration, U.S. Public Health Service, (2) the American Nurses' Foundation, (3) the Committee on Research, The University of Texas Medical Branch, (4) the Research Advisory Council of the UTMB School of Nursing, and (5) the Triservice Nursing Research Program.

presented in the Introduction (Chapter 1). The focus of Chapter 1 is twofold: (1) to present the research foundations for the psychophysiological correlates of prenatal psychosocial adaptation and the seven prenatal personality dimensions with progress in labor and birth outcomes, and particularly (2) to present the theory underlying the seven dimensions of prenatal psychosocial adaptation, which are further analyzed in the following seven chapters.

Chapters 2–8 present a content analysis of the interview responses to the seven significant prenatal personality dimensions that are predictive of pregnancy adaptation, progress in labor, birth outcomes, and postpartum maternal psychosocial adaptation, and they include: (1) Acceptance of Pregnancy, (2) Identification with a Motherhood Role, (3) Relationship with Mother, (4) Relationship with Husband, (5) Preparation for Labor, (6) (Prenatal) Fear of Pain, Helplessness, and Loss of Control in Labor, and (7) (Prenatal) Fear of Loss of Self-Esteem in Labor. There is no other comparable comprehensive, in-depth, prenatal personality research or empirical and content analysis of pregnancy-specific dimensions of maternal psychosocial adaptation to pregnancy.

Chapter 9 provides the findings and discussion of a longitudinal military research project that followed 421 wives of military service members and active duty women through each trimester of pregnancy and delivery. The chapter presents the impact of family flexibility and emotional-esteem building support from a community network on prenatal maternal psychosocial adaptation. The impact of military deployment on maternal adaptation is briefly discussed. Lastly, 113 women from the original 421 were followed through 6 months postpartum. The capability of the Prenatal Self-Evaluation Questionnaire to predict 6-month maternal postpartum satisfaction and confidence with being a mother is presented.

Chapter 10 provides a discussion of the particular developmental and adaptive characteristics of multigravid women pregnant with their second or subsequent child, in contrast to the developmental and adaptive characteristics of primigravidas, women pregnant for the first time. This chapter is a summary of findings from a longitudinal prenatal research project with multigravid women that replicated and extended the initial research project with primigravidas presented in Chapter 1, and of a subsequent large, longitudinal research project with both primigravidas and multigravidas focusing on the quantitative questionnaire assessment of psychosocial adaptation in all the three trimesters of pregnancy. Both quantitative and qualitative results are presented. The presentation of the qualitative content analysis in Chapter 10 was written with the assistance of Fran Holmes.

Chapter 11 presents methods that can be used by professional health care personnel to assess the status of gravid women on each of the personality dimensions. A questionnaire developed to serve as a parallel measure of the interview measures of the seven personality dimensions, the Prenatal Self-Evaluation Questionnaire, also is discussed in Chapter 11, and reliability and validity data of results obtained in research projects are presented. Chapter 1 focuses on early and continued research findings supporting the theory and significance of maternal adaptation to pregnancy, while Chapter 11 focuses on a presentation of psychometric data supporting the questionnaire assessment of maternal prenatal psychosocial adaptation with the Prenatal Self-Evaluation Questionnaire; the difference in the foci of Chapter 1 and Chapter 11 is not entirely precise and may be considered as a fine line rather than a sharp distinction. A section in Chapter 11 also provides recommendations for the clinical and academic researcher.

The method utilized in the original research study of psychophysiological correlates of progress in labor (in primigravidas) was a descriptive analysis based on interview responses recounted to the researcher during meetings with the women who participated in the project. The instruments used in the research project, the interview schedules, and the detailed rating scales for the assessment of personality dimensions are in Appendices A and B. The authors suggest that the readers first peruse the interview questions and the rating scales to become acquainted with the scope of inquiry and the method of assessment that underlies the content analysis of the personality dimensions presented in Chapters 2–8.

The analysis of each personality dimension and the identification of subfactors provide a theoretical framework for each developmental construct. Within this framework, it is possible to distinguish adaptive and maladaptive behavior, the manifestations of behavior, and progress in development. Thus, the text provides a model for continued study and guidance in assessment and evaluation, which can be incorporated into clinical practice and research investigations. The book also provides more than a descriptive narrative of pregnancy adaptation. It includes results and discussion of stress and anxiety in labor, progress in labor, and postpartum maternal and newborn health status. The results of the correlational analysis of the pregnancy, labor, and postpartal data in Chapters 1 and 11 support the significance of each personality dimension, and demonstrate a measure of validity for the interview schedules and the rating scale instrument, as well as the Prenatal Self-Evaluation Questionnaire, all developed to assess and evaluate the seven prenatal personality dimensions. Taken together, the interview and questionnaire assessments constitute empirically established and scientifically based methods of distinguishing maternal low, moderate, and high psychosocial adaptation to pregnancy.

A prospective design was used in the initial research project, which permitted correlational analyses of pre- and postpartum maternal adaptation. However, long-term follow-up of the gravid women, beyond 2–3 years after birth, was not possible within the scope of the project; our curiosity also was roused regarding how the women and their children fared over the years.

Fathers were not directly assessed to determine paternal adaptation. However, some light was shed on this subject by the mothers' narrative concerning their perception of paternal adaptive responses. An added section in Chapter 5 on Relationship to Husband presents a discussion of the transition to fatherhood. References on the paternal adaptive experience are provided for the readers.

Since nurses and health care professionals in a prenatal care setting have extensive contact with pregnant women, the book is primarily intended for nurse practitioners, midwives, and students in maternal and child health. The book will be especially useful to midwives who provide continuous care throughout the reproductive phases, and who will benefit from the increased knowledge and understanding provided by a theoretically informed and scientifically based standard measurement of prenatal psychosocial adaptation. This additional information will enable nurses and nurse-midwives to better understand the relationship between prenatal and parturitional maternal behavior and to provide more informed and individualized maternal care in pregnancy and childbirth. The text will aid Lamaze and other pre-natal educators in their efforts to promote pregnancy adaptation and preparation for labor. Psychologists, psychiatrists, social workers, marriage and family therapists, and professional counselors who work with the expectant family also will benefit from the content. Likewise maternity nurses in England who provide extensive psychosocial clinical and home visit services throughout pregnancy to expectant women will find the book a considerable asset to their assessments and health care delivery services. In addition, the general public can make use of the information in the book, especially considering the current emphasis in health care on self-regulation and on increasing personal health awareness. Expectant women, in par-ticular, actively seek solutions to the psychosocial challenges of pregnancy through personal reading and prenatal education. Thus, this book supplements the educa-tional focus on adaptation to the physiological processes of labor offered by child-birth preparation classes and literature.

We have reviewed and culled the literature to include the best references that are available, and some are dated, but valuable original references that have made sig-nificant contributions. This is a reflection of the state of the science and the spo-radic versus consistent development in a component of the research literature on psychosocial adaptation to pregnancy.

Thanks are due to many colleagues and graduate students who assisted in the collection of data, and especially to the women who consented to participate in the project, many of whom did so out of an altruistic concern for the welfare of other expectant mothers and their families. Those and subsequent expectant women have frequently commented on the interest and knowledge accrual of the investigators regarding the expectant women's trials and challenges, which were not assessed or acknowledged elsewhere in the health care system.

Galveston, TX   Regina Lederman
Brooks-City Base   Karen Weis

Acknowledgments

To my mother: Selma Juliet Lump Placzek for the gifts she passed on to me, and her love.

– Regina Lederman

To my husband: Michael Dean Weis for his loving devotion and support.

– Karen L. Weis

Contents

Chapter 1
Psychosocial Adaptation in Pregnancy: Assessment of Seven Dimensions of Maternal Development

1.1 Introduction

The impetus for this book originated from research on the relationship between psychosocial conflicts during pregnancy and selected complications that arise during labor. It became apparent during the interviews with expectant mothers that all the women experienced some conflict in relation to pregnancy and childbearing, and that the patterns of response to conflict could be identified as either adaptive or maladaptive. These patterns of adaptive responses were observed to be progressive in nature in that the gravid woman advanced toward an orientation to a maternal parenting role. When responses were maladaptive, the mother-to-be struggled with her ambivalence about pregnancy and motherhood, and little progress was made in role clarification in the current or in future pregnancies (based on our separate research projects with both primigravid and multigravid women).

This book is an attempt to explicate the dimensions of maternal role development that are paramount during pregnancy, and to illustrate adaptive and maladaptive responses within each dimension. The prenatal dimensions, when assessed with parallel questionnaire scale items, yield statistically reliable results with numerous different populations, including multiethnic, lower socioeconomic, single and/or partnered women, employed and unemployed women, and teenage gravidas, as well as gravid women over 40 years. The questionnaire scales for the assessment of the prenatal dimensions were constructed to measure broad or universal components of each personality construct, and the consistent reliability results with diverse populations (presented in Chapters 1 and 11) and in several foreign countries provide evidence of the extent to which this goal was achieved, and of the utility of the original definition of each dimension as a personality construct. The results suggest that the framework of experience, as measured by these personality dimensions, is the same for many populations of gravid women on this continent and others. Therefore, the original work serves as a useful foundation to explicate each prenatal dimension and to relate replicated and new work.

Each of the developmental dimensions may be conceived of as adaptive challenges that incur some anxiety, and which occur and can be measured on a continuum from

R. Lederman and K. Weis, *Psychosocial Adaptation to Pregnancy*,
DOI 10.1007/978-1-4419-0288-7_1, © Springer Science+Business Media, LLC 2009

low to high conflict and anxiety. The prenatal dimensions analyzed in the following chapters are:

1. The gravida's acceptance of and adaptation to pregnancy. (Chapter 2)
2. The gravida's development in formulating a parental role and relationship with the coming child. (Chapter 3)
3. The gravida's past and present relationship with her mother. (Chapter 4)
4. The impact of the gravida's relationship with her husband or partner to her adaptation to pregnancy. (Chapter 5)
5. Knowledge of and reasonable (prenatal) preparation by the gravida for the events of labor. (Chapter 6)
6. The gravida's (prenatal) anticipation of mechanisms for coping with fears involving pain, helplessness, and loss of control in labor. (Chapter 7)
7. The way(s) the gravida copes with (prenatal) fears involving loss of self-esteem in labor. (Chapter 8)

Three chapters provide additional pertinent research results. Chapter 9 presents prenatal psychosocial adaptation processes in military women and wives of military men in four branches of the United States military; predictive relationships to birth outcomes—length of gestation and newborn birth weight, and to postpartum adaptation. Chapter 10 presents the specific adaptive responses of multigravid women; contrasts with primigravid responses are examined. Chapter 11 presents additional results to support the reliability and validity of the assessment instruments in predicting to labor events and outcomes, and to postpartal adaptive responses. Recommendations for conducting interview and questionnaire assessments are also provided.

Several of the prenatal developmental dimensions cited were found to correlate with the measures of progress in labor in the original research project conducted by Lederman, Lederman, Work, and McCann (1978, 1979). Furthermore, some prenatal dimensions also correlated with the assessed health status of the fetus and the newborn in the immediate postpartum period (Lederman, Lederman, Work, & McCann, 1981). In a subsequent project with multigravid women, several of these research results were replicated and additional results were presented. Prenatal personality dimensions were again related to the woman's postpartal adaptation to her expanded motherhood role (Lederman & Lederman, 1987). Other research projects with both primigravidas and multigravidas explored prenatal trimester differences and ethnic differences in adaptation to pregnancy (Lederman, Harrison, & Worsham, 1992; Lederman & Miller, 1998), and associations between prenatal psychosocial adaptation and complications in pregnancy and labor (Lederman, Weis, Camune, & Mian, 2002). Thus, taken as a set, the gravid woman's status on these prenatal development dimensions is predictive of progress in labor, complications in labor, birth outcomes, and postpartum adjustment to parenthood. Some differences in emphasis are given to particular dimensions for different types of predictions.

Data from the research study with primigravidas have been replicated in subsequent projects remaining relevant today and thus form the foundation for the chapters that follow. A summary of the relevant theory, design, and results of the research project is provided in this chapter to help the reader understand the foundational relationships among the variables investigated in the study. Subsequent Chapters 2–8 serve the following purposes:

1. To identify and describe the major components of each prenatal personality dimension.
2. To provide descriptive detail based on scientific results of the type and extent of conflict and adaptation, with illustrations from the responses of primigravid women.
3. To identify the correlates of high, moderate, and low conflict and anxiety and the factors influencing conflict resolution.
4. To provide instruments for the assessment of the seven dimensions of prenatal development.

Based on additional studies conducted with both primigravid and multigravid women, this revised third edition includes an expansion of Chapters 1–11 in order to present results from pregnancy and labor research and additional research projects. A chapter also has been added that focuses on assessment of the psychosocial adaptation in military women.

1.2   Foundation Research Projects for Theory Development of the Seven Dimensions of Maternal Prenatal Adaptation

In this section we present both published and recent unpublished research results.

1.2.1   Maternal Psychological and Physiological Correlates of Progress in Labor and Fetal/Newborn Health

1.2.1.1   Theory and Design

The prospective psychophysiological project was designed to investigate three main research questions:

1. Are developmental conflicts in pregnancy predictive of maternal anxiety and plasma catecholamine and cortisol levels in labor?
2. Are prenatal developmental conflicts (or personality dimensions) related to prolonged labor and fetal-newborn health status (perinatal cardiopulmonary function)?
3. Is maternal prenatal adaptation, as measured by the seven prenatal personality dimensions, predictive of postpartum adaptation? (These results are presented and discussed in Chapter 11).

We first present the initial and subsequent research project results that serve as a foundation for the theory pertaining to prenatal psychosocial adaptation and the seven dimensions of prenatal maternal adaptation that are the focus of this third edition textbook. We also present additional research results and references relevant to the relationship between prenatal maternal anxiety and birth outcomes.

Psychophysiological Relationships Regarding Biochemical Stress-Related Substances and Reproductive Outcomes

Epinephrine, norepinephrine, and cortisol are recognized in the research literature as stress-related biochemical measures. Exogenous epinephrine administration during labor results in decreased uterine activity; it also has been observed to result in fetal heart rate (FHR) deceleration, attributable to arterial vasoconstriction and decreased blood flow and oxygen transport to the fetus (Carter & Olin, 1972; Costa et al., 1988; Eskes, 1973; Falconer & Lake, 1982; Jones & Greiss, 1982; Marshall, 1977; Ohno et al., 1986; Paulick, Kastendieck, & Wernze, 1985; Pohjavuori, Rovamo, Laatikainen, Kariniemi, & Pettersson, 1986; Roman-Ponce, Thatcher, Caton, Barron, & Wilcox, 1978; Rosenfeld, Barton, & Meschia, 1976). High levels of epinephrine, in association with high levels of prenatal stress, have also been implicated in precipitating preterm labor (Institute of Medicine, 1985) and low birth weight (Hobel et al., 1995). Norepinephrine has been associated with increased or incoordinate uterine activity (Zuspan, Cibils, & Pose, 1962) and fetal stress (Paulick et al., 1985; Pohjavuori et al., 1986), and cortisol levels have been shown to correlate with the length of labor (Burns, 1976; Oakey, 1975) and the rate of cervical dilation (Tuimala, Kauppila, & Haapalahti, 1975; Ohrlander, Gennser, & Eneroth, 1976). Increases of corticotrophin-releasing hormone in the hypothalamus in stressful situations inhibit the release of oxytocin, which may disrupt parturition as well as lactation (Laatikainen, 1991). Infants, both human and primate, also show effects from stressed pregnancy (Herrenkohl, 1986; Lederman, 1986). Infants from chronically stressed primate pregnancies show impaired performance, specifically greater irritability, poorer motor coordination, impaired balance, and shorter attention spans (Schneider & Coe, 1993; Schneider, Coe, & Lubach, 1992). In a review of the literature Herrenkohl (1986) reported mounting evidence that maternal prenatal stress adversely affects the subsequent reproductive behavior and physiology of rat offspring, with stressed animals showing significantly higher percentages of stillbirths and neonatal deaths. In human subjects, problem pregnancies resulting from marital difficulties and ambivalence about having a child were associated with postpartum depression and lower ratings on maternal–infant interaction (Field, Sandberg, Garcia, Vega-Lahr, Goldstein, & Guy, 1985). And Ward (1991) provides evidence to show that chronic prenatal stress and anxiety, associated with unplanned pregnancy, rejection of pregnancy, and family discord, are risk factors for the later development of childhood psychopathology.

1.2.1.2   Methods

Thirty-two expectant, married, primigravid women, aged 20–32 years, and with no medical or obstetrical complications participated in the initial 4-year project. Their educational levels ranged from completion of high school to completion of graduate studies, with most participants and their husbands (80%) having had some college education. Thirty of the participants were Caucasian, and two were African-American. Various religions were represented in the study population. The socioeconomic status of the participants was predominantly middle class. The names of all participants who took part in the project have been changed to provide anonymity. The prenatal personality dimensions presented in Chapters 2–8 were based on a content analysis of the interview data collected from the sample of gravid women in this project.

Three semistructured interviews were held during the last trimester of pregnancy to obtain demographic data, and the measures of psychosocial variables relevant to pregnancy and labor (quality of the relationship with the husband, mother, and father; acceptance of the pregnancy; identification with a motherhood role; the amount and kind of preparation for labor; and the anticipation of fears of pain, helplessness, loss of control, and self-esteem in labor, reproductive adequacy, injury, and death in labor). The available psychological, psychosocial, and psychoanalytic literature and Lederman's obstetrical clinical experience served as the basis for selection and development of the prenatal psychosocial variables. The interview schedules for assessment of the seven personality dimensions are presented in Appendix A, and were developed to provide content on each of these variables; they were reviewed by several nurses and psychologists to enhance content validity.

Rating scales were developed to quantify the data obtained from interviews. Ratings were based primarily on data obtained during interviews. The expectant mothers were asked to maintain a diary and dream record. These records were incorporated into the assessments to the extent that they were elaborated on and used to elucidate responses in interviews. All psychosocial variables were evaluated on a scale of 1–5 by the first author, R. Lederman, and additionally by a trained research assistant to determine interrater reliability. The median correlation obtained for the two sets of ratings was 0.93. Low scores for each variable indicated low conflict or fear and high scores indicated high conflict or fear.

A measure of trait (general) anxiety in pregnancy and state (present) anxiety in labor was obtained with the Spielberger, Gorsuch, and Lushene (1970) State-Trait Anxiety Inventory (STAI). All the women attended childbirth preparation classes, and all received health supervision in a large university-affiliated health care setting. Thus, several different measures of maternal anxiety and stress were repeatedly obtained both in pregnancy and subsequently in labor, as will be noted later. We used a multidimensional and multimethod approach which has been strongly advocated in literature reviews conducted in this field of research (Lobel, 1994; Lobel & Dunkel-Shetter, 1990).

Measures of duration of labor were obtained in two phases: (1) active phase or Phase 2 labor: from 3- to 10-cm cervical dilatation, and (2) second-stage or Phase 3 labor: from full cervical dilatation to delivery. At the onset of each phase of labor, measures were obtained on anxiety, plasma biochemical substances (Lederman et al., 1978; Lederman, McCann, Work, & Huber, 1977), and uterine activity. Taped records of uterine activity were obtained from a uterine monitor and two consecutive Montevideo units at the onset of each phase of labor were computed from them. Montevideo units are the product of the intensity and frequency of contractions in a 15-min interval. Based on information provided in the patient record and from FHR tape recordings, which were reviewed by an obstetrician and perinatologist (Dr. Bruce Work), the principal investigator (R. L.) assigned ratings to all recordings to provide separate measures of FHR patterns for Phases 2 and 3 of labor. FHR was coded from 0 to 3, based on evidence of normal or deviant FHR response patterns. FHR pattern was coded as follows: 0 = no FHR deceleration; 2 = mild to moderate late and variable FHR deceleration; 3 = severe variable and late deceleration.

1.2.1.3   Results

Data in Labor

Figure 1.1 summarizes the significant relationships of the measures in Phase 2 or active phase labor. The anxiety measure was obtained within a few minutes of the onset of the phase by asking participants to read or listen to short questionnaire statements; the response to how well the statement described their feelings was indicated on a scale from low to high.

As Fig. 1.1 indicates, the self-report anxiety measure had a significant positive correlation with epinephrine ($r = 0.60$) and cortisol ($r = 0.59$), but not with norepinephrine. The negative relationship of epinephrine with the Montevideo units ($r = -0.64$) and the positive relationship of epinephrine with length of active labor ($r = 0.60$) indicate that as epinephrine (a biochemical measure of anxiety) increases, uterine contractile activity in labor decreases and the duration of labor is prolonged. Cortisol, another well-established biochemical measure of stress and anxiety, showed a moderate, negative correlation of $r = -0.44$ with uterine activity, indicating a relationship with uterine activity similar to that of epinephrine. Several patterns of relationships similar to those in Phase 2 were observed in Phase 3 labor.

Later measures of uterine activity in Phase 3 (second-stage labor) also were observed to correlate negatively with the earlier Phase 2 measures of both cortisol ($r = -0.42$) and anxiety ($r = -0.38$), and positively with norepinephrine ($r = 0.32$). In addition, the anxiety measure in Phase 2 correlated positively with the type of delivery, demonstrating that higher anxiety in early labor was associated with deliveries that required the assistance of low or midforceps, while low anxiety was associated with spontaneous vaginal deliveries.

Overall, the specific results and correlational patterns support the theory that anxiety is related to progress in labor–that is, to both uterine contractile activity and the duration of labor. Moreover, the data suggest that anxiety manifested in early labor is predictive of progress in second-stage labor and of the likelihood of a forceps-assisted delivery.

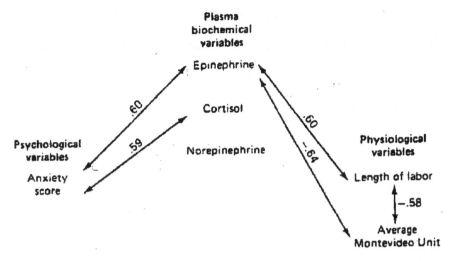

Fig. 1.1 Relationships among Phase 2 labor variables with five subjects deleted. Numbers adjacent to arrows are correlation coefficients. Variables not joined by an arrow showed no significant correlation. All correlation coefficients have $p < 0.01$, except -0.58 where $p < 0.05$ (Data from Lederman et al., 1978.)

Interrelationships Among the Variables During Pregnancy

Examination of the intercorrelations of the interview variables in pregnancy served to identify a cluster of eight moderately interrelated variables (see Table 1.1). The highest relationships were among the four core variables in the cluster: fears of pain, helplessness, and loss of control (later combined into one factor), and loss of self-esteem. Four additional variables: history of psychological counseling or psychiatric treatment, identification with a motherhood role, relationship with mother, and acceptance of pregnancy, have some relationships to the four core variables and to each other; the relationship suggests they are part of a cluster and separate from the other variables.

There generally was a low relationship between the variables in Table 1.1 and demographic variables, such as age and education of the expectant woman and her husband. Preparation for labor correlated positively ($r = 0.51$) with relationship with husband and relationship with mother. These correlations suggest that relationships with significant others (i.e., the subwoman's mother, and particularly her husband) were important factors influencing childbirth preparation. Preparation for labor had a moderate correlation to fear of pain ($r = 0.46$), but low correlations to fears of loss of control, loss of self-esteem, or helplessness in labor, and are not further presented in table format. For this reason, relationship to husband and preparation for labor were retained as part of the prenatal personality dimensions in the subsequent development of the Prenatal Self-Evaluation Questionnaire.

Table 1.1 Intercorrelations among Prenatal Development Dimensions in Primigravid Women ($n = 32$)

Prenatal dimensions	ACCPREG	RELMOTH	IDMORO	HELP	CONTR	PAIN	S-EST	PSYHX
Acceptance of pregnancy (ACCPREG)	0.33	0.36	0.35	0.43	0.37	0.33	0.11	
Relationship with mother (RELMOTH)		0.62	0.33	0.40	0.42	0.51	0.46	
Identification with a motherhood role (IDMORO)			0.58	0.70	0.47	0.62	0.48	
Fear of helplessness (HELP)				0.80	0.59	0.64	0.38	
Fear of loss of control (CONTR)					0.52	0.70	0.42	
Fear of pain in labor (PAIN)						0.58	0.54	
Fear of lots of self-esteem (S-EST)							0.35	
History of psychological counseling or psychiatric treatment (PSYHX)								

Data from Lederman et al., 1979. Copyright by Nursing Research. Reprinted with permission

Trait or general anxiety in last trimester pregnancy was measured by the trait scale of the Spielberger STAI and was the first scale measured in interviews with participants. For the 32 participants in the study, the mean and standard deviation on the trait scale are comparable to the mean and standard deviation reported in the STAI manual (Spielberger et al., 1970) for the normative sample of 231 female undergraduates. The trait anxiety scale had only low positive relationships with other variables (and are not presented). Correlations of the Table 1.1 variables with the remaining psychologic or demographic variables in most cases were only low to moderate, and also are not presented.

Interrelationships Between Pregnancy and Labor

Table 1.2 shows the correlations of prenatal variables that were significantly related to Phase 2 (3–6 cm cervical dilatation) labor measures of anxiety and progress in labor. The data show that the seven prenatal variables in Table 1.1 had consistent negative correlations with the Montevideo units and consistent positive correlations with length of labor, most of which were statistically significant. The correlations, similar to those reported in Fig. 1.1 during labor between anxiety-based measures

Table 1.2 Correlations of Prenatal Dimensions with Phase 2 Labor Variables In Primigravidas ($n = 27$)

Phase 2 labor variables

Prenatal psychosocial variables[a]	Montevideo unit 1 (mmHg)	Montevideo unit 2 (mmHg)	Plasma epinephrine (pg/mL)	Plasma norepinephrine (pg/mL)	Plasma cortisol (ng/mL)	State anxiety score	Duration of labor (Hours)
Acceptance of pregnancy	−0.70**	−0.52*	0.59**	−0.09	0.21	0.39*	0.58**
Identification with a motherhood role	−0.59**	−0.53*	0.37*	−0.20	0.15	0.34	0.41*
Relationship with mother	−0.53*	−0.32	0.07	−0.15	0.05	0.16	0.30
Fears about labor							
Loss of control	−0.67**	−0.71**	0.19	−0.16	0.37*	0.21	0.41*
Helplessness	−0.49*	−0.60**	0.07	−0.31	0.40*	0.35*	0.28
Pain	−0.60**	−0.43	0.30	−0.16	0.18	0.40*	0.48**
Loss of self-esteem	−0.66**	−0.66**	0.31	−0.26	0.10	0.33	0.31

Note: Of the 32 subjects, 5 received early labor medications that could affect the biochemical measures and duration of labor and were therefore deleted from this analysis. The remaining 27 subjects were included in the analysis. Some data are missing for some of the variables. For the precise n for each correlated pair, see Lederman et al. (1979)

*$p < 0.05$; one-tailed

**$p < 0.01$; one-tailed

[a]Montevideo units 1 and 2: uterine activity calculated in Montevideo units for the first and second 15-min interval in a half-hour period at the onset of labor; State Anxiety Score: the State Scale of the Spielberger State-Trait Anxiety Inventory; Duration of labor: from 3 to 10 cm cervical dilatation

Data from Lederman et al. (1979). Reprinted with permission

and progress in labor, indicate that conflicts and fears identified during pregnancy were associated with longer labor due to lower uterine contractile activity during labor (Lederman et al., 1979).

Four prenatal psychosocial variables showed correlations of 0.30 or higher with epinephrine in Phase 2; the highest relationship was between conflict in the acceptance of pregnancy and epinephrine. There were two significant relationships to cortisol but none to norepinephrine. All relationships between the psychosocial variables and norepinephrine were negative, as was expected. Five prenatal variables had correlations that were above 0.30 with respect to state anxiety in Phase 2 labor. Three of these correlations were significant. Of the prenatal psychosocial measures, four of the positive correlations with length of labor were significant, two at the $p = 0.01$ level.

Among the seven psychosocial variables, acceptance of pregnancy produced the most significant relationships to the Phase 2 labor variables, with correlations of -0.70 and -0.52 with the Montevideo units (uterine activity), 0.58 with length of labor, 0.39 with anxiety, and 0.59 with epinephrine. Montevideo units were measured in two consecutive 15-min intervals. Identification with a motherhood role also was significantly related to the Montevideo units, epinephrine, and duration of labor. The significant and consistent pattern of correlations suggests that psychological factors in pregnancy are predictive of progress in labor and provide support for the theory that conflict, fear, and anxiety during pregnancy are related to and predictive of biochemical measures and progress in labor.

Other prenatal variables were measured, but few showed significant relationships to the measures of progress in labor. It is noteworthy that trait anxiety measured during pregnancy generally had low correlations with other prenatal measures, as well as with the length of labor. It appears, therefore, that trait anxiety is not as predictive of the specific fears concerning labor, that were revealed in prenatal interviews, or of the duration of labor. Other researchers, however, most of whom have used larger sample sizes, have found significant correlations with length of labor and the broader prenatal measure of state anxiety (Crandon, 1979; Falorni, Fornasarig, & Stefanile, 1979; Norbeck & Anderson, 1989b; Zax, Sameroff, & Farnum, 1975) or trait anxiety (Beck, Siegel, Davidson, Kormeier, Breitenstein, & Hall, 1980; Levi, Lundberg, Hanson, & Frankenhaeuser, 1989; Pilowsky, 1972).

In our study, only the measures of conflict in the relationship with the husband and preparation for labor showed a significant correlation with length of labor; in addition, these two factors were moderately related. A closer examination of the prenatal interview ratings showed that five participants who had received sedatives and tranquilizers in early labor were among those that showed the highest conflict ratings in the relationship with their husbands as well as poor preparation for labor. Thus, the data demonstrated that a poor relationship with the husband was associated with poor preparation for labor, and that these factors were predictive of early admission to the labor unit and reliance on medication during labor.

In Phase 3 labor (Stage 2 or descent phase) fewer consistent relationships were noted between the prenatal and labor variables. Several women had received analgesia prior to this point in labor, and almost all received some form of anesthesia by the time of delivery. Half of the study sample was delivered by forceps. It is probable that these events–the administration of analgesia and anesthesia and forceps intervention–affected the measures of progress in labor. Nevertheless, all seven psychosocial variables had negative relationships to uterine activity indicating that psychosocial conflict also was related to lower uterine activity in Phase 3. The highest relationship was observed between uterine activity and fear of loss of control ($r = -0.40$). Of particular interest were the significant relationships of the two variables, identification with a motherhood role and acceptance of pregnancy, with duration of labor in Phase 3 ($r = 0.32$ and $r = 0.36$, respectively); these were the only two psychosocial factors to correlate consistently and significantly with duration of labor in Phases 2 and 3, and thus may have had the greatest impact on progress throughout labor.

Measures of FHR response in labor and Apgar scores for newborn respiratory-cardiac adjustment were obtained for the infants. Of 31 FHR patterns for Phase 2, 24 were classified as normal, 3 as early deceleration, and 4 as variable or late deceleration. The FHR pattern ratings had significant negative correlations of -0.50 ($p < 0.01$) with the Apgar 1-min score and -0.47 ($p < 0.01$) with the 5-min score, indicating a relationship between fetal distress in labor and immediate newborn cardiopulmonary response at birth (Lederman et al., 1981). The two sets of Apgar scores had a significant positive correlation ($r = 0.67$, $p < 0.01$).

Maternal epinephrine, measured at the onset of active labor, had a significant positive correlation with the FHR pattern during Phase 2 labor ($r = 0.37$, $p < 0.05$), suggesting that women with high epinephrine levels were more likely to have fetuses that experienced abnormal FHR deceleration than those women with low epinephrine levels. Maternal anxiety, which had a relatively high correlation with the concurrent measure of epinephrine ($r = 0.57$, $p < 0.01$), also was significantly correlated with the FHR pattern ($r = 0.33$, $p < 0.05$).

Reviews of the research literature (Levinson & Shnider, 1979; Myers & Myers, 1979) have offered evidence of the detrimental effect of maternal excitement or anxiety on FHR and newborn health status. Elevated maternal epinephrine level, resulting from stress, has been shown to affect blood flow to the fetus through an alpha-adrenergic constrictive effect on the uterine vasculature (Roman-Ponce et al., 1978; Rosenfeld et al., 1976).

Two of the maternal pregnancy variables, conflict in the acceptance of pregnancy and fear of loss of self-esteem in labor, also had significant correlations with the Apgar 5-min score ($r = -0.38$, $p < 0.05$, and $r = -0.30$, $p < 0.05$, respectively). The two pregnancy variables had significant positive correlations with measures of anxiety and epinephrine in labor and consistently correlated in a negative direction with the newborn Apgar scores. Another repeated measures study of prenatal support in 129 low-income women (Collins, Dunkel-Schetter, Lobel & Scrimshaw, 1993) found that pregnant women who received more prenatal support had better progress in labor and also delivered newborns who had higher 5-min Apgar ratings; in particular, support which was task, material, or informational in nature appeared to be most the significant in predicting Apgar scores. Likewise, Pagel, Smilkstein, Regen, and

Montano (1990) found significant correlations between measures of state anxiety at 21- and 36-week gestation and 5-min Apgar scores at birth.

A subsequent 5-year project, with a subject sample of 73 multigravid women, was conducted to determine whether these findings could be replicated and to investigate additional research questions. Specifically, the sample size was increased and questionnaires were written to assess prenatal and postnatal maternal adaptation, and to supplement interview assessment of the prenatal personality dimensions. Measures of maternal anxiety and FHR in labor were expanded. In addition, postpartum maternal adaptation was assessed after delivery and again at 6–8 weeks, to determine whether maternal prenatal development was predictive of the gravida's actual adjustment to her motherhood role.

The women participating in this project were 20–42 years old, married, and had normal obstetrical histories in the current and previous pregnancies. The project was similarly conducted, except that Phase 1 of labor was from 3 to 6 cm and Phase 2 from 7 to 10 cm cervical dilation. The measure of anxiety in labor was revised to assess anxiety about labor specifically. Three separate anxiety factors were identified upon cluster factor analysis and were measured by patient self-report at the onset of each phase of labor. The three anxiety subscales were: (1) maternal coping behavior during and between contractions (COPING), (2) concerns about a safe maternal and fetal outcome (SAFETY), and (3) fears concerning pain in labor (PAIN). The internal consistency of the three anxiety scales, as measured by Cronbach's alpha, ranged from 0.7 to 0.9 for all measures in Phases 1 and 2 of labor. In addition, a nurse–researcher unobtrusively rated observed stress of each woman prior to her self-report of anxiety. The rating included assessments of the women's stress responses and somatic reactions, and their general appearance and behavior during and between contractions. FHR deceleration patterns were defined and rated on a scale of 1–3, with "1" indicating no or very low deviation from normal and "3" indicating severely abnormal patterns. Since this was a normal sample of women, only 13 fetuses in Phase 1 labor and 27 in Phase 2 had patterns of FHR deceleration.

The results for relationships among the variables in labor are shown in Table 1.3. The results support and add to those of the prior project with primigravid subjects.

The mean duration of labor in Phase 1 (previously designated as Phase 2) was 2.7 hrs. The results show that higher epinephrine and norepinephrine levels, measured at the onset of Phase 1, were significantly associated with a longer duration of Phase 1 labor ($r = 0.29$ and 0.42, respectively) and lower uterine activity ($r = -0.26$ and 0.40, respectively). Anxiety Scale 2, on maternal concerns about safety for herself and the infant, also was significantly related to duration of labor ($r = 0.34$) and to FHR ($r = 0.39$), indicating that higher maternal anxiety at the onset of labor was associated with longer Phase 1 labor and greater FHR deceleration, or fetal distress. Moreover, several relationships among measures were obtained when the onset of Phase 1 labor variables was correlated with subsequent FHR in Phase 2. Significant relationships were found between epinephrine ($r = 0.34$), and an observed stress scale rating ($r = 0.26$), Anxiety Scale 1: COPING ($r = 0.25$), Anxiety Scale 2: SAFETY in Phase 1 and FHR in Phase 2. The results indicate that higher anxiety in labor is associated with FHR deceleration patterns in the subsequent

Phase 2 of labor. The results further support the findings that maternal anxiety is related to duration of labor and fetal well-being. A lengthier discussion of related research findings is presented in another publication (Lederman, Lederman, Work, & McCann, 1985).

Further analysis of the relationships of the prenatal dimensions, using the interview ratings and a prenatal questionnaire with parallel scales (presented in Chapter 11), with the anxiety measures in labor showed the following relationships. Preparation for labor, in both the interview ($r = 0.49$, $p < 0.01$) and questionnaire ($r = 0.34$, $p < 0.01$) measures were related to maternal anxiety about coping during labor. Prenatal concerns about well-being and pain anticipated in labor were related to maternal fears of safety during labor. In findings presented in the paragraphs above, it was shown that maternal concerns about safety were associated with a longer duration of labor, as well as with deviant FHR deceleration patterns. The same prenatal fears concerning pain and well-being were correlated with fear of pain in labor. However, a multiple regression analysis showed that a pregnancy variable cluster containing Acceptance of Pregnancy, Identification of a Motherhood Role, and Relationships with Mother and Husband was the highest predictor of fear of pain in labor. A more extensive presentation and discussion of the relationships between the prenatal dimensions and the anxiety measures in labor is presented in Chapter 11. Additional research results supporting the reliability and validity of the prenatal instruments are also presented in Chapter 11.

In summary, data from the initial two projects suggest that unresolved conflicts and fears during pregnancy are predictive of fetal-newborn health status as well as progress in labor, due to their association with elevated anxiety and epinephrine levels during labor. The results highlight the significance of psychosocial development and adaptation during pregnancy, and underscore a need for a better understanding of the challenges and conflicts of expectant parenthood.

1.2.2   Relationship of Maternal Prenatal Psychosocial Adaptation and Family Functioning to Pregnancy Outcomes

This research project sought to determine relationships of prenatal personality dimensions and family functioning with pregnancy outcomes: length of gestation, newborn weight, newborn Apgar scores, and complications in pregnancy and labor.

1.2.2.1   Background and Theory

Significant differences in the outcomes of pregnancy for women experiencing high prenatal state anxiety and psychosocial or developmental conflict have been reported in the research literature (DaCosta, Brender, & Larouche, 1998; Paarlberg,

Vingerhoets, Passchier, Dekker, Heinen, & van Geijn, 1999; Wadhwa, Porto, Garite, Chicz-DeMet, & Sandman, 1998; Dole, Savitz, Hertz-Picciotto, Siega-Riz, McMahon, & Buekens, 2003; Jesse, Seaver, & Wallace, 2003; Pryor et al., 2003; Ruiz, Fullerton, & Dudley, 2003) and reviews of literature (Fogel & Lewallen, 1995; Lederman, 1984, 1995). Substantial empirical evidence also indicates that high levels of maternal stress are consistently and deleteriously related to length of gestation (Lederman et al., 1978, 1979). For antepartum complications, high levels of life-change stress and maternal anxiety increase a woman's risk of reporting at least one complication during pregnancy. DaCosta, Larouche, Dritsa, and Brender (1999) found that women who reported higher levels of state anxiety, daily hassles, and pregnancy-specific stress beginning in first trimester, subsequently reported gestational complications. Leeners, Neumaier-Wagner, Kuse, Stiller, and Rath (2007) impressively showed that emotional stress during pregnancy was associated with a 1.6-fold increased risk for hypertensive disease in pregnancy. Wadhwa, Sandman, Porto, Dunkel-Schetter, and Garite (1993) found significant relationships between life-event stress and infant birth weight, and between a measure of pregnancy-related anxiety (adapted from Lederman's measures, 1984) and gestational age at birth; both results occurred independent of subjects' biomedical risk. Wadhwa (2005) in a review of the literature concluded that there is a significant and independent role for prenatal maternal stress and anxiety in the etiology of preterm birth (PTB) outcomes. Peacock, Bland, and Anderson (1995) reported significant relationships of PTB with lower social class, single marital status, and little contact with neighbors. Other researchers and reviewers also have found an association between maternal stress/anxiety and preterm uterine contractions (Facchinetti, Ottolini, Fazzio, Rigatelli, & Volpe, 2007) and PTB (Hedegaard, Henrihen, Secher, Hatch, & Sabroe, 1995; Nordentoft et al., 1996; Mancuso, Dunkel-Schetter, Rini, Roesch, & Hobel, 2004; Orr, Reiter, Blazer, & Sherman, 2007). Paarlberg, Vingerhoets, Passchier, Dekker, and van Geijn (1995) concluded that the most consistent finding in their review of the literature was the relationship between PTB and highly stressful or major life events.

The predictors of low birth weight appear to have a greater association with already altered physical states. Paarlberg et al. (1999) found that first trimester smoking, severity of daily stressors, and depressive mood were significant risk factors, as well as maternal height, weight, and educational level. Dejin-Karlsson, Hanson, Ostergren, Lindgren, Sjoberg, and Marsal (2000) also found that first trimester psychosocial resources influenced intrauterine growth and the risk of giving birth to a small-for-gestational-age infant; these factors were independent of background, lifestyle, and biological risk factors. Thus, prior studies suggest that maternal anxiety and coping responses have more associations with preterm labor, whereas smoking and other physical conditions (height, weight, hypertension), and persistent chronic stress or major life stress may be more consistently related to low birth weight, although these are relative rather than precise determinants. Researchers consistently found that first and third trimester measures of psychosocial status are reliable predictors of pregnancy outcomes.

Social support also has been examined in the research literature in relation to birth outcomes. Constructs of social support have included network size, types of support (e.g., emotional, instrumental), and the specific persons offering support. Lieberman (1986) found that women received most support from their partner/ husband and their (the women's) mothers, and these persons also provided most types of support. He underscored the centrality of the marital or partner relationship as a critical source of support. Lieberman suggested focusing measurement of social support on those persons closest to the woman (i.e., her partner and/or her mother) vs. other extended support systems. Several investigators attest to the importance of kin relationships to pregnancy outcomes, particularly of marital or partner support (Fogel & Lewallen, 1995; Longo, Kruse, LeFevre, Schramm, Stockbauer, & Howell, 1999). In a review of literature by Hoffman and Hatch (1996), intimate support from a partner or family member appeared to improve fetal growth, even for women with little life stress, and the association appeared stronger among lower-income women. Dejin-Karlsson et al. (2000) reported that lack of social stability, social participation, and emotional and instrumental support increased the mother's likelihood of giving birth to small-for-gestational-age infants. In another study (Kalil, Gruber, Conley, & Sytniac, 1993), women who were married, or had an emotional confidante or supportive husbands, reported lower state anxiety. Majewski (1986) further reported that maternal marital satisfaction correlated with ease of transition to the maternal role.

Studies on socially supportive community intervention during pregnancy suggest that such support may have near-term and long-term beneficial maternal-child effects. A home-visit program by registered nurses to African-American pregnant women with inadequate social support was effective in substantially reducing the rate of low birth weight (Norbeck, DeJoseph, & Smith, 1996). In another study (Oakley, Hickey, Rajan, & Rigby, 1996), pregnant women who received social support from midwives had fewer very low birth weight infants, and other favorable maternal-child health outcomes. At a 7-year follow-up, there were still significant health and development benefits for the children, as well as for the mothers' physical and psychosocial health. Another supportive nurse home-visitation program (Olds, Henderson, Kitzman, Eckenrode, Cole, & Tatelbaum, 1998) yielded beneficial maternal-child results as much as 15 years later, including improvement in women's health behaviors and the quality of child caregiving.

Prenatal personality dimensions, as previously discussed, also have been related to higher plasma epinephrine, lower uterine contractility, a longer duration of labor, and increased FHR deceleration during labor in normal primigravid and multigravid women (Lederman et al., 1978, 1979, 1985; Lederman, 1996). Other research findings shed additional light on the significance of maternal acceptance of pregnancy or anxiety related to unmarried status and unwanted pregnancy. Sable, Stockbauer, Schramm, and Land (1990); Albrecht, Miller, and Clarke (1994); and Gazmararian et al. (1995) report that women who are poor, and who had an unwanted pregnancy and more prenatal stress also had inadequate prenatal care. Women with unwanted or mistimed pregnancies reported higher rates of physical violence, and they accounted for 70% of the women who reported physical violence (Gazmararian et al., 1995). Myhrman (1988) found that women who reported at birth that they did not want their infants were more likely to have lower birth weight newborns and higher rates of infant mortality. Bustan and Coker (1994) also report that parents with an unwanted pregnancy had more than a twofold-increased risk of neonatal death. Retrospective prenatal chart review by Ward (1991) showed that children who developed psychopathology were more likely to be born to mothers who were unmarried and had unwanted children. Thus, conflict and anxiety regarding acceptance of pregnancy may have far-reaching health effects, including low birth weight, neonatal mortality, and maternal physical abuse. Such abuse also is associated with maternal depression, anxiety, low prenatal weight gain, infection, and anemia (McFarlane, Parker, & Soeken, 1996a, 1996b).

Pertaining to motherhood role identification, two studies (Fonagy, Steele, & Steele, 1991; Williams et al., 1987) indicate that maternal attachment and parenting confidence showed consistent and stable responses when measured across prenatal and postpartum periods. Similar results were reported by Lederman (1996) and Deutsch, Ruble, Fleming, Brooks-Gunn, & Stangor, (1988. Deutsch et al. (1988) also found that the woman's relationship with her mother during pregnancy strongly correlated with self-definition of her maternal role. In a multiethnic sample of 689 gravid women (Lederman et al., 1992), higher anxiety about motherhood role was significantly related to lower newborn birth weight.

Family Functioning also appears related to pregnancy adaptation and birth outcomes. Ramsey, Abell, and Baker (1986) showed that family structure and family functioning are significantly and independently related to birth weight. Women living in dysfunctional families (Olson, Sprenkle, & Russell, 1979; Olson, Russell, & Sprenkle, 1983) had the greatest risk of having a lower birth weight infant, while married women living with their husbands had the least risk. A subsequent study (Abell, Baker, Clover, & Ramsey, 1991) also found a negative relationship between family functioning and birth weight. In another study (Reeb, Graham, Zyzanski, & Kitson, 1987) family functioning emerged as the only biopsychosocial predictor of intrapartum complications and low birth weight. Albrecht et al. (1994) found that structure of the household—living arrangements and marital status—was a key determinant of the level of prenatal care. Women living with their spouse had the lowest probability of receiving inadequate care.

Thus, factors pertaining to maternal prenatal stress and anxiety, specific prenatal personality dimensions, social support, and family functioning appear to be associated with pregnancy complications, particularly PTB, and low birth weight.

1.2.2.2   Design and Methods

It is well recognized that PTB and low birth weight are multifaceted health problems that include psychosocial and behavior factors, and that occur most often in lower socioeconomic and African American populations (Office of the Surgeon General and the Eunice Kennedy Shriver National Institute of Child Health and Human

Development, 2008). Due to the heterogeneous etiology of PTB, the Surgeon General's Conference on the Prevention of Preterm Birth (2008) recommended quantitative and qualitative studies of risk factors that include lifestyle and sociodemographic factors, and the development of personalized, specific interventions and therapies. Additional recommendations included improvement in the screening and measurement of psychosocial risk factors and responses. Thus, the research project we present focuses on the recommendations underscored by the Surgeon General and the Institute of Medicine, and include assessment of psychosocial and behavioral factors for PTB. Furthermore, the Surgeon General's panel recommended that measurement of stress include specific constructs such as anxiety. Most studies on maternal anxiety measure general or perceived anxiety (Mancuso et al., 2004; Roesch, Dunkel-Schetter, Woo, & Hobel, 2004), but fail to identify the roots of anxiety critical to the development of therapeutic interventions. In this project we measured pregnancy-specific anxiety, social support, and family functioning, and determine the strength of their effects on pregnancy complications and birth outcomes.

Questionnaire assessments of adaptation to pregnancy and family functioning were made in the latter half of pregnancy with the Lederman Prenatal Self-Evaluation Questionnaire scales and Olson's Family Adaptability and Cohesion Evaluation Scales-II (FACES-II, Olson et al., 1983). Cronbach's reliability coefficients for the Prenatal Self-Evaluation Questionnaire (PSEQ) scales range from 0.75 to 0.92.

The two FACES-II scales measure: (1) Family Adaptability – the ability of the family to change its roles, rules, and power structure, and the extent to which families are chaotic or rigid (dysfunctional) vs. flexible or adaptable (balanced), and (2) Family Cohesion – the emotional bonding of family members, and the extent to which families are disengaged or enmeshed (dysfunctional) vs. flexibly connected or separated (balanced). Low values indicate extreme (dysfunctional) scores; high values indicate flexibility, adaptability, or balance. Cronbach's reliability coefficients for FACES-II range from 0.83 to 0.88 for Family Cohesion and 0.78 to 0.80 for Family Adaptability (McCubbin, McCubbin, Thompson, & Huang, 1989).

Complications During Antepartum, Intrapartum, and Delivery

Many pregnancy risk assessment systems have been reported in the literature (Gillen-Goldstein, Paidas, Sokol, Jones, & Pernoll, 2003; Institute for Clinical Systems Improvement, 2000). No single model is considered the standard. The differences in the models resides in the focus of risk (psychosocial, interpersonal, physiological, environmental, and behavioral) and the categorization of risk levels (low or high) (Gilbert & Harmon, 2003). Because there is a difference in the risk categorization between models, experienced clinicians (physician and midwives) within our group made reasonable decisions for categorization for our project. These decisions were based on the availability, complexity, and frequency of interventions to rectify the condition or complication, and the gravity of threat to maternal/fetal well-being.

Complications were classified based on their timing in relation to pregnancy, and thus into antepartum, intrapartum, and delivery intervals. Each of these groups was further subdivided based on the seriousness of the complications into mild, moderate, and severe categories.

Mild antepartum complications comprised medical complications not requiring hospitalization. Mild labor complications were related to fetal size and to dysfunctional patterns without fetal distress. Mild delivery complications included conditions requiring expedient intervention but with good expected outcomes.

Moderate antepartum complications included physical threat to the mother and fetal development problems. Moderate intrapartum complications were categorized by threat to fetal well-being (amniotic fluid disorders, abnormal positions, and pregnancy-induced hypertension). Moderate complications during delivery required invasive techniques to deliver the fetus with unknown expected outcomes.

Severe complications posed great threat to the mother and fetus. Severe antepartum complications involved fetal death, severe fetal anemia, and uncontrolled hypertension. Severe intrapartum risks were related to fetal distress. Emergent cesarean birth and large postpartum hemorrhage comprised the severe risks at delivery with poor expected outcomes.

1.2.2.3   Results

Data were analyzed using descriptive statistics and ordinary least squares regression, and presented at professional scientific conferences (Lederman et al., 2002).

The sample included 106 pregnant women: 27 African-Americans, 47 Latin-Americans, and 32 Anglo-Americans. Most participants were 18–36 years old, had ≤12 years' education, low income, and a parity of 0 or 1. Approximately half the women were married and half were single, divorced, or separated. Mean values for Length of Gestation, Apgar scores, and Newborn Weight were within normal parameters. Most participants had either no or mild antepartum, intrapartum, or delivery complications.

Cronbach's alpha coefficients for the Prenatal Self-Evaluation Questionnaire scales all were between 0.72 and 0.92, except for Fear of Pain, Helplessness, and Loss of Control ($\alpha = 0.68$). The intercorrelations among the scales ($r = 0.00$–0.45, not shown in table) are lower than the reliability coefficients, indicating that each scale is measuring unique content. The reliability coefficients for the FACES-II scales are somewhat lower (Family Cohesion, $\alpha = 0.70$; Family Adaptability, $\alpha = 0.63$).

Correlations Among the Demographic, Psychosocial, and Pregnancy
Outcome Variables

Correlations were determined between three sets of data: demographic and psychosocial variables, demographic and outcome variables, and psychosocial and outcome variables.

For the demographic and psychosocial variables, significant correlations were obtained for Age with Acceptance of Pregnancy ($r = -0.24$, $p < 0.05$), Family Cohesion ($r = 0.43$, $p < 0.01$), and Family Adaptability ($r = 0.25$, $p < 0.05$), indicating that for the sample in this project younger women experienced more conflict in the acceptance of pregnancy, and less family cohesion and adaptability.

Women with more education felt better prepared for labor (had less conflict and anxiety) ($r = -0.22$, $p < 0.05$) and had a greater sense of maternal/fetal well-being ($r = -0.26$, $p < 0.05$).

Single gravidas reported more conflict/anxiety in Acceptance of Pregnancy ($r = 0.32$, $p < 0.05$), Relationship with Husband/Partner ($r = 0.37$, $p < 0.05$), Preparation for Labor ($r = 0.23$, $p < 0.05$), and Family Cohesion ($r = -0.21$, $p < 0.05$).

Women who smoked also were more anxious about Acceptance of Pregnancy ($r = 0.27$, $p < 0.01$), Identification with a Motherhood Role ($r = 0.26$, $p < 0.05$), Relationship with Mother ($r = 0.23$, $p < 0.05$), and with Husband/Partner ($r = 0.26$, $p < 0.05$).

Few significant relationships were found among the demographic variables and pregnancy outcomes. Parity was related to Gestational Age at First Prenatal Visit ($r = 0.20$, $p < 0.05$), indicating that primigravidas sought prenatal care earlier than multigravidas. Single status was related to Intrapartum Complications ($r = 0.22$, $p < 0.05$), indicating that single expectant mothers had more intrapartum complications than married women.

More relationships were obtained with the psychosocial variables and pregnancy outcomes. Relationship with Husband correlated with Gestational Age at First Prenatal Visit ($r = 0.28$, $p < 0.01$), and Identification with a Motherhood Role correlated with Length of Gestation ($r = -28$, $p < 0.01$), indicating that better spouse/partner relationships were associated with earlier initiation of prenatal care, and lower anxiety about motherhood role identification was related to longer gestation and less PTB. In addition, Acceptance of Pregnancy was related to Intrapartum Complications ($r = 0.24$, $p < 0.05$), and Identification with a Motherhood Role was related to Antepartum Complications ($r = 0.28$, $p < 0.01$), indicating that higher anxiety on these two dimensions was related to a higher incidence of complications.

Few significant demographic and psychosocial correlations were found with Newborn Weight, Apgar Scores, and Delivery Complications, and they are not presented.

Regression Analyses of Significant Demographic and Psychosocial Variables with Pregnancy Outcomes

Regression analyses were first conducted of the demographic variables with the pregnancy outcome variables, and then for the psychosocial scales (PSEQ and FACES-II) with Pregnancy Outcomes. Final regression analyses were conducted using the statistically significant demographic and psychosocial variables with each pregnancy outcome (Tables 1.4–1.7).

Table 1.3 Multiple Regression with Length of Gestation as Dependent Variable: Model Summary

R	R^2	F	df	p
0.552	0.304	9.294	4, 85	0.000

Regression coefficients				
Independent variable		β	t	p
Identification with a motherhood role		−0.154	−1.477	0.143
Preparation for labor		0.252	2.519	0.014
Relationship with husband		−0.230	−2.251	0.027
Complications during antepartum		−0.363	−3.745	0.000

Table 1.4 Multiple Regression with Gestational Age at First Prenatal Visit as Dependent Variable: Model Summary

R	R^2	F	df	p
0.293	0.086	4.370	2, 93	0.015

Regression coefficients				
Independent variable		β	t	p
Relationship with mother		0.091	0.898	0.372
Relationship with husband		0.260	2.556	0.012

Table 1.5 Multiple Regression with Complications during Antepartum as the Dependent Variable: Model Summary

R	R^2	F	df	p
0.383	0.147	5.287	3, 92	0.002

Regression coefficients				
Independent variable		β	t	p
Identification with a motherhood role		0.289	2.777	0.007
Preparation for labor		−0.264	−2.533	0.013
Maternal well-being		0.171	1.583	0.117

Table 1.6 Multiple Regression with Complications during Intrapartum as the Dependent Variable: Model Summary

R	R^2	F	df	p
0.241	0.058	5.665	1, 92	0.019

Regression coefficients				
Independent variable		β	t	p
Acceptance of pregnancy		0.241	2.380	0.019

Table 1.4 presents the regression analysis for Length of Gestation. Of the four variables from the first regression, two psychosocial variables attained significance with Length of Gestation in the final regression: Preparation for Labor and Relationship with Husband/Partner. Antepartum Complications also had a significant

beta value with Length of Gestation. The total variance explained by the model for Length of Gestation is 0.30.

Table 1.5 presents the final regression analysis for Gestational Age at First Prenatal Visit. Two psychosocial variables, Relationship with Mother and Relationship with Husband/Partner, were retained from the first regression analyses. In the final regression analysis, only Relationship with Husband/Partner was significantly associated with maternal initiation of prenatal care.

Table 1.6 presents the final regression analysis for Complications during Antepartum. Two psychosocial variables retain significance in the final model: Identification with a Motherhood Role and Preparation for Labor.

Table 1.7 presents the final regression analysis for Complications during Intrapartum and shows that only Acceptance of Pregnancy was significantly predictive of Intrapartum Complications in the first and final regression analyses.

In summary, prenatal psychosocial dimensions pertaining to conflict or anxiety in the Relationship with Husband/Partner, Identification with a Motherhood Role, Acceptance of Pregnancy, and Preparation for Labor were predictive of several birth outcomes in the correlation and multiple regression analyses. Of particular interest are the significant multiple regression results for Relationship with Husband/Partner with both Length of Gestation and Gestational Age at First Prenatal Visit. Our findings suggest that single expectant women experience greater prenatal anxiety regarding acceptance of pregnancy, and substantive deficits in personal and financial support, as well as other types of support, while married or partnered women more likely welcome the pregnancy and receive greater support and encouragement, which is reflected in earlier initiation of prenatal care. Research reports from other investigators support this interpretation. Giblin, Poland, and Ager (1990) report that intimate support from a husband, partner, or other family member was related to obtaining adequate prenatal care and to positive attitudes and behaviors, such as an initial happy feeling about the pregnancy, feeling hopeful about the future, and not using drugs while pregnant. Kalil et al. (1993) found that married women and those who had an emotional confidante or supportive partners reported lower anxiety. DaCosta et al. (1999) found that marital adjustment was the strongest predictor of higher pregnancy anxiety and psychosocial stressors. Low partner support in combination with high life stress may engender high maternal anxiety (Norbeck & Anderson, 1989a). Poor partner or marital relationships during pregnancy have been associated with preterm uterine contractions (Facchinetti et al., 2007), maternal emotional distress, and subsequent postpartum depression (Dimitrovsky et al., 1987; O'Hara, 1986; Watson et al., 1984). Social support and stress also have been associated with maternal postpartum behavior. Crnic, Greenberg, Ragozin, Robinson, and Basham (1983) reported that mothers with greater stress were less positive in their attitudes and behavior toward the infant. Intimate support from the husband had the most positive effects. Our data indicate that the partner relationship and the quality of support can influence pregnancy adaptation and health outcomes. The data are also consistent with the suggestion offered by Fogel and Lewallen (1995) that marital status itself may be an indicator of risk, since mortality and morbidity rates are higher for nonmarital than marital births.

Another psychosocial dimension, maternal Preparation for Labor, had a significant beta weight in the model for Length of Gestation, and two dimensions were significant in the model for Complications during Antepartum–Identification with a Motherhood Role and Preparation for Labor. In this project, Preparation for Labor correlated with Relationship with Husband/Partner ($r = 0.35$, $p = 0.000$), suggesting that a woman concerned about her partner relationship also may be anxious about the support available to her in labor. Or, she may be too preoccupied about her personal circumstances to consider preparing for labor and, thus, may be in a lesser state of readiness for childbirth.

Several of the psychosocial dimensions measuring developmental conflict or adaptation anxiety were significantly related to maternal smoking in the correlation analyses, including Acceptance of Pregnancy, $r = 0.27$ ($p < 0.01$), Identification with a Motherhood Role, $r = 0.26$ ($p < 0.01$), and Relationship to Husband/ Partner, $r = 0.26$ ($p < 0.01$), and to Mother, $r = 0.23$ ($p < 0.01$). However, maternal smoking was not a correlate of any pregnancy outcome in the multiple regression analyses. Although maternal smoking has been a correlate of newborn weight in some studies (Orr et al., 1996; Kramer, 1998) and not others (Ounsted, Moar, & Scott, 1981), our data suggest that psychosocial factors may have a more significant bearing on maternal risk status and health outcomes.

Investigators (Hedegaard, Henriksen, Sabroe, & Secher, 1993; Norbeck & Anderson, 1989b) also report that measures of anxiety are consistent and stable throughout pregnancy, indicating that early measures may be useful as screening tools to identify women who might benefit from counseling.

Correlation analyses showed several significant relationships of the demographic data and FACES-II with the pregnancy outcome variables, but none of these results survived the multiple regression analyses. The reliability coefficient for Family Cohesion was low, which may partially account for our results. In another study (Reeb et al., 1987), a composite score derived from three different family functioning measures was the best predictor of subsequent low birth weight and intrapartum complications. The construct of family functioning may require more comprehensive measurement than is possible with a two-dimension instrument.

The foregoing research results show that psychosocial measures of developmental conflict and adaptation anxiety are warranted in the analysis of reproductive health outcomes. Our results indicate that prenatal psychosocial anxiety pertaining to partner or husband support, the gravida's conflict concerning acceptance of the pregnancy, psychosocial preparation for motherhood, and preparedness for labor and childbirth have an influence on birth outcomes.

The results indicate that psychosocial dimensions pertaining to developmental and adaptive responses to pregnancy are significant predictors of pregnancy outcomes and pregnancy complications, even in the presence of antepartal complications, and warrant inclusion in prenatal assessment and health care intervention.

1.2.3   Maternal Prenatal Psychosocial Adaptation Predictors of Infant Birth Weight and Gestational Age [1,2]

1.2.3.1   Theory and Background

The rate of PTBs (12.7%) and low birth weight births (8.2%) continues to rise despite decreases in the overall birth rate, decreases in teen births for all races, decreases in smoking during pregnancy, and increases in the percentage of women who begin prenatal care in the first trimester (all predictors of gestational age and/or low birth weight (Hamilton, Minino, Martin, Kochanek, Strobino, & Guyer, 2007; Arias, MacDorman, Strobino, & Guyer, 2003).

Prenatal life is a period of increased vulnerability for the stress system (Charmandari, Kino, Souvatzoglou, & Chrousos, 2003). Studies indicate that pregnant women with high stress and anxiety levels are at increased risk for preterm labor and delivery of low birth weight infants (Hobel, Dunkel-Schetter, Roesch, Castro, & Arora, 1999; Misra, O'Campo, & Strobino, 2001). Few investigations, however, conduct assessments of the gravida's level of stress or anxiety in the first trimester (Dunkel-Schetter, Gurung, Lobel, & Wadhwa, 2001). The stress the woman experiences as she accepts the pregnancy and begins to identify with her imminent role as a mother may have profound effects on the health of the fetus, and subsequent birth outcomes. Importantly, the greatest anxiety concerning acceptance of pregnancy and identifying with the role of being a mother occurs during the first and second trimesters of pregnancy (Weis, 2006). This study followed women from the first through third trimester of pregnancy in order to obtain individual maternal adaptive trajectories for the psychosocial dimensions of adaptation to pregnancy. Notably, these trajectories are an indication of pregnancy-specific anxiety and conflict.

1.2.3.2   Design and Methods

Individual growth models for prenatal maternal psychosocial variables were followed across all trimesters of pregnancy and regressed on gestational age at birth and on infant birth weight for 421 military wives from two large military treatment facilities providing care to Army, Navy, and Air Force personnel and their family members. Following approval by the appropriate institutional review boards, all women attending obstetrical orientation classes from September 2002 through April 2003 were invited to participate in the study. The target population was all primigravid and multigravid women between the ages of 18–35 years having a

---

[1] The content and conclusions expressed here are those of the authors and do not necessarily reflect the views of TriService Nursing Research Program, the Department of Defense, or the U.S. Government.

[2] The military-related results discussed in Chapters 1 and 9 were the findings from a project sponsored by the TriService Nursing Research Program, MDA-905–00–1–0039.

singleton pregnancy of less than 20 weeks' gestation upon entry into the study. The women could have no preexisting medical conditions such as diabetes, hypertension, cardiac or collagen diseases, or chronic anemia. A total of 1,324 women were provided information regarding the project. Of this number, 504 consented to participation (64% of eligible women), 279 declined (37% of eligible), and 541 women did not meet inclusion criteria for participation.

In each trimester of pregnancy, the women were given Lederman's (1996) PSEQ. The gestational age for every newborn was determined from the last menstrual period or from documented ultrasound prior to 20 weeks' gestation. A nearly continuous measure of birth weight for gestational age by race was calculated from tables generated from multiple reference percentiles of birth weight for each completed week of gestation from 22 to 44 weeks by Oken, Kleinman, Rich-Edwards, and Gillman (2003).

The specific questions that guided the analyses were:

1. Do individual growth curves measuring dimensions of maternal prenatal anxiety related to Acceptance of Pregnancy, Identification with a Motherhood Role, Preparation for Labor, and Concerns about Well-Being of Self (mother) and Infant in Labor have a direct main effect on gestational age after controlling for parity, infant gender, smoking history, and age of mother?
2. Do prenatal individual growth curves measuring dimensions of anxiety related to Acceptance of Pregnancy, Identification with a Motherhood Role, Preparation for Labor, and Concerns about Well-Being of Self (mother) and Infant in Labor have a direct main effect on infant birth weight after controlling for gestational age, parity, infant gender, smoking history, and age of mother?

1.2.3.3   Results

The majority of the sample were married (90%), white, non-Hispanic (62%) and were wives of enlisted members between the ranks of E1–E7 (84%). The only unmarried women in this sample were active duty members ($n = 4$). The sample was slightly higher educated than the overall Air Force, Army, or Navy populations. The figures provided are fairly representative of the overall Air Force military population. The sample was composed of approximately 55% Air Force wives and active duty women.

Prenatal Psychosocial Adaptation and Gestational Age

Individual growth curves for six of the seven dimensions of the PSEQ were modeled on gestational age at birth. The Relationship with Mother dimension was not used in the analysis as a number of the participants did not have a mother figure in their lives due to death and there was significant missing data. A two-level unconditional linear growth model was applied, with the level-1 model representing the linear growth, and the level-2 model expressing variation in parameters from the growth model as random effects for each six dimensions of prenatal maternal adaptation by individual across the three trimesters. The results from the multilevel model (the slopes of each of the six dimensions of prenatal adaptation) were then entered into a regression model with the covariates of infant sex, smoking history during pregnancy, participant age, and parity. Results regarding the effect of the individual growth models (change over time for individual prenatal maternal adaptation to pregnancy) on gestational age at birth indicated a significant intercept ($\beta = 39.74$, $p \leq 0.001$) and a significant linear slope for *Acceptance of Pregnancy, Identification with a Motherhood Role, Preparation for Labor, and Concerns about Well-Being of Self and Baby in Labor*. The trajectories indicating anxiety related to *Fear of Pain, Helplessness, and Loss of Control* and *Relationship with Husband* did not significantly affect gestational age at birth (Table 1.7).

Prenatal Psychosocial Adaptation and Birth Weight

The same analysis as described earlier was used to assess the effect of individual growth curves for prenatal psychosocial adaptation on birth weight. Results for this question regarding the effect of the individual growth models to infant birth weight

Table 1.7 Coefficients from Regression of Change across Time for Prenatal Maternal Adaptive Dimensions and Covariates on Gestational Age at Birth

Variables	Model 1	
	β coeff.	S.E.
ACCPREG[a]	−0.15***	0.04
IDMORO[b]	0.20***	0.05
PREPLAB[c]	0.10**	0.04
WELLBE[d]	−0.12***	0.04
HELPL[e]	−0.06	0.05
RELHUS[f]	−0.00	0.03
INFSEX	0.08	0.09
SMOKER	0.04	0.06
AGE	−0.03**	0.01
PARITY	0.02	0.06
Intercept	39.74***	0.29
Critical value	5.41***	
Degrees of freedom	10	
R^2	0.04	

$*p \leq 0.05$; $**p \leq 0.01$; $***p \leq 0.001$
[a] Acceptance of Pregnancy
[b] Identification with a Motherhood Role
[c] Preparation for Labor
[d] Concerns for Well-Being of Self and Baby
[e] Fear of Pain, Helplessness, and Loss of Control
[f] Relationship with Husband

after controlling for gestational age indicated a significant intercept, and significant linear slopes for *Preparation for Labor,* and *Fear of Helplessness and Loss of Control in Labor.* The trajectories indicating anxiety related to *Acceptance of Pregnancy, Identification with a Motherhood Role Well-Being of Self and Baby,* and *Relationship with Husband* did not significantly affect infant birth weight after controlling for gestational age (Table 1.8).

1.2.3.4 Discussion

The findings provide evidence for change over time in anxiety related to prenatal maternal adaptation directly predicting gestational age at birth and infant birth weight. Clearly, the anxiety a woman experiences prenatally related to her acceptance of pregnancy, identification of her motherhood role, preparation for labor, and concerns she has over her safety and the safety of her unborn fetus directly predict gestational age at birth. The dimensions directly affecting infant birth weight varied from those found to affect gestational age. The change over time in anxiety related to preparation for labor and concerns about feelings of helplessness or loss of control in labor significantly affected infant birth weight after controlling for the gestational age of the infant at birth. Additionally, variables known to impact infant birth weight, infant sex, history of smoking during pregnancy, and parity also significantly affected infant birth weight. The results for the change across trimesters for the various dimensions of prenatal adaptation to pregnancy do not all indicate a

Table 1.8 Coefficients from Regression of Change Across Time for Prenatal Maternal Adaptive Dimensions and Covariates on Infant Birth Weight

	Model 1	
Variables	β coeff.	S.E.
ACCPREG[a]	0.03	0.03
IDMORO[b]	0.03	0.03
PREPLAB[c]	−0.05*	0.02
WELLBE[d]	−0.03	0.03
HELPL[e]	0.07**	0.03
RELHUS[f]	−0.00	0.02
INFSEX	−0.29***	0.05
SMOKER	−0.13***	0.04
PARITY	0.13***	0.03
Intercept	0.29***	0.08
Critical value	9.75***	
Degrees of freedom	9	

*$p \leq 0.05$; **$p \leq 0.01$; ***$p \leq 0.001$
[a] Acceptance of Pregnancy
[b] Identification with a Motherhood Role
[c] Preparation for Labor
[d] Concerns for Well-Being of Self and Baby
[e] Fear of Pain, Helplessness, and Loss of Control
[f] Relationship with Husband

negative relationship to estimated gestational age or infant birth weight. For women with decreasing anxiety across pregnancy related to acceptance of pregnancy an increase in gestational age of the newborn was observed. The gravida's acceptance of pregnancy requires a complex, introspective contemplation in which she weighs the costs and benefits of pregnancy. The anxiety related to accepting pregnancy changes significantly during the course of pregnancy (Weis, Lederman, Lilly, & Schaffer, 2008). The results indicate that increased anxiety related to accepting pregnancy predicts gestational age at birth. Identifying with a maternal role, unlike acceptance of pregnancy, is an intellectual task in which the gravida either recognizes that she does not want to be like her maternal role models (yet does not know where or how to initiate change), or she is comfortable with her impending role and feels free to face changes she deems appropriate without conflict or anxiety. Importantly, while there was a significant intercept ($\beta = 18.79$, $p \leq 0.001$) for *Identification with a Motherhood Role* (IDMORO), the linear and curvilinear slopes were nonsignificant ($\beta = 0.48$, $p \leq 0.07$; $\beta = -0.23$, $p \leq 0.06$), indicating that the developmental trajectory of IDMORO began in the first trimester with little change across the trimesters. For *Preparation for Labor* (PREPLAB), there was a significant intercept ($\beta = 18.12$, $p \leq 0.001$) and significant curvilinear slope ($\beta = -0.55$, $p \leq 0.05$). The linear slope of PREPLAB was nonsignificant indicating that the developmental trajectory specifically for preparation for labor changed very little during pregnancy. There was, however, a decrease of 0.55 in PREPLAB from the first to the second and the second to the third trimester (the curvilinear slope). The nonsignificant linear change for both IDMORO and PREPLAB indicates that the feelings a woman has regarding her anticipated role as a mother and potentially her concerns regarding labor are fairly constant throughout pregnancy, yet have a significant impact on gestational age at birth. The anxiety the gravida feels related to her well-being and the safety of herself and her unborn baby have a significant negative predictive effect to gestational age at birth.

Patterns of adaptation are complicated (Sameroff, 2000) and socialization processes throughout the course of the women's life are integral to her development as a mother (Cairns & Rodkin, 1998). Rubin described giving of oneself as the most "intricate and complex task of childbearing and childbirth" (1984, p. 66). Giving of oneself refers to a mother's willingness and ability to make personal sacrifices (Sleutel, 2003). This ability is not learned during pregnancy but throughout life through continual experiences and reflections. Similarly, the anxiety women feel related to labor preparation emanates partly from the overall fantasies and dreams related to the anticipated birth experience. Additionally, fears or concerns regarding the medical system or provider availability may have an impact on anxiety. Obtaining information through prenatal classes, books, magazines, and from family members and friends helps to alleviate anxiety, hence the significant decrease in concerns about preparedness for labor as pregnancy progresses. The anxiety women experience related to preparation for labor and concerns about helplessness change very little across pregnancy; however, the level of anxiety women experience overall regarding this dimension of adaptation to pregnancy and motherhood does predict infant birth weight. Findings by Lederman (2008) indicate that the anxiety women feel across pregnancy for these particular dimensions can be decreased through supportive and informational interventions.

Summary

The research results presented thus far show that pregnancy-specific dimensions of psychosocial conflict and anxiety are related to plasma measures of epinephrine and cortisol, and are predictive of decreased uterine activity in labor, a longer duration of labor, and lower newborn Apgar scores. Higher epinephrine in labor also was associated with increased FHR deceleration patterns, and higher anxiety was associated with more low- and midforceps deliveries. In another foundation research project with low to high risk gravidas of mixed parity several of the pregnancy personality dimensions were predictive of length of gestation, antepartum complications, and intrapartum complications.

The research project conducted with military women showed that pregnancy-specific anxiety related to prenatal personality dimensions directly predicted gestational age at birth and infant birth weight. Anxiety related to acceptance of pregnancy, identification with a motherhood role, preparation for labor, and concerns the expectant mother has over her safety and the safety of her unborn fetus directly predicted gestational age at birth. The dimensions directly and significantly predicting infant birth weight were anxiety related to preparation for labor and concerns about feelings of pain, helplessness or loss of control in labor. Importantly, these results indicate that the developmental trajectory that began in first trimester changed significantly across the trimesters for most prenatal psychosocial dimensions and at the same time remain relatively constant throughout pregnancy. These are complex results in an emerging area of science that is now supported by both the Institute of Medicine and the Surgeon General of the United States. The findings presented in this chapter indicate there is considerable potential for early and accurate assessment of pregnancy-specific dimensions in first trimester and the initiation of supportive intervention strategies to enhance maternal prenatal psychosocial adaptation. Additional research findings supporting the theory and validity of the seven prenatal psychosocial personality dimensions of adaptation to pregnancy will be presented in Chapter 11 which focuses predominantly on assessment of prenatal psychosocial adaptation and the psychometric properties of the assessment instruments.

1.3   Theoretical Foundations of the Seven Dimensions of Adaptation to Pregnancy

The following section describes the theory inherent in each of the seven dimensions of adaptation to pregnancy. Selection of the seven psychosocial variables relevant to the woman's experience of pregnancy resulted from a conceptual model which views pregnancy as a period of transition between two lifestyles, two states of being: the woman-without-child and the woman-with-child, and the important aspects of such a change.

Transition between the two lifestyles can be viewed as a paradigm shift, paradigm being understood here as a constellation of current self-image, beliefs, values, priorities, behavior patterns, relationships with others, and set of problem-solving skills. According to Kuhn (1970), a paradigm shift is stimulated when life change occurs – in this case, the fact of pregnancy – which will result in the birth of a child who cannot be easily integrated into the old paradigm. Throughout the 9-month gestation period, there is a reassessment of the self and significant others, a discarding of some old ways, and a replacement with new ways. Pregnancy is a period of preparation for the emergence of the new paradigm, with the newborn infant as an integral and crucial part.

The paradigm shift can be thought of as a change in perception. The woman-without-child looks at the world differently than the woman-with-child. The shift takes place in an evolutionary framework, for pregnancy-childbirth is a developmental process with several incremental steps in which there can be no return to the former self. It is expected that there will be some personal conflict and critical resistance to change before any fundamental adjustment to the new paradigm takes place. The developmental and adaptive process of the pregnancy and childbirth experience has been recognized by others (Grossman, Eichler, & Winickoff, 1980). Trad (1991) refers to the "developmental transformations" set in motion by pregnancy and that occur throughout pregnancy as exerting powerful and encompassing effects on the lives of women.

Pregnancy often is described as a life crisis, one in which growth takes place through crisis resolution, although Leifer (1980) and Wolkind and Zajicek (1981) reported that few subjects in their studies experienced pregnancy as a crisis. During the course of our several research projects, it was discerned that a sense of crisis is felt only when the two paradigms are far apart, when the two lifestyles cannot be reconciled, and when the developmental step is too large to make in 9 months. In these cases, pregnancy may indeed be a period fraught with intense conflict and ambivalence. What often seems to have happened, however, is that, before becoming pregnant, the woman has consciously or unconsciously prepared herself for motherhood; she has moved toward the new paradigm and the developmental step is not so difficult to make in 9 months. Therefore, it would seem more appropriate to conceptualize the normal course of childbearing as a test which comes as part of growth, and as a challenge rather than a crisis. This represents a more optimistic view of childbirth, one that better recognizes the complexity and creativity of the childbearing event.

In the model proposed here, the mother considers the child, as she does other significant people in her life, a unique being apart from herself. This assumption implies respect for the child and recognition of the child's integrity and rights. Unless this respect exists, a woman cannot truly give to or nurture the child. Giving is the defining characteristic of motherhood. The woman is no longer self-contained; she is now concerned with her child's welfare as well as her own.

Almost inevitably the new child cannot be easily integrated into the former paraigm. The mother's former lifestyle, priorities, and self-image are no longer feasible; modification is required if the new paradigm, the mother-and-child, is to flourish. When the loss of a former lifestyle is not counterbalanced by clearly perceived satisfaction in the expected child, then ambivalence mounts and the transition is resisted. A greater level of conflict and anxiety results. Near term pregnancy, the expectant mother may be in a state of upheaval when confronted with the imminent appearance of the infant for which she had difficulty preparing – an upheaval that may be intensified by social pressures and expectations. The woman near term may become more and more distraught and feel trapped with no apparent escape. Excessive anxiety can affect the course of labor, as the project findings demonstrate, with possible implications for the well-being of the mother and child. Women who feel this way may still make the paradigm shift, but it is reasonable to expect that it will be more traumatic. Actually, progressive variations in the paradigm shift occur over time and the process of maturation continues as the child grows or as other children are born.

The mother-to-be performs certain developmental tasks while making the paradigm shift. Initially, the woman's task is to accept the idea of pregnancy and assimilate it into her way of life. Reactions of anticipation, perhaps euphoria, are common if the gravid woman has been looking forward to motherhood. At the same time, she may be assailed by doubts, weighing the pros and cons, and rethinking her motives and the ultimate consequences of a changed reality. She may, for example, worry about how well she will manage both her career and caring for a child, and when or if she should continue working; she may also anticipate problems with finances. Some degree of ambivalence and vacillation is expected throughout pregnancy even when clear choices have been made. Emotions such as anger, fear, and loneliness occur during the transition to motherhood (Trad, 1990). The motives for pregnancy influence how well the pregnancy is accepted and tolerated. The desire for motherhood and a child of one's own, however, may or may not be central to the mother's motivation for pregnancy, although they often are among the numerous motives expressed. Variations in the themes of acceptance, as well as important areas for assessment, are discussed in Chapter 2.

Two developmental tasks – the identification with a motherhood role and the renewal and deepening of the mother–daughter relationship – often are complementary in pregnancy. When speculating about what it will be like to be a mother, the primigravida naturally reflects back on her own mother and reevaluates the quality of her early nurturing in terms of her own future role. The primigravida tends to reassess her present relationship with her mother and considers the possibility of empathic reconciliation if conflict existed before, because she now recognizes her mother as a human being with limits. This process of reworking the mother–daughter relationship can continue throughout the pregnancy. An analysis of the interrelationships of this variable with others in pregnancy indicates that a good relationship with one's mother helps build a solid foundation for identifying a motherhood role of one's own. A good mother–daughter relationship also is associated with a reasonable degree of self-confidence regarding motherhood, and with less fear and anxiety in pregnancy and childbirth. Steps in the developmental process of identifying a motherhood role are presented in Chapter 3, while factors enhancing and hindering the mother–daughter relationship are analyzed in Chapter 4.

During the course of her pregnancy, the woman becomes preoccupied not only with her own future role, but also with the role her husband/partner will assume as both husband/partner and father. In focusing her thoughts on her husband/partner, it is not unusual for a pregnant woman to undertake a reevaluation of the marital/ couple relationship or even of sex roles. She may wonder whether her husband/ partner will indeed give her support when she needs it most. The mother-to-be often notices that she, as well as her husband/partner, feels an increased sense of vulnerability during her pregnancy. Mood swings, on the one hand, are often precipitated by contemplation of the challenges of parenthood and, on the other hand, by its anticipated rewards. Elements of the marital/couple relationship impinging on maternal adaptation during pregnancy are discussed in Chapter 5.

In the third trimester, when the woman's focus often shifts to the imminent reality of and preparation for childbirth, fears and anxieties about pain, about how well she will cope, about possible injury to herself or to her child, and about death precipitate readiness for educational preparation for childbirth. Consequently, another salient task of pregnancy is the expectant mother's preparation for labor, which is effected through various means such as attending classes, reading books, and discussions with others. Such efforts are sparked by fears of the unknown – how she will perform in labor, how she will get to the hospital, and whether she will arrive at the hospital in due time. Since labor and delivery are a journey into the unknown and no one can predict the outcome, the woman faced with mounting anxiety and uncertainty about this journey learns to balance these emotions through positive anticipation; in other words, preparation for labor assumes acquisition of knowledge as well as a reasonable degree of self-confidence. Adaptive and maladaptive steps in the preparation for labor are discussed in Chapter 6.

As a woman learns about and prepares for the events of labor, she is faced with yet another paradox. Even though she has no control over her contractions, she still must take a certain degree of responsibility for the course of events. She must listen to her body and actively work with it. She must perform as well as she can on her own, and yet be willing to accept help when she needs it. The fear of loss of control can be adaptive or it can be maladaptive if it becomes too diffuse. Associations of pain can trigger fears about loss of control and a subsequent loss of self-esteem. In our society, the concept of control has special significance and this element is manifested in women's concerns and fears about labor. The many meanings of control and mastery of control, as well as confidence and dependency during pregnancy and childbirth, are discussed in Chapter 7. Factors precipitating fears of loss of self-esteem are described in Chapter 8.

In summary, the transition to parenthood – the paradigm shift – is a psychological process of unfolding that keeps pace with and complements the physical development of the fetus inside – a transition that carries with it variable amounts of resistance and progress.

An analogy may be made between childbirth and the creation of a work of art. The creative act requires a dramatic shift of perspective, a different way of seeing the world. Creation is essentially active, for the creative personality does not merely follow in the footsteps of others, but permits his or her mind to touch the borders of the unknown. To carry the analogy further, the preparatory process for creation almost always involves periods of withdrawal, brooding introspection, and intensified sensibility, and it is close to the indescribable world of the unconscious, because creation is an inner process. The creating person is, therefore, essentially alone – despite all the encouragement and adulation she might receive–and what she does necessarily carries some degree of stress and tension. She works and waits for the work of art to take on a life of its own, and at a certain moment puts it forth for the world to see. The creative act also requires that the creating person separate herself from her production; and, in terms of both figures in the analogy, mother and child, the creating person feels a sense of accomplishment.

To make this paradigm shift and to change perspective means taking an untried path, a path both unsettling and exhilarating, fraught with dangers, and invested with unexpected rewards. The ensuing chapters attempt to elucidate some of the challenges and psychological work inherent in expectant parenthood, as well as the developmental steps associated with adaptation to and progress in labor. The work of other theorists and researchers is integrated into chapter discussions.

The book focuses on objective, reliable, and valid assessment and interpretation. The use of interview assessment as a first-line intervention is discussed in Chapter 11. We include novel research on intervention to promote psychosocial adaptation to pregnancy. However, much of the research on intervention still needs to be conducted. Where it was deemed appropriate, the ensuing chapters have been expanded to include implications for practice and identification of circumstances when referral to counseling is warranted for expectant mothers who are experiencing difficulty in adapting to pregnancy and the advent of motherhood. Recommendations for future research also are presented.

References

Abell, T. D., Baker, L. C., Clover, R. D., & Ramsey, C. N., Jr. (1991). The effects of family functioning on infant birthweight. *Journal of Family Practice, 32,* 37–44.

Albrecht, S. L., Miller, M. K., & Clarke, L. L. (1994). Assessing the importance of family structure in understanding birth outcomes. *Journal of Marriage and Family, 56,* 987–1003.

Arias, E., MacDorman, M. F., Strobino, D. M., & Guyer, B. (2003). Annual summary of vital statistics – 2002. *Pediatrics, 112*(6 Pt 1), 1215–1230.

Beck, N. C., Siegel, L. J., Davidson, N. P., Kormeier, S., Breitenstein, A., & Hall, D. G. (1980). The prediction of pregnancy outcome: Maternal preparation, anxiety, and attitudinal sets. *Journal of Psychosomatic Research, 24,* 343–351.

Burns, J. K. (1976). Proceedings: Relation between blood levels of cortisol and duration of human labour. *Journal of Physiology, 254,* 12P.

Bustan, M. N., & Coker, A. L. (1994). Maternal attitude toward pregnancy and the risk of neonatal death. *American Journal of Public Health, 84,* 411–414.

Cairns, R. B., & Rodkin, P. C. (1998). Phenomena regained. In R. B. Cairns, L. R. Bergman, & J. Kagan (Eds.), *Methods and models for studying the individual: Essays in honor of Marian Radke-Yarrow* (pp. 245–265). Thousand Oaks, CA: Sage.

Carter, A. M., & Olin, T. (1972). Effect of adrenergic stimulation and blockade on the uteroplacental circulation and uterine activity in the rabbit. *Journal of Reproductive Fertility, 29,* 251–260.

Charmandari, E., Kino, T., Souvatzoglou, E., & Chrousos, G. P. (2003). Pediatric stress: Hormonal mediators and human development. *Hormone Research, 59,* 161–179.

Collins, N. L., Dunkel-Schetter, C., Lobel, M., & Scrimshaw, C. M. (1993). Social support in pregnancy: Psychosocial correlates of birth outcomes and postpartum depression. *Journal of Personality and Social Psychology*, 65, 1243–1258.

Costa, A., De Filippis, V., Voglino, M., Giraudi, G., Massobrio, M., Benedetto, C., et al (1988). Adrenocorticotropic hormone and catecholamines in maternal, umbilical and neonatal plasma in relation to vaginal delivery. *Journal of Endocrinological Investigation*, 11, 703–709.

Crandon, A. J. (1979). Maternal anxiety and obstetric complications. *Journal of Psychosomatic Research*, 23, 109–111.

Crnic, K. A., Greenberg, M. T., Ragozin, A. S., Robinson, N. M., & Basham, R. B. (1983). Effects of stress and social support on mothers and premature and full-term infants. *Child Development*, 54, 209–217.

DaCosta, D., Brender, W., & Larouche, J. (1998). A prospective study of the impact of psychosocial and lifestyle variables on pregnancy complications. *Journal of Psychosomatic Obstetrics and Gynaecology*, 19, 28–37.

DaCosta, D., Larouche, J., Dritsa, M., & Brender, W. (1999). Variations in stress levels over the course of pregnancy: Factors associated with elevated hassles, state anxiety and pregnancy-specific stress. *Journal of Psychosomatic Research*, 47, 609–621.

Dejin-Karlsson, E., Hanson, B. S., Ostergren, P., Lindgren, A., Sjoberg, N., & Marsal, K. (2000). Association of a lack of psychosocial resources and the risk of giving birth to small for gestational age infants: A stress hypothesis. *British Journal of Obstetrics and Gynaecology*, 107, 89–100.

Deutsch, F. M., Ruble, D. N., Fleming, A., Brooks-Gunn, J., & Stangor, C. (1988). Information-seeking and maternal self-definition during the transition to motherhood. *Journal of Personality and Social Psychology*, 55, 420–431.

Dimitrovsky, L., Perez-Hirshberg, M., & Itskowithz, R. (1987). Depression during and following pregnancy: Quality of family relationships. *The Journal of Psychology*, 121(3), 213–218.

Dole, N., Savitz, D. A., Hertz-Picciotto, I., Siega-Riz, A. M., McMahon, M. J., & Buekens, P. (2003). Maternal stress and preterm birth. *American Journal of Epidemiology*, 157, 14–24.

Dunkel-Schetter, C., Gurung, R., Lobel, M., & Wadhwa, P. (2001). Stress processes in pregnancy and birth: Psychological, biological, and sociocultural influences. In A. Baum, T. A. Revenson & J. E. Singer (Eds.), *Handbook of health psychology* (pp. 495–518). Mahwah, NJ: Lawrence Erlbaum Associates.

Eskes, T. K. A. B. (1973). The influence of B-mimetic catecholamines upon uterine activity in human pregnancy and labor. In J. B. Josimovich (Ed.), *Uterine contraction – Side effects of steroidal contraceptives* (pp. 265–286). New York: Wiley.

Facchinetti, F., Ottolini, F., Fazzio, M., Rigatelli, M., & Volpe, A. (2007). Psychosocial factors associated with preterm uterine contractions. *Psychotherapy and Psychosomatics*, 76, 391–394.

Falconer, A. D., & Lake, D. M. (1982). Circumstances influencing umbilical-cord plasma catecholamines at delivery. *British Journal of Obstetrics and Gynaecology*, 89, 44–49.

Falorni, N. L., Fornasarig, A., & Stefanile, C. (1979). Research about anxiety effects on the pregnant woman and her newborn child. In L. Carenza & L. Zichella (Eds.), *Emotion and reproduction*, Proceedings of the Serono Symposia at the Fifth International Congress of Psychosomatic Obstetrics and Gynecology, Rome, Italy (Vol. 20B, pp. 1147–1153). New York: Academic.

Field, T., Sandberg, D., Garcia, R., Vega-Lahr, N., Goldstein, S., & Guy, L. (1985). Pregnancy problems, postpartum depression, and early mother-infant interactions. *Developmental Psychology*, 21, 1152–1156.

Fogel, C. I., & Lewallen, L. P. (1995). High-risk childbearing. In C. I. Fogel & N. F. Woods (Eds.), *Women's health care: A comprehensive handbook*. Thousand Oaks, CA: Sage.

Fonagy, P., Steele, H., & Steele, M. (1991). Maternal representations of attachment during pregnancy predict the organization of infant-mother attachment at one year of age. *Child Development*, 62, 891–905.

Gazmararian, J. A., Adams, M. M., Saltzman, L. E., Johnson, C. H., Bruce, F. C., Marks, J. S., et al. (1995). The relationship between pregnancy intendedness and physical violence in mothers of newborns. *Obstetrics and Gynecology*, 85, 1031–1038.

Giblin, P. T., Poland, M. L., & Ager, J. W. (1990). Effects of social supports on attitudes, health behaviors and obtaining prenatal care. *Journal of Community Health*, 15, 357–368.

Gilbert, E. S., & Harmon, J. S. (2003). *Manual of high-risk pregnancy.* St. Louis: Mosby.

Gillen-Goldstein, J., Paidas, M. J., Sokol, R. J., Jones, T. B., & Pernoll, M. L. (2003). Methods for assessment for pregnancy at risk. In A. H. DeCherney & L. Nathan (Eds.), *Current obstetric & gynecologic diagnosis & treatment* (9th ed., pp. 261–271). New York: McGraw-Hill Companies.

Grossman, F. K., Eichler, L. S., & Winickoff, S. A. (1980). *Pregnancy, birth and parenthood.* San Francisco, CA: Jossey-Bass.

Hamilton, B. E., Minino, A. M., Martin, J. A., Kochanek, K. D., Strobino, D. M., & Guyer, B. (2007). Annual summary of vital statistics: 2005. *Pediatrics, 119,* 345–360.

Hedegaard, M., Henriksen, T. B., Sabroe, S., & Secher, N. J. (1993). Psychological distress in pregnancy and preterm delivery. *British Medical Journal, 307,* 234–239.

Hedegaard, M., Henriksen, T. B., Secher, N. J., Hatch, M. C., & Sabroe, S. (1996). Do stressful life events affect duration and risk of preterm delivery? *Epidemiology, 7,* 339–345.

Herrenkohl, L. R. (1986). Prenatal stress disrupts reproductive behavior and physiology in offspring. *Annuals of the New York Academy of Sciences, 474,* 120–128.

Hobel, C. J., Castro, L. C., Woo, G., Dunkel-Schetter, C., Roll, C., et al. (1995). Individual and interactive effects of mental stress and physical strain in late pregnancy on urinary catecholamine excretion. *Journal for Society of Gynecological Investigations, 2,* Mar/Apr 1995, Abstract No. P354.

Hobel, C. J., Dunkel-Schetter, C., Roesch, S. C., Castro, L. C., & Arora, C. P. (1999). Maternal plasma corticotropin-releasing hormone associated with stress at 20 weeks' gestation in pregnancies ending in preterm delivery. *American Journal of Obstetrics and Gynecology, 180*(1 Pt 3), S257–S263.

Hoffman, S., & Hatch, M. C. (1996). Stress, social support and pregnancy outcome: A reassessment based on recent research. *Paediatric and Perinatal Epidemiology, 10,* 380–405.

Institute for Clinical Systems Improvement. (2000). Health care guidelines: Routine prenatal care. Retrieved February 24, 2003 from http://www.icsi.org/knowledge/detail.asp?catID=29&itemID=191

Institute of Medicine. (1985). *Preventing low birthweight.* Washington, DC: National Academy.

The Institute of Medicine Report. (2007). Preterm birth: Causes, consequences, and prevention. In R. E. Behrman & A. S. Butler (Eds.), *Committee on understanding premature birth and assuring healthy outcomes.* Washington, DC: The National Academies.

Jesse, D. E., Seaver, W., & Wallace, D. C. (2003). Maternal psychosocial risks predict preterm birth in a group of women from Appalachia. *Midwifery, 19,* 191–202.

Jones, C. M.III, & Greiss, F. C., Jr. (1982). The effect of labor on maternal and fetal circulating catecholamines. *American Journal of Obstetrics and Gynecology, 144,* 149–153.

Kalil, K. M., Gruber, J. E., Conley, J., & Sytniac, M. (1993). Social and family pressures on anxiety and stress during pregnancy. *Pre- and Perinatal Psychology Journal, 8,* 113–118.

Kramer, M. S. (1998). Socioeconomic determinants of intrauterine growth retardation. *European Journal of Clinical Nutrition, 52*(Suppl. 1), S29–S33.

Kuhn, T. S. (1970). *The structure of scientific revolutions* (2nd ed.). Chicago: University of Chicago Press.

Laatikainen, T. J. (1991). Corticotropin-releasing hormone and opioid peptides in reproduction and stress. *Annals of Medicine, 23,* 489–496.

Lederman, R. (1984). Anxiety and conflict in pregnancy: Relationship to maternal health status. In H. H. Werley & J. J. Fitzpatrick (Eds.), *Annual review of nursing research* (vol. 2). New York: Springer.

Lederman, R. (1986). Maternal anxiety in pregnancy: Relationship to fetal and newborn health status. In H. H. Werley, J. J. Fitzpatrick, & R.L. Taunton (Eds.), *Annual review of nursing research* (vol. 4, pp. 3–19). New York: Springer.

Lederman, R. P. (1995). Relationship of anxiety, stress, and psychosocial development to reproductive health. *Behavioral Health, 21,* 101–112.

Lederman, R. P. (1996). *Psychosocial adaptation in pregnancy: Assessment of seven dimensions of maternal development* (2nd ed.). New York: Springer.

Lederman, R. P. (March 22–25, 2008). *Effectiveness of maternal prenatal psychosocial support for decreasing anxiety in experimental and control groups.* Paper presented at the 28th Annual Meeting of the Society of Behavioral Medicine, San Diego, CA.

Lederman, R., Harrison, J., & Worsham, S. (1992). Progressive prenatal personality changes: Patterns of maternal development, anxiety, and depression. Paper presentation at the Sigma Theta Tau International Nursing Research Conference, Columbus, OH.

Lederman, R., & Lederman, E. (1987). Dimensions of postpartum adaptation: Comparisons of multiparas 3 days and 6 weeks after delivery. *Journal of Psychosomatic Obstetrics and Gynaecology, 7*, 193–203.

Lederman, R., Lederman, E., Work, B. A., Jr., & McCann, D. S. (1978). The relationship of maternal anxiety, plasma catecholamines, and plasma cortisol to progress in labor. *American Journal of Obstetrics and Gynecology, 132*, 495–500.

Lederman, R., Lederman, E., Work, B. A., Jr., & McCann, D. S. (1979). Relationship of psychological factors in pregnancy to progress in labor. *Nursing Research, 28*, 94–97.

Lederman, R., Lederman, E., Work, B. A., Jr., & McCann, D. S. (1981). Maternal psychological and physiological correlates of fetal-newborn health status. *American Journal of Obstetrics and Gynecology, 139*, 956–958.

Lederman, R., Lederman, E., Work, B. A., Jr., & McCann, D. S. (1985). Anxiety and epinephrine in multiparous women in labor: Relationship to duration of labor and fetal heart rate pattern. *American Journal of Obstetrics and Gynecology, 153*, 870–877.

Lederman, R. P., McCann, D. S., Work, B., Jr., & Huber, M. J. (1977). Endogenous plasma epinephrine and norepinephrine in last trimester pregnancy and labor. *American Journal of Obstetrics and Gynecology, 129*, 5–8.

Lederman, R. P., & Miller, D. (1998). Adaptation to pregnancy in three different ethnic groups: Latin-, Africa-, and Anglo- American. *Canadian Journal of Nursing Research, 30*, 37–51.

Lederman, R. P., Weis, K., Camune, B., & Mian, T. S. (2002). Prediction of pregnancy outcomes from measures of adaptation to pregnancy and family functioning. Paper Presentation at the VIII Nursing Research Pan American Colloquium, Mexico City, Mexico.

Leeners, B., Neumaier-Wagner, P., Kuse, S., Stiller, R., & Rath, W. (2007). Emotional stress and the risk to develop hypertensive diseases in pregnancy. *Hypertension in Pregnancy, 26*, 211–226.

Leifer, H. (1980). *Psychological effects of motherhood: A study of first pregnancy.* New York: Praeger.

Levi, R., Lundberg, U., Hanson, U., & Frankenhaeuser, M. (1989). Anxiety during pregnancy after the Chernobyl accident as related to obstetric outcome. *Journal of Psychosomatic Obstetrics and Gynecology, 10*, 221–230.

Levinson, G., & Shnider, M. (1979). Catecholamines: The effects of maternal fear and its treatment on uterine function and circulation. *Birth and the Family Journal, 6*, 167–174.

Lieberman, M. A. (1986). Social supports-the consequences of psychologizing: A commentary. *Journal of Clinical and Consulting Psychology, 54*, 461–465.

Lobel, M. (1994). Conceptualizations, measurement, and effects of prenatal maternal stress on birth outcomes. *Journal of Behavioral Medicine, 17*, 1–48.

Lobel, M., & Dunkel-Shetter, C. (1990). Conceptualizing stress to study effects on health: Environmental, perceptual, and emotional components. *Anxiety Research, 3*, 213–230.

Longo, D. R., Kruse, R. L., LeFevre, M. L., Schramm, W. F., Stockbauer, J. W., & Howell, V. (1999). An investigation of social class differences in very-low-birth-weight outcomes: A continuing public health concern. *Journal of Health Care Finance, 25*, 75–89.

McCubbin, H., McCubbin, M. A, Thompson, A., Huang, S. T. (1989). Family assessment and self-report instruments in family medicine research. In C. N. Ramsey, Jr. (Ed.), *Family systems in medicine.* New York, Guilford Press, pp. 181–214.

McFarlane, J., Parker, B., & Soeken, K. (1996a). Abuse during pregnancy: Associations with maternal health and infant birth weight. *Nursing Research, 45*(1), 37–41.

McFarlane, J., Parker, B., & Soeken, K. (1996b). Physical Abuse, smoking, and substance use during pregnancy: prevalence, interrelationships, and effects on birth weight. *Journal of Obstetric, Gynecologic, and Neonatal Nursing, 25*(4), 313–320.

Majewski, J. L. (1986) Conflicts, satisfaction, and attitudes during transition to the maternal role. *Nursing Research, 34*(1), 10–14.

Mancuso, R. A., Schetter, C. D., Rini, C. M., Roesch, S. C., & Hobel, C. J. (2004). Maternal prenatal anxiety and corticotropin-releasing hormone associated with timing of delivery. *Psychosomatic Medicine, 66,* 762–769.

Marshall, J. M. (1977). Modulation of smooth muscle activity by catecholamines. *Federation Proceedings, 36,* 2450–2455.

Misra, D. P., O'Campo, P., & Strobino, D. (2001). Testing a sociomedical model for preterm delivery. *Paediatric Perinatal Epidemiology, 15,* 110–122.

Myers, R. E., & Myers, S. E. (1979). Use of sedative, analgesic, and anesthetic drugs during labor and delivery: Bane or boon? *American Journal of Obstetrics and Gynecology, 133,* 83–104.

Myhrman, A. (1988). The Northern Finland cohort, 1966–82: A follow-up study of children unwanted at birth. In H. P. David, Z. Dytrych, Z. Matejcek, & V. Schuller (Eds.), *Born unwanted* (pp. 103–110). New York: Springer.

Norbeck, J. S., & Anderson, N. J. (1989a). Psychosocial predictors of pregnancy outcomes in low-income black, Hispanic, and white women. *Nursing Research, 38,* 204–209.

Norbeck, J. S., & Anderson, N. J. (1989b). Life stress, social support and anxiety in mid- and late-pregnancy among low income women. *Research in Nursing & Health, 12,* 281–287.

Norbeck, J. S., DeJoseph, J. F., & Smith, R. T. (1996). A randomized trial of an empirically-derived social support intervention to prevent low birth weight among African-American women. *Social Science and Medicine, 43,* 947–954.

Nordentoft, M., Lou, H. C., Hansen, D., Nim, J. Pryds, O., Rubin, P., et al (1996). Intrauterine growth retardation and premature delivery: The influence of maternal smoking and psychosocial factors. *American Journal of Public Health, 86,* 347–354.

Oakey, R. E. (1975). Serum cortisol binding capacity and cortisol concentration in the pregnant baboon and its fetus during gestation. *Endocrinology, 97,* 1024.

Oakley, A., Hickey, D., Rajan, L., & Rigby, A. S. (1996). Social support in pregnancy: Does it have long-term effects? *Journal of Reproductive and Infant Psychology, 14,* 7–22.

Office of the Surgeon General and the Eunice Kennedy Shriver National Institute of Child Health and Human Development (NICHD). (2008) *The Surgeon General's Conference on the Prevention of Preterm Birth,* webcast on June 16 and June 17, 2008.

O'Hara, M. W. (1986). Social support, life events, and depression during pregnancy and the puerperium. *Archives of General Psychiatry, 43*(6), 569–573.

Ohno, H., Yamashita, K., Yahata, T., Doi, R., Kawamura, M., Mure, K., et al (1986). Maternal plasma concentrations of catecholamines and cyclic nucleotides during labor and following delivery. *Research Communications in Chemical Pathology and Pharmacology, 51,* 183–194.

Ohrlander, S., Gennser, G., & Eneroth, P. (1976). Plasma cortisol levels in human fetus during parturition. *Obstetrics and Gynecology, 48,* 381–397.

Oken, E., Kleinman, K. P., Rich-Edwards, J., & Gillman, M. W. (2003). *A nearly continuous measure of birth weight for gestational age using a United States national reference.* Retrieved May 12, 2004, from http://www.biomedcentral.com/1471-2431.

Olds, D., Henderson, C., Jr., Kitzman, H., Eckenrode, J., Cole, R., & Tatelbaum, R. (1998). The promise of home visitation: Results of two randomized trials. *Journal of Community Psychology, 26,* 5–21.

Olson, D. H., Bell, R., & Portner, J. (1992). *FACES II.* Minneapolis, MN: Life Innovations.

Olson, D. H., Russell, C. S., & Sprenkel, D. H. (1983). Circumplex model of marital and family systems: VI. Theoretical update. *Family Process, 22,* 69–83.

Olson, D. H., Sprenkle, D. H., & Russell, C. S. (1979). Circumplex model of marital and family system: I. Cohesion and adaptability dimensions, family types, and clinical applications. *Family Process, 18,* 3–28.

Orr, S. T., James, S. A., Miller, C. A., Barakat, B., Daikoku, N., Pupkin, M., et al. (1996). Psychosocial stressors and low birth weight in an urban population. *American Journal of Preventive Medicine, 12,* 459–466.

Orr, S. T., Reiter, J. P., Blazer, D. G., Sherman, J. (2007). Maternal prenatal pregnancy-related anxiety and spontaneous preterm birth in Baltimore, Maryland. *Psychosomatic Medicine, 69*, 566–570.

Ounsted, M., Moar, M., & Scott, W. A. (1981). Perinatal morbidity and mortality in small-for-dates babies: The relative importance of some maternal factors. *Early Human Development, 5*(4), 367–375.

Paarlberg, K. M., Vingerhoets, A. J. J. M., Passchier, J., Dekker, G. A., Heinen, A. G. J. J., & van Geijn, H. P. (1999). Psychosocial predictors of low birth weight: A prospective study. *British Journal of Obstetrics and Gynaecology, 106*, 834–841.

Paarlberg, K. M., Vingerhoets, A. J. J. M., Passchier, J., Dekker, G. A., & van Geijn, H.P. (1995). Psychosocial factors and pregnancy outcome: A review with emphasis on methodological issues. *Journal of Psychosomatic Research, 39*, 563–595.

Pagel, M. D., Smilkstein, G., Regen, H., & Montano, D. (1990). Psychosocial influences on new born outcomes: A controlled prospective study. *Social Science & Medicine, 30*, 597–604.

Paulick, R., Kastendieck, E., & Wernze, H. (1985). Catecholamines in arterial and venous umbilical blood: Placental extraction, correlation with fetal hypoxia and transcutaneous partial oxygen tension. *Journal of Perinatal Medicine, 13*, 31–42.

Peacock, J. L., Bland, J. M., & Anderson, H. R. (1995). Preterm delivery: Effects of socioeconomic factors, psychological stress, smoking, alcohol, and caffeine. *British Medical Journal, 311*, 531–535.

Pilowsky, I. (1972). Psychological aspects of complications of childbirth: A prospective study of primiparae and their husbands. In N. Morris (Ed.), *Psychosomatic medicine in obstetrics and gynaecology* (pp. 161–165). Basel, Switzerland: Karger.

Pohjavuori, M., Rovamo, L., Laatikainen, T., Kariniemi, V., & Pettersson, J. (1986). Stress of delivery and plasma endorphins and catecholamines in the newborn infant. *Biological Research in Pregnancy and Perinatology, 7*, 1–5.

Pryor, J. E., Thompson, J. M., Robinson, E., Clark, P. M., Becroft, D. M. Pattison, N. S., et al. (2003). Stress and lack of social support as risk factors for small-for-gestational-age birth. *Acta Paediatrica, 92*, 62–64.

Ramsey, C. N., Jr., Abell, T. D., & Baker, L. C. (1986). The relationship between family functioning, life events, family structure, and the outcome of pregnancy. *Journal of Family Practice, 22*, 521–527.

Reeb, K. G., Graham, A. V., Zyzanski, S. J., & Kitson, G. C. (1987). Predicting low birthweight and complicated labor in urban black women: A biopsychosocial perspective. *Social Science Medicine, 25*, 91–98.

Roesch, S. C., Dunkel-Schetter, C. D., Woo, G. & Hobel, C. J. (2004). Modeling the types and timing of stress in pregnancy. *Anxiety, Stress & Coping: An International Journal, 17*, 87–102.

Roman-Ponce, H., Thatcher, W. W., Caton, D., Barron, D. H., & Wilcox, C. J. (1978). Effects of thermal stress and epinephrine on uterine blood flow in ewes. *Journal of Animal Science, 46*, 167–174.

Rosenfeld, C. R., Barton, M. D., & Meschia, G. (1976). Effects of epinephrine on distribution of blood flow in the pregnant ewe. *American Journal of Obstetrics and Gynecology, 124*, 156–163.

Rubin, R. (1984). *Maternal identity and the maternal experience.* New York: Springer.

Ruiz, R. J., Fullerton, J., & Dudley, D. J. (2003). The interrelationship of maternal stress, endocrine factors and inflammation on gestational length. *Obstetrical & Gynecological Survey, 58*, 415–428.

Sable, M. R., Stockbauer, J. W., Schramm, W. F., & Land, G. H. (1990). Differentiating the barriers to adequate prenatal care in Missouri, 1987–88. *Public Health Reports, 105*, 549–555.

Sameroff, A. J. (2000). Developmental systems and psychopathology. *Development and Psychopathology, 12*, 297–312.

Schneider, M. L., & Coe, C. L. (1993). Repeated social stress during pregnancy impairs neuromotor development of the primate infant. *Developmental and Behavioral Pediatrics, 14*, 81–87.

Schneider, M. L., Coe, C. L., & Lubach, G. R. (1992). Endocrine activation mimics the adverse effects of prenatal stress on the neuromotor development of the infant primate. *Developmental Psychobiology, 25,* 427–439.

Sleutel, M. R. (2003). Intrapartum nursing: integrating Rubin's framework with social support theory. *Journal of Obstetrics, Gynecology, and Neonatal Nursing, 32,* 76–82.

Spielberger, C. D., Gorsuch, R. L., & Lushene, R. E. (1970). *Manual for the state-trait anxiety inventory (self-evaluation questionnaire).* Palo Alto, CA: Consulting Psychologists.

Trad, P. (1990). On becoming a mother: In the throes of developmental transformation. *Psychoanalytic Psychology, 7,* 341–361.

Trad, P. (1991). Adaptation to developmental transformations during various phases of motherhood. *Journal of the American Academy of Psychoanalysis, 19,* 403–421.

Tuimala, R. J., Kauppila, A. J., & Haapalahti, J. (1975). Response of pituitary-adrenal axis on partal stress. *Obstetrics and Gynecology, 46,* 275–278.

Wadhwa, P. D. (2005). Psychneuroendocrine processes in human pregnancy influence fetal development and health. *Psychneuroendocrinology, 30,* 724–723.

Wadhwa, P. D., Porto, M., Garite, T. J., Chicz-DeMet, A., & Sandman, C. A. (1998). Maternal corticotrophin-releasing hormone levels in the early third trimester predict length of gestation in human pregnancy. *American Journal of Obstetrics and Gynecology, 179,* 1079–1085.

Wadhwa, P. D., Sandman, C. A., Porto, M., Dunkel-Schetter, C., & Garite, T. J. (1993). The association between prenatal stress and infant birthweight and gestational age at birth: A prospective investigation. *American Journal of Obstetrics and Gynecology, 169,* 858–865.

Ward, A. J. (1991). Prenatal stress and childhood psychopathology. *Child Psychiatry and Human Development, 22,* 97–110.

Watson, J. P., Elliott, S. A., Rugg, A. J., & Brough, D. I. (1984). Psychiatric disorders in pregnancy and the first postnatal year. *British Journal of Psychiatry, 144*(5), 453–462.

Weis, K. L. (2006). *Maternal identity formation in a military sample: A longitudinal perspective.* Unpublished Dissertation, University of North Carolina, Chapel Hill, NC.

Weis, K. L., Lederman, R. P., Lilly, A. E., & Schaffer, J. (2008). The relationship of military imposed marital separations on maternal acceptance of pregnancy. *Research in Nursing & Health, 31,* 196–207.

Williams, A. M., Joy, L. A., Travis, L., Gotowiec, A., Blum-Steele, M., Aiken, L., et al. (1987). Transition to motherhood: A longitudinal study. *Infant Mental Health Journal, 8,* 251–265.

Wolkind, S., & Zajicek, E. (1981). *Pregnancy: A psychological and social study.* New York: Grune & Stratton.

Zax, M., Sameroff, A. J., & Farnum, J. E. (1975). Childbirth education, maternal attitudes, and delivery. *American Journal of Obstetrics and Gynecology, 123,* 185–190.

Zuspan, F. P., Cibils, L. A., & Pose, S. V. (1962). Myometrial and cardiovascular responses to alterations in plasma epinephrine and norepinephrine. *American Journal of Obstetrics and Gynecology, 84,* 841–851.

Chapter 2
Acceptance of Pregnancy

In a broad sense, acceptance of pregnancy refers to a woman's adaptive responses to the changes inherent in prenatal growth and development. Data presented in Chapter 1 suggest that acceptance of pregnancy is associated with the gravida's adaptation to and her gratification with being pregnant. The results further indicate that the gravida is less prepared for childbirth and motherhood when acceptance of the pregnancy is low, and she is more likely to have conflicts and fears concerning labor, and to have a longer duration of labor. Anxiety about acceptance of pregnancy also was related to greater Intrapartum Complications and lower Gestational Age at Birth. Recent data from the National Survey of Family Growth show that half (49%) of all US pregnancies are unplanned (Finer & Henshaw, 2006), a factor in acceptance of pregnancy that may substantially contribute to the findings noted above.

Questionnaire and interview data from the aggregate research projects presented in Chapter 1 indicate that if the gravida wants to be a mother, she usually accepts being pregnant. However, the reverse is not necessarily true; if a woman accepts being pregnant, it cannot be assumed that she accepts the child and motherhood. The woman's satisfaction with the pregnancy may mean that she feels a sense of biological, feminine, or societal role fulfillment (Flapan, 1969; Pohlman, 1969; Wenner et al., 1969) without wanting the baby. It also is possible that the baby and motherhood are desired, but that the pregnancy itself is resisted. Therefore, although acceptance of the pregnancy usually is associated with desires for motherhood and a child, the study assessments distinguished between the motivation for pregnancy and the motivation for motherhood.

Of particular interest in evaluating a woman's acceptance of the pregnancy, was the extent to which the expectant mother exhibited the following characteristics:

1. Consciously planned and wanted the pregnancy,
2. Was predominantly happy versus depressed during the pregnancy,
3. Had discomfort during the pregnancy and addressed that discomfort,
4. Accepted or rejected changes in her body, and
5. Was ambivalent and experienced conflict about the pregnancy near term.

A woman may express overt acceptance of her pregnancy, but her behavior may belie this attitude. If she generally was distressed and irritable during the 9 months

R. Lederman and K. Weis, *Psychosocial Adaptation to Pregnancy*,
DOI 10.1007/978-1-4419-0288-7_2, © Springer Science+Business Media, LLC 2009

because she had discomforts, often felt depressed, detested her changed appearance, or was burdened with conflict, it was assumed that she partly rejected the pregnancy. But it may not have been possible for her to express the rejection directly. Such factors were considered in evaluating the gravida`s acceptance of the pregnancy.

It also should be kept in mind that women generally may feel lower self-acceptance during pregnancy (Bailey & Hailey, 1986–1987) and a somewhat lower capacity for independent thinking, as they experience a stronger introverted personality change. These paradoxical changes occur at a time when the need for self-acceptance may be pivotal, and individual conflict resolution and progress are paramount for maternal development.

In all the sections that follow in which the five concepts cited above on Acceptance of Pregnancy are discussed, the narrative progresses from descriptions and examples of high adaptation to moderate and low maternal adaptation. This pattern is repeated in all the seven chapters on dimensions of maternal adaptation to pregnancy.

2.1 Planning and Wanting the Pregnancy

The women's reactions to pregnancy varied. Many women had planned to have a baby and when the pregnancy was confirmed they were elated. Ms. Inis and her husband had planned for 5 years.

> Ed just graduated in December, and we knew that we would wait until he graduated. It got kind of hard near the end. I got really anxious… to have a baby. And he's really excited about it too, even more so than I thought he would be.

Ms. Aaron stated that this was a good time for her pregnancy.

> We're probably more settled now than we have been in all of the years we were married, even though we just moved. This is a perfect time. I'm looking forward to it. I wish it would have been a little earlier…. I would have been even happier to have the baby a year ago.

Several women who were approaching 30 wanted the baby very much because they feared that they might become too old to have children. For example, Ms. Carre said:

> But I am so old. I can't start any later than this, because I don't believe in only children. Only children think it's just fine…, but I am married to an only child…and I'm not going to have an only child. Which means I've got to get busy with this business because I don't believe in having them after 35. This is, in my opinion, courting disaster…. We have put it off as long as I think we can put it off.

Nevertheless, Ms. Carre had some qualms about having the baby because her husband did not have a job at the time. She had fantasies and dreams of returning to school and to her premarital state. Wanting the baby because she was approaching 30, may have indicated that Ms. Carre was quite ready to take the step into motherhood, but she also could have been motivated by family or community pressure or by the fear of missing one of the major experiences in a woman's life.

Thus, a planned pregnancy is not necessarily associated with the desire to be a mother. Interestingly, other researchers have reported that planning is not related to a woman's attitude toward being pregnant (Entwisle & Doering, 1981; Klerman, 2000) or to adaptation to pregnancy (Shereshefsky & Yarrow, 1973), while still others have reported that planning is associated with less depression during pregnancy (Lips, 1984). Lawrence, Rothman, Cobb, Rothman, and Bradbury (2008) conducted pre- and post-pregnancy marital satisfaction assessments and found that couples with pre-pregnancy planned pregnancies had higher pre-pregnancy marital satisfaction scores. They also found that the decline in marital satisfaction that many couples experience post-pregnancy was diminished in couples with planned pregnancies.

In many instances the woman's pregnancy was unplanned. Some women, no longer taking the contraceptive pill for fear of deleterious side effects, found themselves "caught" unaware. Others became pregnant through contraceptive carelessness. All of these women claimed that they wanted the baby even though they initially may have contemplated abortion. No woman stated explicitly that she did not want the baby and would reject it once born. In most cases of unplanned pregnancy, the woman came to accept the pregnancy and used the 9 months to resolve conflicts and develop her motherhood role. When resolution of psychosocial conflict occurred slowly or not at all, even a planned pregnancy was difficult to accept. If residual conflict still seemed unresolved by the third trimester, it was expressed more indirectly – for example, in dreams and in intense fears about labor, responses also reported by Trad (1991) and Cohen (1988). Examples of this are provided in the following sections.

2.2 Happiness Versus Depression During Pregnancy

In the study, it was assumed that if a woman was happy during the pregnancy and expressed a sense of well-being, then she accepted being pregnant. As found in our studies, others (Sable & Libbus, 2000; Peacock et al., 2001) also found that not all woman with unintended or unplanned pregnancies were unhappy about them. Thus, a distinction is made in the literature between pregnancy attitudes and planned pregnancy or intendedness (Klerman, 2000). Several women saw pregnancy as a happy period in their lives. Not only was Ms. Xana's pregnancy planned, but she stated that she had become pregnant more quickly than she had expected and was "very happy" about it.

> We both wanted children, and we were talking about it…very seriously and I wanted kids really bad, and I felt my husband did too. And that same month…presto, I found out that I was pregnant.

There seemed to be correspondence between feeling happy during pregnancy and having made long-term plans that included a baby. Ms. Inis said that her pregnancy had "been really nice."

I haven't had very many physical discomforts, and I'm really happy about it. I've been wanting to quit work and have a baby and go back to school; the whole big plan has been in my head for a couple of years. And it's all working out now, so it seems really nice.

Some women claimed that they enjoyed their pregnancy not only because it fulfilled a plan or because of a lack of discomfort, but also for its own rewards. Several women were reassured, as well as delighted, with fetal movement. In her diary Ms. Aaron wrote:

All I seem to think about is the baby. I think I could spend all my money on baby clothes. I'm so excited. I'd love to have the baby right now. Somehow this week I feel on top of the world. I love watching my whole tummy move. I keep telling Charles ours will be the most beautiful baby on the block.

For some women, it was possible to enjoy being pregnant despite considerable discomfort. Ms. Fair experienced morning sickness and some vomiting through the 5th month; these episodes occasionally triggered short-lived negative feelings, but she still enjoyed being pregnant. She derived pleasure from the extra attention she received from others, although she denied this feeling. In her diary she wrote:

In my own opinion I can't wait to get out of the center of attention..... I don't [want to] have ten people worried if I'm all right. People (men especially) act like pregnant women are a piece of china. I'd like to get out and move! I do enjoy being pregnant though. It's fun.

Ms. Fair's pregnancy was planned, and the baby was very much wanted. Fetal movement gave her pleasure. On one occasion when she was worried and not feeling well, she recorded in her diary the following:

I decided to take a bath…and watch my stomach move with the baby. I do that a lot, in the tub or lying down, I get a feeling of enjoyment and satisfaction out of seeing the baby move. I also wondered if it had all of it's [sic] fingers and toes and a healthy body.

Ms. Fair's pleasure stemmed from the reassurance that she derived from knowing that her baby was alive. Fetal movement was particularly important to her because she had greatly feared that her baby might be abnormal; her fears of abnormality were prevalent throughout the pregnancy. In Ms. Fair's case, acceptance of the pregnancy appeared somewhat equivocal insofar as it was contingent on confidence in the well-being of the fetus.

A few women enjoyed being pregnant, but dreaded labor and delivery. Ms. Meta felt "great" throughout her pregnancy, which was unplanned, but wished that she did not have to go through labor and delivery. She was ready for her baby, but not for labor and delivery. Ms. Bode was enjoying a planned "easy pregnancy," but she also feared labor and delivery. Because of marked doubts about her mothering skills and a pronounced motherhood-career conflict, she was not ready for her baby or for labor and delivery. In cases like these, the women were enjoying their pregnancies not only out of a sense of biological fulfillment, but also out of a desire to postpone labor and delivery. The desire for postponement of childbirth may therefore be viewed as a product either of ambivalence about the forthcoming child, or of fears and anxieties about the risks of childbirth.

Ms. Bode enjoyed being pregnant, but her enjoyment was lessened by her concerns about sustaining herself both as a mother and in a career. She read obsessively about childbirth which made her feel "creative," but at the same time caused her to dwell on imagined problems. When she had a pain in her side, for example, she was afraid that she had a tubal pregnancy. She was extremely concerned about birth defects and her ability to sustain her career after the baby was born. The extent to which her fears were based on her own perceived ability to give as a mother, rather than on a realistic concern about birth defects, was difficult to determine. She reported no family history of or recent acquaintance with birth defects.

Quite a few women were not happy about being pregnant, but were happy at the thought of having a child. For these women, pregnancy was seen chiefly as the vehicle to obtain the baby. Ms. Hayes did not suffer much physical discomfort, but she would have rather not gone through the pregnancy. She said that she was "happy to be having a baby."

> Pregnancy is not bad for me at all, and I'm having an easy time, but I know that I would feel more energetic and...more comfortable in the summer if I wasn't pregnant. It's funny because it's not an ordeal, but I'm not enjoying being pregnant.... I don't hate the idea of being pregnant. I haven't cried because of it or been depressed because of it. It's just that afterwards you think about having to lose weight and exercise and get yourself back in shape, and that's a lot of energy.

It should be noted that Ms. Hayes had considerable difficulty in evolving a motherhood role and feared postpartum depression. She obviously was disconcerted by her awkward body. She also was frightened of labor and delivery, and her fear affected the way she viewed pregnancy. She had heard people talking "about all the terrible things in labor" and had read a book that seemed to have reinforced her fears.

> I thought if I had read that [the book] first, I would never be pregnant now. You know, you hear that women scream during labor and all that and the idea of doing that and creating horrible scenes and making things worse probably scared me the most.

Although Ms. Hayes truly wanted a child, she was troubled by the numerous sacrifices that she would have to make during pregnancy and childbirth.

Mood swings, commonly associated with pregnancy, were prevalent during the last trimester. The less extreme these swings, the easier they were for the women to manage. Ms. Uman admitted to having periods of depression and was aware that she felt less sociable at such times, but she appeared confident in her ability to handle such situations. She even expected some depression after the birth of her child. "If it [depression] happens, I think I'll understand why I am tending to feel depressed, but I'll be able to overcome it."

A characteristic expression of lability is reflected in an entry in Ms. Santa's diary.

> I don't know if this is really considered a problem or not, but at times it seems like a problem. I'm really subjective to drastic mood changes. That or I'll be extremely emotional. For no reason at all I'll start crying or just laugh till I can hardly breathe. I don't know why; and if I can't understand it, it's twice as hard for John, especially if I'm bummed out or crying. It don't [sic] seem normal for a person to cry for no reason, and I never did it before.

Many women felt foolish about finding themselves so emotionally unstable. A few had difficulty in handling their increased lability. Ms. Vale, for example, said: "This is the weirdest pregnancy because I've been pretty much like a yo-yo through it." Later, she complained of passivity mixed with "anxiety fits.: I've been really sort of non-anything lately, non-aggressive. I've been really passive..... If I don't have the drive, it's just great. But then I get these anxiety fits. I feel really useless, like I'm not doing anything." Typically, the mood swings were occasioned by anticipation of maternal fulfillment, followed by fear of failure as a mother; they tended to be short-lived, with depression readily assuaged by reassurance and support.

Several women were depressed above and beyond the expected mood swings during their pregnancies; when depression occurred in these cases, it was not short-lived. These women may have been prone to depression before pregnancy. The conflicts precipitated by pregnancy may have triggered a depressed state of mind or deepened an already existing depression. Because proneness to depression often is associated with low self-esteem (Beck, 1967), it was expected that those women suffering from low self-esteem and guilt would tend to be more doubtful about their ability to cope with labor and delivery, or their ability to mother. Therefore, they might be depressed more often during their pregnancy. For instance, Ms. Lash wanted her baby and had a good relationship with her husband, but she had rather low self-esteem. She had difficulty in handling her depressed feelings. She was extremely anxious about possible injury to herself or her baby during labor and delivery. Although her acceptance of pregnancy was high, her 9 months were weighted with challenge and intense introspective questioning.

On the other hand, Ms. Aaron, who also suffered from low self-esteem and was ambivalent about being a mother and frightened of labor, did not complain about being depressed. She stated that her pregnancy had been "great" and that she had enjoyed it. So, it is not necessarily the case that low self-esteem and difficulty in establishing a motherhood identity lead to depression and unhappiness during pregnancy. Instead, pregnancy can enhance a sense of worth in some women, particularly those with low self-esteem (Young, 1984).

In contrast to women with low self-esteem, a woman of high self-esteem who experiences a great deal of ambivalence and conflict about motherhood might also tend to be depressed during pregnancy (Lips, 1984). Such a state of mind could be considered reactive. Ms. Dann, for example, had considerable self-confidence, yet she experienced conflict about her ability to sustain her profession and mother her child. Her conflict was compounded by a disintegrating marriage and depression. She described her first reaction to learning of her pregnancy.

> I was just generally depressed, but really bad. As a matter of fact it was the only time I had morning sickness symptoms like that.... The morning sickness was more due to just plain general feeling terrible about myself than to the really physical things.... Then I toyed with the idea of an abortion; I decided that I couldn't. That was that.

Ms. Dann also felt resentful that the constraints of pregnancy, particularly fatigue, were interfering in her life.

As discussed previously, another situation that sparks conflict and depression is one in which the woman perceives herself as isolated at home alone, when she previously has been active in a career or in the community. Ms. Bode's depression was preceded by thoughts of being at home all day with the baby.

I think I, in a sense, have a prepartum depression – already!... Over Easter when I was home from teaching, it just really hit me how I would be home like that all the time.... I was very depressed one day just kind of anticipating it and realizing how much of a change it was going to be, because I had been really active with my teaching, and it has been a pretty major part of my life now for 4 years.

Her depression did not last long. A sense of isolation, however, can easily lead to depression for many women who have difficulty handling loneliness; isolation tends to intensify dependency needs. Other research has shown that depression tends to increase the most from the 6th to the 9th month of pregnancy (Lips, 1985). This appears to parallel the period of time principally associated with the anticipation of and preparation for childbirth, as well as the imminent prospect of motherhood and its trials. The work of Shereshefsky and Yarrow (1973) support such an interpretation.

Guilt, closely associated with depression (Kiloh, Andrews, Bianchi, & Neilson, 1972), also can spoil the pleasure of being pregnant. Ms. Wooly became pregnant before marriage and, in the third trimester, still was embarrassed by her pregnant body, which outwardly symbolized her guilt. "I felt like they look at me funny in school sometimes.... Maybe it's because I was pregnant before I got married. I think it's guilt feelings projected on other people.

Ms. Wooly especially experienced "guilt feelings" when she was with her family. "You know it's like I'm back in the family again and being punished for something bad."

In summary, the women who generally were happy had planned and/or wanted the pregnancy. They perceived it as the unfolding of their life plan for a family. Gratification from biological fulfillment and the desire for a child characterized these women. They enjoyed fetal movement and other aspects of pregnancy associated with creativity and life. Discomforts were either minimal or tolerated well. Anticipated childbirth and motherhood were experienced as a challenge, and were assumed with relative self-confidence regarding outcomes for the baby, themselves, and their careers. It is noteworthy that other investigators (Blake, Kiely, Gard, Ayman, & El-Mohanedes, 2007) found that happiness about pregnancy was a stronger predictor of psychosocial and behavioral risk factors, (such as smoking, drinking alcohol, using illicit drugs, depression, being without a partner or having a partner that did not want the baby) than intendedness [planning] of pregnancy. Happy women also reported better coping strategies.

Women who generally were unhappy frequently were plagued with intense anxiety about motherhood, the trials of labor and delivery, depression concerning bodily changes, possible infant anomalies, isolation in their new role, and career interruption. They tended to experience guilt and lower self-esteem, as well as sustained depression. A similar factor structure for pregnancy attitude was found by Reading, Cox, Sledmere, and Campbell (1984), who discovered that positive maternal feelings were associated with feeling happy and fulfilled, and negative feelings embodied worry, uncertainty, and stress. Other researchers have reported higher state and trait anxiety (Kalil, Gruber, Copley, & Sytniac, 1993) as well as greater depression (Messer, Dole, Kaufman, & Savitz, 2005; Najman, Morrison, Williams, Anderson, & Keeping, 1991) when a pregnancy was unwanted.

2.3   Discomfort During Pregnancy

The degree of discomfort experienced during pregnancy can be another indicator of a woman's acceptance of the pregnancy. The prevalence of pregnancy symptoms has been associated with levels of anxiety (Green, 1973; Lubin, Gardener, & Roth, 1975) and stress (Georgas, Giakonmaki, Koumandakis, & Kaskarelis, 1984), the desire for pregnancy (Klein, Potter, & Dyk, 1950), the woman's emotional health (Grossman, Eichler, & Winickoff, 1980), the incidence of personality problems and the overall reaction to pregnancy (Shereshefsky & Yarrow, 1973), and the acceptance of pregnancy (Kuo, Wang, Tseng, Jian, & Chou, 2007). Discomfort can spoil the pleasure of being pregnant, although it need not. Most women experience fatigue, bodily awkwardness, mood swings, and other problems or limitations (Lips, 1984, 1985). It is important to evaluate the following factors: (1) the intensity of the discomfort, (2) how much discomfort interferes with normal activity, and (3) how the discomfort is managed and tolerated. The prevalence of pregnancy symptoms also has been associated with current life stress, as well as a past suscep-tibility to illness or experiencing symptoms (Fagley, Miller, & Sullivan, 1982).

Some women declared that they had no discomfort at all. Ms. Carre said that she had no nausea and no problems. She said that she felt "terrific." "I'm so lucky. Everyone says to me things like,'Oh, I was throwing up so much my first three months. I lost 17 pounds,' and all this…. I have had no problems, none."

Ms. Tell said that she felt better than she ever had felt. She had a long history of psychiatric problems and suffered from acute anxiety and self-denigration during pregnancy; yet she insisted that she "never felt better." She may have been an example of the way conception and childbearing can render a temporary sense of self-importance (Young, 1984).

In a minority of cases, neither discomforts nor differences from the non-pregnant state were observed. Ms. Carre reported no mood swings. According to her husband, she hardly looked different. She had no physical difficulties, felt that she had not acted differently, and had little or no problem adjusting to her pregnant state. Ms. Carre did, in fact, complete pregnancy with relative ease.

Most women reported some nausea in the first trimester, but by the second and third trimester it usually was negligible. Ms. Uman had what she called "severe cases of morning sickness."

> I could barely make it out of bed in the morning. Nothing stayed down; I threw up for a whole month straight and lost 15 pounds. It wasn't very pleasant for either of us, but since then it's been fine.

Ms. Aaron stated that she felt "great" despite some initial "queasy spells" and fatigue in the first trimester. She said that she had been "healthy as an ox really." "The first three months I couldn't get enough to eat and I slept a lot, but since… about the fourth month, I've felt really terrific."

Ms. Zeff experienced nausea in the first months that was a "horror." Then her nausea diminished.

All the last semester I had sickness really bad in the morning and all day, and a lot of foods just completely turned me off. I threw up a lot...and it was hard to drive myself to class,... when I look back on it, it wasn't all that horrible. It seems like after Christmas, all the really bad feelings started going away, and I've been more tired and had little backaches...that I can remedy right away by lying down and propping my feet up.... I had a hard time keeping up with my homework because I was sleepy all the time, but the teachers are really understanding.... I took very easy classes on purpose because I knew what a rough time I had the first semester.

Ms. Zeff's enterprising ways of finding relief from her discomfort and altering her schedule so that attending classes would not be too much of a strain, indicated that she was adjusting well to the physiological changes brought on by pregnancy. Similarly, Ms. Xana did not resent the fatigue that she experienced. Adjustment to fatigue depended on each woman's general ability to adapt to new situations, to compensate, to search for new alternatives, and to lower self-expectations for the duration of pregnancy.

Some women were not very adaptable and had a difficult time with pregnancy. Ms. North, for example, declared that she had significant nausea and vomiting, was sick all the time, had "a lot of pain and stuff" with quickening, and was not enjoying her pregnancy at all. She had had a previous traumatic abortion and was frightened of labor. Nevertheless, she wanted a baby very much. Pregnancy for her mostly was a requisite for the desired baby. In another study (Kuo et al., 2007) the severity of nausea and vomiting was significantly associated with the Acceptance of Pregnancy scale from the Chinese translated Lederman Prenatal Self-Evaluation Questionnaire.

In summary, the data demonstrated that the discomforts commonly associated with pregnancy are not universal. Discomforts, even if mild or short-lived, may mar a pregnancy. Severe discomforts and discomforts that may be magnified due to association with a previous traumatic experience, may indicate rejection of the pregnancy; however, the expression of discomfort does not necessarily represent rejection of the forthcoming child. When the child is happily anticipated, discomforts tend to be perceived as an irritating imposition, and measures to minimize them usually meet with success.

In other cases, the frequent complaint of discomforts may be a sign of conflict regarding mothering ability, childrearing responsibilities, or feminine biological functions, also noted by Trad (1991) and Cohen (1988). Such cases required extended assessment in other areas of role adaptation. Generally, a report of the absence of discomforts may indicate acceptance of the pregnancy. However, the achievement of a higher level of physical well-being in the last trimester, relative to the pre-pregnant state, is suspect. Although rare, a high level of well-being during pregnancy may suggest a weak self-concept, one dependent on ulterior sources of recognition. Such a situation demands further exploration of attitudes, and of the extent of confidence or conflict about motherhood and childrearing. When these cases are encountered, the accuracy of an interpretation of adaptation to pregnancy, grounded predominantly on an assessment of discomforts and symptoms (as in the research study by Kirgis, Woolsey, & Sullivan, 1977), is questionable; more extensive assessment of coping measures and tolerance is required.

2.4 Body Change During Pregnancy

There is a relationship between the way a woman thinks about her body and her attitude toward pregnancy (McConnell & Daston, 1961) and attachment to the fetus (Haedt & Keel, 2007), and later to toddler attachment security (Ipsa, Sable, Porter, & Csizmadia, 2007). In general, women who accepted their pregnancies were little troubled by their altered state; they tended to accept their larger size. No woman expressed pride in body size during the third-trimester interviews. Such expression may be more common in the second trimester.

In her diary, Ms. Zeff admitted feeling miserable about her stretch marks. She felt "unsightly" and disfigured. "I must say that I am disappointed. It seems that you can never be the same after having children." She clearly expressed the sense of losing her old self, and a sense that she would never be the same again. Loss, in this case, was experienced with a depth of remorse that went beyond a vacillating ambivalence. Ms. Zeff admitted that she tended to avoid people while she was pregnant out of a sense of shame.

> Especially when I started to show, I was so mad…because I couldn't get into my clothes, and I didn't want a lot of my male friends to see me at all…. I just wished it wasn't happening to me and that I could still flit around in my fashionable clothes…. And it took a lot of getting used to, people seeing me like this….Vainness, that's all, total vainness.

Later, in her diary, she recounted a dream. "I was around lots of people at my parents' and in-laws' houses. I felt like a circus animal. Everybody watches you, asks questions, makes stupid remarks.

Ms. Zeff's unhappiness with her pregnant body manifested itself in anger at the fetus and newborn infant. In another dream she hid her baby in a neighbor's garden, expressing her anger at the pregnancy/baby and her wish to be rid of it. She also entered some recollections in her diary about a movie she had seen.

> There were pictures and shots of unborn fetuses throughout the movie. All the time I watched, I thought that awful looking junk was inside me. It actually turned my stomach. I felt very queasy all night imagining what was inside me…. I couldn't sleep all night; I felt like some kind of monster.

Her non-acceptance of her changed body size reflected her unresolved ambivalence about motherhood, and fear that she might lose control over her life. She became angry at circumstances involving disorder and disruption; she was compulsive about details. Pregnancy, and possibly the baby, meant disruption of her well-ordered life as well as her body.

In contrast, Ms. Acton came to terms with her altered body size, although it was difficult.

> The biggest thing for me has been the changes in my body…. I've had some real kind of psychological effects over my body changes because when I did get pregnant, I was a little heavier than I like to be anyway, and then I think that that was a little psychological too because I had this desire to get pregnant before that…. I kept thinking, Well, I don't look so good. I didn't fit into my clothes so well…. So it was an ego thing, but then once it

started to look like I was pregnant, then I felt better about it. But I still think…when I look in the mirror, God, you're wide.

Ms. Santa felt "ugly" because she had "this bulge in front of me." Her delivery date signaled the time when her shape would return to normal. As her delivery date approached she said:

I don't feel so pregnant as I used to. I'm not as moody or sensitive about when the baby is coming. I'm more socially minded and conscious about my personal appearance. I guess it's because I know it has to be any day, and to sit back and brood won't help. I like looking at regular clothes for the Spring. I even tried my old jeans on, which still fit except of course around the tummy. That made me feel good.

Ms. Xana reported feeling quite depressed about her appearance and wrote in her diary that she "started crying for no reason at all." She explained further: "Looking at myself I felt so big and clumsy that I guess I just felt that…[no one] could see me and not think I'm a big huge pig." Once her husband comforted her, she "felt fine."

Ms. Eaden, who experienced a high acceptance of pregnancy and high self-esteem, also had trouble accepting her changed shape. In a diary entry she stated that she was "mainly concerned about regaining my shape after the baby comes."

The loss of my figure is on my mind at times, but I know the result will be worth it. At least John doesn't think I'm FAT (or says he doesn't!), so that keeps my morale up! I also like to dress neatly, get lots of sun and get enough rest. Being tan gives me SUCH a lift makes me feel wonderfully healthy!

In handling her concern with being "fat," Ms. Eaden worked toward acceptance by telling herself that the result would be worth it. She felt reassured by her husband and used what means she had to make herself more attractive.

In many instances, the desire for a trim body may well be an expression of "binding out of the pregnancy," a developmental task associated with pregnancy near term (Rubin, 1975). When assessing acceptance of body changes, it is necessary to separate cultural factors from psychological factors. American society tends to admire a trim female figure. When an American woman is pregnant, she is likely to feel some embarrassment over not fitting the norm (Young, 1984). An extreme reaction to her changed body, such as a feeling of hatred or inability to accept the change, however, can indicate either low self-esteem or intense conflict about motherhood; such feelings are not ameliorated by a husband's reassurance of a return to normal size after birth. Haedt and Keel (2007) found that body dissatisfaction during pregnancy moderated a positive relationship between maternal attachment and weeks of pregnancy, i.e., greater gestational age predicted greater maternal attachment for women who reported low or moderate body dissatisfaction, but in women with high body dissatisfaction the association between maternal attachment and weeks gestation was lower. These researchers also found that body mass index correlated positively with maternal-fetal attachment, and suggested that high body dissatisfaction may contribute to poorer maternal health and poorer fetal outcomes through blunted growth of maternal attachment during pregnancy.

2.5   Ambivalence Toward Pregnancy

Even for women who plan, accept, and enjoy pregnancy, there may be some ambivalence at first. Surprise or shock often is the initial reaction to the validation of pregnancy. Caplan (1959) originally reported that initial rejection of pregnancy is common, but that rejection generally is followed by acceptance at the end of the first trimester. Ambivalence is repeated occasionally throughout pregnancy as a wish not to be pregnant; it is associated particularly with speculation about the immensity of the step into motherhood. In evaluating ambivalence, it is important to assess the following factors:

1. How honestly ambivalence is expressed,
2. The reason for ambivalence,
3. The intensity of ambivalence, and
4. How sustained the ambivalence is.

Ambivalence is widely recognized as normal, but in this project ambivalence was evaluated on a continuum from low to high, and it was not necessarily considered normal throughout pregnancy. If ambivalence still is prevalent and intense in the third trimester, it is indicative of unresolved conflicts. Other researchers have reported that the level of ambivalence has significant consequences for the gravida's overall response to the 9 months of pregnancy, and that pronounced ambivalence is tantamount to rejection of the pregnancy (Klein, Potter, & Dyk, 1950). Pohlman (1968) indicated that although some progress in acceptance may occur throughout pregnancy, there is general stability in parental attitudes. He asserted that for some women with an unwanted pregnancy, a large proportion of change from rejection to acceptance is accomplished by repression of rejection, rationalization, or resignation. A related finding was reported by another investigator (Lips, 1984), who found that a woman's positive expectation of pregnancy at 3–5 months was related to a lower level of depression in every trimester of pregnancy. When ambivalence is high and progress in conflict resolution does not occur, it can presage poor attachment to (Reading et al., 1984) or rejection (Zemlick & Watson, 1953) of the newborn, as well as later lower toddler attachment security (Ipsa, Sable, Porter, & Csizmadia, (2007). Reading et al. (1984) discovered that positive feelings about the fetus/neonate at delivery were associated with lower levels of ambivalence or concern about the neonate.

Some women experienced little or no ambivalence; that is, they never wished that they were not pregnant, but most, as expected, had some ambivalence. Ms. Jabon admitted:

> There are moments and times when I am very ambivalent about being pregnant, in part because it's such a deviant thing to be in dance, and it certainly does cut down on your ability to play your professional role, at least temporarily…. Then, of course, feeling ambivalent about the tremendous responsibility and the change in lifestyle once the baby comes. There are times I do feel uncomfortable and feel like a big house, and other women are so much more attractive and everyone starts looking very thin to you, and you feel like this big mountain.

The ambivalence resulted from interference with her profession, an altered life-style, and the feeling that a pregnant body is an unattractive body. However, this reaction is not unreasonable for a dancer in American society.

During pregnancy, many women had dreams in which they saw themselves back in school or college before they had ever married or conceived. Such dreams expressed the desire to return to the past in order to avoid the developmental challenges of expectant motherhood. Ms. Carre reported a dream in which she was struggling to get to the home of an old college friend, and trying to get her bearings in Washington, D.C. 20 years ago. She was thoroughly disoriented, but eventually reached her friend's house. This dream not only expressed a wish to return to the past, but also demonstrated the difficulty of returning.

Ms. Uman recognized that she was ambivalent and handled it well. She was concerned about whether there had been enough time to stabilize her marriage. When she occasionally wished that she was not having a baby, she experienced "guilt feelings afterwards."

> There are times when I wonder whether or not we're actually prepared to have a child now. We've only been married a year and a half. You wonder if a year and a half is really long enough to know another person. There are certain questions about how unstable our future is right now, and we sometimes hope and wish that we'd have a more secure future ahead, and anticipate what was going to happen.

Ms. Uman's ambivalence stemmed from her thoughts about whether it was fair to bring a baby into such an uncertain world. She was aware of the reason for her guilt.

> I tend to think sometimes that I, perhaps, am blaming the baby for things that it's not responsible for.... I don't want to put any blame on the child. I really don't regret being pregnant.... I'm guilty because there I am regretting it and feeling sorry for myself when really I shouldn't feel sorry for myself. It's kind of a vicious circle I guess.

She chose an optimistic way out of the "circle: "But then again you kind of figure that things will work out for the best; they always have. The future has a way of sorting itself out for you. Her sense of relative hope and self-confidence instead of persistent despair and anxiety is characteristic of a healthy adjustment, and has been cited by other researchers (Wenner et al., 1969).

Financial worries, especially if based on realistic circumstances, also seem to raise feelings of ambivalence about the pregnancy (Georgasm, Giakoumaki, Georgoulias, Koumandakis, & Kaskarelis, 1984). The future was unstable for Ms. Uman because of financial insecurity. Ms. Raaf had some concern about finances and realized that it led to her ambivalence. "I wish sometimes that I wasn't pregnant because of the fact that we have just bought a house, and we could use the money if I wasn't pregnant. She thought that her ambivalence was "just natural" and that "everything will work out." She did not experience guilt as did Ms. Uman.

Ms. Santa was concerned about her husband's unemployment.

> Tom's unemployment runs out some time in February. If he don't [sic] get called back to work we'll have about $40.00 a week to live on. Even if we get public assistance, life still would be tough, and with a new baby yet. I guess it won't do any good to worry now; take one day at a time.

Ms. Santa's worries were realistic, but did not become pervasive and interfere with the enjoyment of her pregnancy. Similarly, Ms. Carre was concerned because her husband had been laid off, but, again, it did not seem to spoil her excitement about the coming child. Ms. Dann admitted some concern about finances, but seemed to handle it well.

> I'd rather have it [the baby] a year from now when I'm finished with school.... If my husband had tons of money, I wouldn't care. I'd probably quit school, or finish school just for the heck of it. But in a way I say the timing is right because at least we can both take care of the baby, and we can both spend time with the baby and get involved with it.

Ms. Dann used rationalization in an adaptive way.

In contrast, Ms. Lash did not feel well during her pregnancy and seemed to harbor constant worries about money. She said that she and her husband had been having "some pretty bad times coping with things that are happening because we're almost out of money."

> And we're worrying about whether we'll make it until the end of the month when supposedly his check is coming, which I hope is coming. And we've been sort of getting on each other's nerves and having a lot of heated discussion about what we're doing.

Ms. Lash admitted feeling ambivalent, especially when she was angry with her husband; she thought that this ambivalence stemmed mainly from her awareness of the financial obligations that they would incur with the baby. She continued to suffer from doubts about her ability to manage other life situations, especially her career as an actress and her responsibility as a mother. She found it difficult to control the intensity of her anxiety concerning financial security, but this anxiety did not seem to diminish her acceptance of the baby. "I want the baby; I do want it. So I have doubts at some points – which I'm sure everybody does – but they don't change the fact that I'm very glad that I'm having one." Financial concerns then, even if realistic, need not undermine a young woman who has a few doubts about being a mother. She still may enjoy her pregnancy.

A further cause of ambivalence is the prospect of anticipated changes in lifestyle. If faced honestly and worked through, these changes need not be a serious hindrance to a woman's preparation for motherhood, or to her enjoyment of pregnancy. Ms. Jabon, for example, had good reason to be concerned about how the pregnancy would affect her performance as a dancer, and she admitted being ambivalent. She adapted by adjusting her expectations. Ms. Eaden was concerned about the disruption of her special "twosome" relationship with her husband and had initially considered abortion, but she had worked through her conflicts by the third trimester. Ms. Banor admitted a similar ambivalence, but felt it was not serious. She thought of ambivalence as "natural," because there were so many adjustments to make at once. Ms. Banor admitted that she sometimes wished she were not pregnant.

> Especially in the beginning, you feel all sick and everything.... There's really nothing positive going on because you can't feel it move or anything.... You look fat and...just feeling bad about yourself really.... I think it's also being newly married and newly having a baby – all those adjustments all at once – all tied up together.

Having summed up all the reasons for feeling ambivalent, Ms. Banor then stated that her negative feelings had never been strong enough to upset her.

Overall, it was assumed that the greater the ambivalence, the lower would be the acceptance of the pregnancy. No woman totally rejected her pregnancy. Ambivalence often was expressed indirectly when the gravida was not happy and did not enjoy her pregnancy – for example, when she reported considerable physical discomforts and constraints, excessive mood swings, considerable difficulty in accepting life changes, frequent and prolonged depression, a desire to be pregnant at some later time, or extreme displeasure with her changed body shape. Most women with a low acceptance of their pregnancy displayed some of these characteristics, and many had considerable motherhood-career conflicts. These women often reported high conflict on the prenatal dimension: Identification with a Motherhood Role. Their preoccupation with the concerns cited could have interfered with their orientation toward this important task.

2.6 Summary

The task, acceptance of pregnancy, pervaded the gravidas' overall behavior. In general, low acceptance was associated with unplanned pregnancy, greater conflicts and fears, more physical discomforts, and depression. Acceptance was characterized by feelings of happiness and enjoyment of the pregnancy, relatively little physical discomfort or high tolerance of the discomfort by the third trimester, moderate mood swings, and relatively little reported ambivalence during the third trimester. The challenges precipitated by pregnancy were readily acknowledged and a general sense of hope and self-confidence prevailed. Brown (1988) also found that pregnancy included simultaneous positive and negative responses, but that feelings of well-being prevailed, and others found that women who were happier about the pregnancy used a greater range of cognitive and behavioral coping strategies to deal with negative moods or affect (Blake et al., 2007; Facchinetti, Ottolini, Fazzio, Rigatelli, & Volpe, 2007).

The generalization can be made that if a woman accepts the pregnancy, then she typically is in a happy state of mind despite bodily discomfort, altered body shape, mood swings, or financial worries. If she does not accept the pregnancy, she tends to despair and to be depressed, and both physical and emotional disruptions loom large. It also should be noted that, in some instances, acceptance of pregnancy can be unhealthy – for example, if a woman enjoys being pregnant but does not want the baby. Some rejection is expected, such as when a woman is acutely aware that she currently is unprepared to have a child because of a disintegrating marriage, or because she feels emotionally unprepared. Actually, total acceptance is rare. Some women pointed out that they felt some ambivalence was "normal." When ambivalence was excessive and sustained, there was a tendency to displace the emotional concerns of pregnancy and motherhood onto the physical aspects of pregnancy and childbirth, such as the bodily changes and discomforts of pregnancy, and the pain of labor, also noted by Trad (1991). Persons conducting assessments of pregnancy acceptance need to be cognizant of this type of displacement.

Ambivalence was found to be expressed overtly in two main areas: financial security and changed lifestyle, which includes motherhood-career conflict. The women seemed to find it easier to talk about their ambivalent feelings regarding these areas of concern. Heinicke (1984) found that maternal ambivalence also was expressed by intense concerns about an abnormal baby. Ambivalence was expressed indirectly when a woman complained excessively about physical discomfort, being depressed, and feeling that she had an "ugly" shape – in short, if she said simply, "This is not a good time to be pregnant." Evidence further suggested that initial reactions and early responses concerning acceptance versus ambivalence of the pregnancy may be relatively stable, even though wide fluctuations in mood occurred. Other investigators also report that decisions regarding "wantedness" of pregnancy almost always remain stable or constant (Cohan, Dunkel-Shetter, & Lydon, 1993). Using an individual growth model perspective to look at a woman's prenatal maternal identity formation, Weis (2006) found that conflict about acceptance of pregnancy was significantly higher in the first trimester and then decreased over the course of pregnancy. Additionally, there were significant individual differences in the intercepts and rate of change over the three trimesters of pregnancy for the mothers in her study. More importantly, the rate of change was impacted by community support and family adaptability. Acceptance of Pregnancy was not impacted by parity or age of the gravida.

References

Bailey, L., & Hailey, B. (1986–1987). The psychological experience of pregnancy. *International Journal of Psychiatry in Medicine, 16*, 263–274.

Beck, A. (1967). *Depression: Clinical, experimental, and theoretical aspects.* New York: Harper & Row.

Blake, S. M., Kiely, M., Gard, C. C., El-Mohandes, A. A., & El-Khorazaty, M. N. (2007). Pregnancy intentions and happiness among pregnant black women at high risk for adverse infant health outcomes. *Perspectives on Sexual and Reproductive Health, 39*, 194–205.

Brown, M. (1988). A comparison of health responses in expectant mothers and fathers. *Western Journal of Nursing Research, 10*, 527–549.

Caplan, G. (1959). *Concepts of mental health and consultation.* Washington, DC: Superintendent of Documents, U.S. Government Printing Office.

Cohan, C. L., Dunkel-Shetter, C., & Lydon, J. (1993). Pregnancy decision-making: Predictors of early stress and adjustment. *Psychology of Women Quarterly, 17*, 223–229.

Cohen, R. L. (1988). Developmental tasks of pregnancy and transistion to parenthood: An approach to assessment. In R. L. Cohen (Ed.), *Psychiatric consultation in childbirth settings: Parent- and child-oriented approaches* (pp. 51–70). New York: Plenum Medical Book Co.

Entwisle, D. R., & Doering, S. G. (1981). *The first birth.* Baltimore: Johns Hopkins University Press.

Facchinetti, F., Ottolini, F., Fazzio, M., Rigatelli, M., & Volpe, A. (2007). Psychosocial factors associated with preterm uterine contractions. *Psychotherapy and Psychosomatics, 76*, 391–394.

Fagley, N., Miller, P., & Sullivan, J. (1982). Stress, symptom proneness, and general adaptational distress during pregnancy. *Journal of Human Stress, 8*, 15–22.

Finer, L. B., & Henshaw, S. K. (2006). Disparities in rates of unintended pregnancy in the United States, 1994–2001. *Perspectives in Sexual and Reproductive Health, 38*, 90–96.

Flapan, M. (1969). A paradigm for the analysis of childbearing motivations of women prior to birth of the first child. *American Journal of Orthopsychiatry, 39*, 402–417.

Georgas, J., Giakoumaki, E., Georgoulias, N., Koumandakis, E., & Kaskarelis, D. (1984). Psycholosocial stress and its relation to obstetrical complications. *Psychotherapy and Psychosomatics, 41*, 200–206.

Green, R. T. (1973). *Perceived styles of mother–daughter relationship and the prenatal adjustment of the primigravida.* Doctoral dissertation, The George Washington University, Washington, DC. *Dissertation Abstracts International* (University Microfilms No. 73–25, 094).

Grossman, F.K., Eichler, L.S., & Winickoff, S. A. (1980). Pregnancy, birth, and parenthood. San Francisco: Jossey-Bass.

Haedt, A., & Keel, P. (2007). Maternal attachment, depression, and body dissatisfaction in pregnant women. *Journal of Reproductive and Infant Psychology, 25*, 285–295.

Heinicke, C. (1984). The role of pre-birth parent characteristics in early family development. *Child Abuse and Neglect 8*, 169–181.

Ipsa, J. M., Sable, M. R., Porter, N., & Csizmadia, A. (2007) Pregnancy acceptance, parenting stress and toddler attachment in low income black families. *Journal of Marriage and Family, 69*, 1–13.

Kalil, K. M., Gruber, J. E., Conley, J, & Sytniac, M. (1993). Social and family pressures on anxiety, and stress during pregnancy. *Pre- and Perinatal Psychology Journal 8*, 113–118.

Kiloh, L. G., Andrews, G., Bianchi, G. N. & Neilson, M. (1972). On studying depression. *Australian and New Zealand Journal of Psychiatry, 6*, 85–93.

Kirgis, C. A., Woolsey, D. B., & Sullivan, J. J. (1977). Predicting infant Apgar scores. *Nursing Research 26*, 439–442.

Klein, H. R., Potter, H. W., & Dyk, R. B. (1950). *Anxiety in pregnancy and childbirth.* New York: Hoeber.

Klerman, L. V. (2000). The intendedness of pregnancy: A concept in transition. *Maternal and Child Health Journal, 4*, 155–162.

Kuo, S., Wang, R., Tseng, H., Jian, S, & Chou, F. (2007). A comparison of different severities of nausea and vomiting during pregnancy relative to stress, social support, and maternal adaptation. *Journal of Midwifery and Women's Health, 52*, E1–E7.

Lawrence, E., Rothman, A. D., Cobb, R. J., Rothman, M. T., & Bradbury, T. N. (2008). Marital satisfaction across the transition to parenthood. *Journal of Family Psychology, 22*, 46–51.

Lips, H. (1984). Personality and attitude variables of women and their spouses as predictors of women's experience of pregnancy. *Zentralblatt Fur Gynakologie, 106*, 1325–1337.

Lips, H. (1985). A longitudinal study of the reporting of emotional and somatic symptoms during and after pregnancy. *Social Science and Medicine, 21*, 631–640.

Lubin, B., Gardener, S. H., & Roth, A. (1975). Mood and somatic symptoms during pregnancy. *Psychosomatic Medicine, 37*, 136–146.

Messer, L. C., Dole, N., Kaufman, J. S., & Savitz, D. A. (2005). Pregnancy intendedness, maternal psychosocial factors and preterm birth. *Maternal and Child Health Journal, 9*, 403–412.

McConnell, O., & Daston, P. G. (1961). Body image changes in pregnancy. *Journal of Projective Techniques, 25*, 451–456.

Najman, J. M., Morrison, J., Williams, S., Anderson, M., &Keeping, D J.(1991). The mental health outcomes of women six months after they give birth to an unwanted baby: A longitudinal study. *Social Science and Medicine, 32*, 241–247.

Peacock, N. R., Kelley, M. A., Carpenter, C., Davis, M., Burnett, G., Chavez, N., et al. (2001). Pregnancy discovery and acceptance among low-income primiparous women: A multicultural exploration. *Maternal and Child Health Journal, 26*, 177–190.

Pohlman, E. (1969). *The psychology of birth planning.* Cambridge, MA: Shenkman.

Pohlman, E. W. (1968). Changes from rejection to acceptance of pregnancy. *Social Science and Medicine, 2*, 337–340.

Reading, A., Cox, D., Sledmere, C., & Campbell, S. (1984). Psychological changes over the course of pregnancy: A study of attitudes toward the fetus/neonate. *Health Psychology, 3*, 211–221.

Rubin, R. (1975). Maternal tasks in pregnancy. *Maternal-Child Nursing Journal, 4*, 143–153.

Sable, M. R., & Libbus, M. K. (2000). Pregnancy intention and pregnancy happiness: Are they different? *Maternal Child Health Journal, 4*, 191–196.

Shereshefsky, P. M., & Yarrow, L. J. (Eds.). (1973). *Psychological aspects of a first pregnancy and early postnatal adaptation*. New York: Raven.

Trad, P. (1991). Adaptation to developmental transformations during various phases of motherhood. *Journal of the American Academy of Psychoanalysis, 19*, 403–421.

Weis, K. L. (2006). *Maternal identity formation in a military sample: A longitudinal perspective*. Unpublished doctoral dissertation, The University of North Carolina, Chapel Hill, NC.

Wenner, N. K., Cohen, M. B., Weigert, E. V., Kvarnes, R. G., Ohaneson, E. M., & Fearing, J. M. (1969). Emotional problems in pregnancy. *Psychiatry, 32*, 389–410.

Young, I. (1984). Pregnant embodiment: Subjectivity and alienation. *The Journal of Medicine and Philosophy, 9*, 45–62.

Zemlick, M. J., & Watson, R. I. (1953). Maternal attitudes of acceptance and rejection during and after pregnancy. *American Journal of Orthopsychiatry 23*, 570–584.

Chapter 3
Identification with a Motherhood Role

The developmental step of the woman-without-child to the woman-with-child is the goal of identification with a motherhood role. Achievement of this identification can be thought of as a process of unfolding characterized by progressive emphasis in the mother's thinking away from the single self and toward the mother–baby unit, and ultimately toward recognizing the separateness and individuality of the coming child (Lederman, 1984; Trad, 1991). Identification with a motherhood role also refers to the mother's attachment orientation and reflective functioning or the capacity to understand the nature of her own patterns of thinking or mental states, as well as those of the developing fetus-baby and newborn infant (Condon & Corkindale, 1997; Haedt & Keel, 2007; Slade, Grienenberger, Bernbach, Levy, & Locker, 2005).

Often a woman comes to the experience of pregnancy with a clearly defined philosophy of motherhood; that is, she sees motherhood as an end in itself or as one of several, perhaps competing, goals (Flapan, 1969). Other women have not considered what motherhood means until they are suddenly forced to confront their new role. Some women give limited thought to any philosophy of motherhood, but simply want the baby.

Data presented in Chapter 1 suggest that anxiety, conflict, or difficulty concerning Identification with a Motherhood Role was found to be related to the woman's acceptance of the pregnancy and, notably, to the woman's relationship with her mother. Anxiety or conflict concerning motherhood was associated with fears about labor related to pain, helplessness, loss of control, and loss of self-esteem, as well as slower progress in labor (Lederman, Lederman, Work, & McCann, 1979). It was also related to antepartum complications, to gestational age at birth (Lederman, Weis, Brandon, Hills, & Mian, 2002), and to lower birthweight in a project with a large (679) sample size (Lederman, Harrison, & Worsham, 1992). Measures of anxiety concerning maternal-fetal safety in labor also correlated with duration of labor and fetal heart rate deceleration patterns in labor (Lederman, Lederman, Work, & McCann, 1985).

Two factors were considered important in assessing a woman's identification with a motherhood role. The first was to learn how motivated the woman was to assume a motherhood role; the second was the extent to which the woman had prepared for a motherhood role.

R. Lederman and K. Weis, *Psychosocial Adaptation to Pregnancy*,
DOI 10.1007/978-1-4419-0288-7_3, © Springer Science+Business Media, LLC 2009

3.1   Motivation for Motherhood

At critical times during the life span, when significant changes occur, individuals are motivated to reflect on and modify their self-concepts and redefine their identities and roles to accommodate the anticipated changes (Ruble, 1983, 1987).

The salience of motivation to prenatal and parental adaptation is well documented (Flapan, 1969; Grossman, Eichler, & Winickoff, 1980; Pohlman, 1969). The rationale for learning the mother's motives for bearing a child is that conflicted motivation may contribute to problems during the reproductive process, such as aberrant somatic reactions during pregnancy, labor and delivery complications, postpartum depressive reactions, and inadequate or maladaptive maternal behavior (Flapan, 1969).

No universal set of motives are assumed to account for reproductive behavior. It is assumed that the woman's appraisal of her current life situation and circumstances have a significant influence on her childbearing motivation. It also is understood that a woman may or may not recognize the multiplicity of diverse meanings that motivate her or make her reluctant to bear children, or that induce childbearing conflicts. These diverse meanings may be revealed in expectations, hopes, values, dreams, fears, and fantasies pertaining to pregnancy, childbirth, motherhood, and childrearing. For a multigravida, the motivations and conflicts for childbearing and motherhood are altered by previous pregnancy, labor, childbirth, and motherhood experiences (Flapan, 1969), whereas those of a primigravida may more abstractly relate to the experiential account of friends and relatives, as well as to her own mothering experiences in childhood and her mother's recollections of childbearing and the childbirth event. In this regard it is noteworthy that increasing parity is associated with lower maternal–fetal attachment (Haedt & Keel, 2007).

The numerous motivations for childbearing and motherhood may include confirmation of femininity, a fondness for children, a wish to reproduce a happy family life, fulfillment of a motherhood wish, and the desire to have someone to nurture for whom love, affection, and tenderness can be expressed. However, childbearing and child rearing also may be viewed as causing boredom and drudgery, loss of freedom, and economic constraints. A woman's appraisal of her own competence may affect her childbearing motivations. If a woman has had positive past experiences with children, she may take it for granted that she will love her own children. On the other hand, if she has experienced children as annoying and demanding, she may wonder whether she will love her own children or whether her children will love her. Nevertheless, her concerns about competence in motherhood may be assuaged somewhat by a supportive, encouraging husband, particularly if she views her husband as a good father (Flapan, 1969). There are numerous other childbearing motivations that relate to the gravida's relationship with her husband and with her mother, her age and career aspirations, her expected fertility, and her anticipations and fears regarding childbirth and a normal newborn infant.

In order to assess the gravida's level of motivation to assume a motherhood role, interviews focused on how much she wanted to become a mother. Her attitude and potential ability to be nurturant and empathic toward a child were assessed, as was her general anticipation for interaction with the child.

Some women were clear about their readiness to have a baby. They wanted the baby, liked children, and were looking forward to motherhood. Ms. Carre said: "The only reason that we are having children is because I enjoy them and I wanted to have children."

Ms. Lash said: "[I have always]...had this mothering instinct and wanting children... and I've been thinking about it a lot and have adjusted myself to it."

Ms. Yuth similarly said: "[I]...always wanted a baby.... I always enjoyed children."

Ms. Inis said that a baby was more important to her than expanding other interests in her life.

> I always think, No, I don't want to wait [for children]; I don't want to work longer and have more money or travel first or anything, although that would be kind of nice. I would rather have the baby than do that.

Closely related to the felt need to nurture a baby was the woman's perception of motherhood, and the development of a sense of herself as a mother (Ballou, 1978). Some women saw motherhood as "fulfilling," as "an extension of life's goals," or as "the most important thing you can do in life." Ms. Lash epitomized the latter point of view.

> The family is a very, very important part of our religion, and probably...the most important thing that you can do is to succeed in raising your children well and in having a very good family situation.

If a woman said that she would be happy to stay at home with the baby or that she wished to be a full-time mother, it was concluded that she wanted the baby very much. Ms. Meta, for example, said: "I will go back [to work] when the child is in school. But as long as the child is at home, I want to be at home."

Although Ms. Banor was a serious student and planned to have a career, staying home did not worry her.

> I'm really looking forward to it because I've been...in school for the past so many years. I'm...looking forward to a different aspect of my life. I'm looking forward to motherhood...to being at home...not as a permanent thing, but as kind of a diversion for a while.... It's a short-term thing, maybe a year or two at the most that I'll be at home the whole time.

The opposite viewpoint was not seen as necessarily ominous; many women viewed the prospect of staying home all day with the baby as difficult to accept. This attitude was particularly true of career women who were accustomed to active roles in the community at large. Ms. Gale gave a response that was typical of this ambivalence about staying at home, but did not reflect ambivalence about the baby itself.

> I wonder how it's going to work out sometimes, but I find that I don't particularly like staying home all day. Like even working half-time now, I'm really enjoying having the work and getting out into the office ...and I think about staying home all day for months, and then I think, 'Oh, my goodness, I'll never stand that!' I really don't know. I will just have to see how I feel, but I have a feeling that I'll be ready to get out in a couple of months and get a job again.

The idea of motherhood as an unpleasant or depressing chore was never expressed directly in the interviews. Some women did have grave doubts about their futures as mothers, however, and some expressed hostility toward the fetus. Ms. Fair stated that she felt she had "no overwhelming maternal instincts." Ms. Penn said that she had been "antichildren" before becoming pregnant, but that she had nonetheless come to accept the idea of having a child. Ms. Penn had a great deal of conflict regarding identification with a motherhood role. She was concerned that the child might interfere with her life and fray her nerves; she generally disliked other people's children. Ms. Hayes categorically disagreed with the notion of fulfillment entirely through motherhood. She said:

> I'm concerned more about picking up my life after…rather than thinking about the glorified part of having a child, and how cute the baby is going to be…. The reality is, what am I going to do with my life? That's where I have rejected this Lamaze thing. I think that women have been so repressed, and they have tried to find an identity, but…motherhood will be a part of my life, but it's not going to be the major part.

Initial role identification was considered to be impeded if thoughts about the child were infrequent or aversive, or if they were avoided or denied. Similar reasoning applied when motivation for motherhood included the desire for pregnancy, but not the wish for a child.

3.2   Preparation for Motherhood

It is not enough for a gravida to want to be a mother or to have established her philosophy of motherhood. She also needs to prepare for her new role by envisioning herself as a mother and contemplating her life as a woman-with-child. Fantasizing and dreaming are two ways in which a woman prepares for her future as a mother (Caplan, 1959; Rubin, 1967a; Trad, 1991), and they may be predictive of her ability to cope with the challenges of motherhood (Trad, 1991). The woman's life experience and the availability of a role model are major determinants influencing preparation for motherhood, and the development of feelings of competence in the new role. In addition, the degree of conflict resolution concerning pregnancy and motherhood affects preparation for a motherhood role. Those women in the project who were well prepared for motherhood tended to have resolved their conflicts about their pregnancies and impending motherhood, and had crystallized a new role for themselves that ultimately was expressed as a need to attach to the baby. Other investigators reported that women who are able to visualize themselves as mothers during pregnancy adapted better postpartally, and reported more satisfaction than those who had difficulty visualizing themselves as mothers or as competent in the role (Deutsch, Ruble, Fleming, Brooks-Gunn, & Stangor, 1986; Shereshefsky & Yarrow, 1973). In a sample of multiparas at 6–8 weeks' postpartum, Lederman (1988) reported that satisfaction with motherhood and infant care tasks was related to how well the mother identified and defined a motherhood role during pregnancy.

3.2.1 Fantasizing

Initial steps in identifying a motherhood role are to:

1. Envision oneself as mother,
2. Think about those characteristics one wishes to have as a mother, and
3. Anticipate future life changes that will be necessary.

Each of these steps is discussed in turn.

3.2.1.1 Envisioning Oneself as a Mother

It was difficult for many women to project themselves as a mother and envision motherhood, but most made some progress throughout the 9 months. Ms. Uman reported that she now "projected" herself more realistically.

> I find myself thinking more in terms of time spent in the labor room as well as trying to picture the actual delivery scene. It is still difficult to imagine myself in the role of a new mother.

Ms. Dann fantasized about herself and her child.

> I actually have those themes go through my mind – with the child doing something similar to the things that my friend's child does, and how I would do in that situation. I think that I act it out in my mind.

Ms. Cole saw herself in a different "world" than the one she had known.

> It's something new. It's a new experience. You know, babies…depend so much upon everybody until they're old enough to take care of themselves. It's just a 24-hour watch that you have to settle here.

Ms. Inis said that she daydreamed about the baby.

> … [I daydream] a lot about having the baby with me some place, all dressed up, cute, you know, going someplace. I think about that a lot… that's what I see the most.

Ms. Fair experienced pleasant daydreams about the baby, illustrated by the following entry from her diary.

> Quite a bit I find myself 'daydreaming,' totally unconscious of everything around me. I think about how it'll feel to finally hold a cuddly, small bundle, and how much I'm going to love it. I imagine reading Winnie the Pooh tales to the baby at night and watching Joe play with the baby – throwing him into the air. I like to think about the toddler stage when the baby is stumbling around uncoordinated on his feet.

These excerpts show the young gravida anticipating the future with eagerness. She anticipated a new and exciting relationship, described as a "love affair with her baby" (Baker, 1966).

On the other hand, excessive doubts and fears can interfere with fantasizing. Ms. Tell was so overwhelmed by fear and anxiety that she did not fantasize in a productive way. In response to the question "How do you think you'll feel about the baby when you're at home alone with him or her?" she said: "I don't know; I never thought of it." Most women tried to picture themselves as mothers, but some found this effort too abstract. Ms. Bode said:

> I can't look ahead so far. It is very difficult even to imagine having the baby, let alone how the child and I will interact. I mean, I haven't planned anything out about it.

The anxieties that commonly inhibited fantasizing included fears of being at home alone with the child, fears of social isolation or entrapment in a traditional housewife role, and fears of establishing a nonstimulating routine.

Some women envisioned their motherhood role in a predominantly negative way. They were fearful of having a screaming baby, of having an overly demanding baby, or of harming or dropping the child when alone with him or her. Such thoughts suggested a lack of confidence in mothering skills and perhaps hostility toward the baby. For example, when Ms. Penn tried to envision what her child would be like, she could only think that she did not want her child to be like two other children she had observed in her circle of friends.

> [They are] constantly underfoot, constantly bombarding you, bugging you, pestering you to do this and do that.... They resort to screaming and hollering when they do something.... The two of them eat like animals.... That's disgusting.

On the whole, the women tried to make progress throughout the 9 months despite their ambivalence. Ms. Carre initially was unable to think about the baby at all, but with quickening she said she was forced to do so. Ms. Vale felt that the pregnancy had "made me think about [the] baby."

> I've never thought about a baby before. In fact, now I find myself thinking of nursing a child, or holding one, or even looking at them. I hated baby-sitting. I... never took that much notice. I'm real excited. But it's taken me months to really feel good about it, really positive about it.

Thus, initial steps in identifying a motherhood role begin during pregnancy, and include attempts to envision oneself as a mother and to contemplate the changes inherent in caring for and relating to an infant. The process begun during pregnancy often continues and is elaborated on in the future (Rubin, 1984).

3.2.1.2   Characteristics Desired as a Mother

Another important preparation for the gravida's new role is thinking about the characteristics that she wishes to have as a mother. All women expressed some desire to be available, warm, loving, and close to their children. Such attitudes were accepted as a matter of course for women who had come from a caring home. Ms. Raaf expressed this idea:

> I want him to know that he can always come to me whenever he wants to. I want him to feel that I really love him.... I want to be fair above all.

(Author's note: Use of a masculine pronoun by the interview subject does not indicate a sexual bias or a preference for a male child).

Ms. Santa believed that an important quality of nurturing was to be available all the time. As a child, she had felt the lack of a supportive, omnipresent figure because her mother worked; she considered this factor responsible for the separation between them.

> I think that one of the reasons that I don't want to work [after the baby comes] is because my mother worked. When I was real little, she was at home, but after I got a little bit older, she went back to work. Like me and my mom, when I lived at home, weren't really close and I couldn't always just really talk to her openly because...she wasn't always there.

Nevertheless, Ms. Santa appreciated her mother's capacity for empathic understanding and wished to emulate her in this respect. "It just seems like she feels just as hurt as I do and I think that that is good, if you can really feel it."

A distinction is made here between nurturing and empathy. Both terms describe a woman's relationship to others. The way a woman relates to significant others in her past and current life has been found to be consistent with the way she perceives and relates to her child (Ballou, 1978; Fonagy, Steele, & Steele, 1991; von Klitzing, Amsler, Schleske, Simoni, & Burgin, 1996; Wilson, Rholes, Simpson, & Tran, 2008). Quality nurturing, as used here, refers to giving with empathy – that is, respecting the needs of others and at the same time respecting one's own needs. Poor nurturing refers to giving without empathy – that is, giving in a possessive or indifferent manner or out of a sense of duty. Poor nurturing also can imply giving without respecting one's own needs and, therefore, allowing oneself to be exploited. Wenner, Cohen, Weigert, Kvarnes, Ohaneson, and Fearing (1969) recognized some loss of an independent identity in mothers who enacted the motherhood role by "merging with" or "subjugating oneself" to their child.

The interview data provided a basis for assessing the gravida's feelings of empathy for her husband and for her parents as they tried to adapt to their anticipated new roles. The potential ability to be nurturant and empathic in relating to a child was assessed in terms of the quality of relationships with others, the expressed motivation to become a mother, the gravida's perception of a baby, and the anticipated interactions in meeting the child's needs.

The gravidas often equated closeness with being open, communicative, and ready to answer their child's questions. Ms. Yuth stressed this point.

> ... parents should spend a lot of time with their children, as much as they can, and answer their questions and play with them, and watch them grow. Because a lot of times, like I've seen where a child will ask a question, and the parents can ignore it or they've got too much to do. I think a mother should spend a lot of time with her babies in answering questions and just show them a lot of love.

Some women hoped to build a close relationship with their child, while still allowing the child to develop in his or her own way. Ms. Lash, for example, said that she wanted to treat her child "as a separate human being, not as something she owns." Rees (1980) also reported a relationship between nurturant or motherly feelings and maternal perception of the fetus as a person – that is, having unique characteristics.

Other women were concerned about setting limits for the child as well as giving love. When the woman's need to discipline the child became a preoccupation, however, she may have been expressing some reservations about the coming child and the demands ultimately placed on her. Ms. Carre, a teacher, was absorbed with the idea of discipline.

> I have this feeling that if you let the kid get away with it once, there is no reason why he shouldn't be able to get away with being obnoxious or whining or all this other business, you know, a million more times…. I see these people [parents] letting their kids drive them crazy, and I say, it's your fault the kid's driving you crazy. I wouldn't let the kid drive [me] crazy.

A few women found it difficult either to think about their baby or to envision the kind of mother that they wished to be. They simply experienced a vague sense of anxiety. Ms. Vale found it difficult to think about the baby and motherhood.

> I hadn't thought about it. I tried and tried to get into thinking about having a baby, and I just wasn't thinking about it at all. Lately I've just started thinking about holding it, keeping it close, and I hope that I just don't worry a whole lot.

Ms. Bode claimed that she had no time to think about such matters because she was working up until the last moment. She said that she did not think about the fact that she was pregnant or even that she was approaching labor and delivery.

> That's why my dream record is zilch…. I was teaching…well, three days past when she was due, still teaching, and of course she still didn't come. So I never – during the course of my pregnancy and the experiment – I never really had the time to sit and think about what was going to happen…. I never wrote anything down because I honestly didn't think about that.

This response seemed to reflect avoidance rather than the stress of professional life alone. In contrast, other women who were still pursuing active careers in their third trimester found some time to consider their roles.

Some women remained confused and anxious about their new roles. When asked "How strong or serious would you say your doubts are about being a mother and caring for a baby?" Ms. Eaden gave the following response:

> I'm sure with the support of my husband, I can manage. I guess I don't feel confident at this point…. Now talk to me in two months, when I've got a baby in my arms, then I'll be losing my mind…. It's easy to say now, but when you've never been a mother, you don't know.

Although she wanted a child, Ms. Lash was uncertain about her maturity in the motherhood role.

> I get really nervous around kids sometimes when they are older, because I don't really know how to deal with them. I guess I feel too much like a child myself, and I don't feel old enough to be having children. I still feel like I'm sort of a freshman in high school or something like that.

Based on doubts commonly expressed during mood swings and the frequent dream record accounts of wishes to return to an earlier life phase, the researchers had reason to believe that this sentiment may have been more prevalent than was apparent, yet it seldom was expressed in such a direct manner.

To help prepare themselves, most women read pertinent materials, talked with other women, and observed how other mothers handled their children. Such information seeking is considered important in the new self-conceptualization of oneself as a mother (Deutsch, Ruble, Fleming, Brooks-Gunn, & Stangor, 1988; Hart & McMahon, 2006). In this process, the mother first constructs an image of herself and then seeks to confirm and validate the constructed image (Deutsch et al., 1988), a process associated with the increasing accrual of mothering characteristics and self-confidence during pregnancy. Previous experience with infants has been identified as an important factor influencing adaptation to parenthood (Oakley, 1980). Interestingly, the information gained about the experience of pregnancy correlates with information sought about motherhood (Deutsch et al., 1988). However, a woman's positive self-definition of herself as a mother postpartally appears to be multiply determined, and also may reflect her relationship with her mother (Deutsch et al., 1988), her self-esteem (Deutsch et al., 1988), and her level of general anxiety (Lederman, 1988).

In addition, Deutsch et al. (1988) showed that information seeking is a means of effective coping with change, i.e., women who are more interested in and gather more information prior to becoming mothers perceive themselves as more likely to possess the characteristics of a good mother, and report greater self-confidence in anticipation of their new role. It is likely that information seeking stimulates the vision of oneself as a mother. Deave (2005) found that women who were more aware of the changes that might accompany motherhood were more likely to have planned their pregnancy and had children with more advanced cognitive development at 2 years of age as measured by the Mental Development Inventory of the Bayley Scales of Infant Development

Thus, thinking about their new role may lead women to more positive self-evaluations in the role of mother. The study by Deutsch et al. (1988) also suggested that positive maternal self-definition contributes to information seeking more than does high self-esteem. Positive maternal self-definition appears to parallel a behavioral commitment to the new role as a mother, and the ultimate integration of the role into the self-concept.

When asked if she thought about the kind of mother she wanted to be, Ms. Inis answered:

> Yes. A lot. We have been sort of observing friends all this time. We're always going home and talking about the way people treat their children and deciding if we like that or not. And I think that that's kind of a preparation for how we are going to discipline too. We have some friends...we like very much the way they raise their child,...and then other friends where we haven't agreed with their ways.

3.2.1.3 Anticipating Future Life Changes as a Mother

Another indicator of a woman's success in crystallizing a motherhood role was her ability to anticipate changes in her life. This activity was complementary to her ability to fantasize about herself as a mother. Most women saw change in terms of more responsibility and less freedom. When a woman has come to terms with her new role this change is accepted. When asked "How do you think having a baby will change your life?" Ms. Uman said:

> There's no question that it's going to. I think…we're going to find that it's a little different in that we'll have to assume more responsibility. We will have someone who will be totally dependent on us for quite a few years, so we're not going to have the independence to come and go as we used to…. We're just going to have to start thinking in terms of two instead of one before…. I can't say that we resent that; I think we're looking forward to it.

When the marital relationship is perceived as ideal by the couple or as mutually warm and satisfying, some misgivings about accommodating a third member of the family have been found to be healthy and augur well for the future. Concern about accommodating the baby does not portend conflict, but rather is indicative of an interest in extending love and incorporating the child into the family.

It was seen as healthy and adaptive when women understood life change in terms of compensations. In discussing this view, Ms. Eaden said:

> I'm sure a baby takes more time than we think it will. And plus…it'll affect us financially. But I think the child itself will make up for any sacrifices we have to make.

A few participants saw the change in lifestyle as developmental. In this regard, Ms. Bode commented:

> I sort of look at it as a further step in my life and not the end. It's a very important one, but I consider my other, my own interests to be strong enough that I want to follow through with them. I am looking forward to it [motherhood].

Change, as she saw it, did not represent a radical shift, but the integration of a new life experience into her life plan. Ms. Yuth thought the change "will mature me a lot because I've always enjoyed children." Similarly, Ms. Santa explained:

> I can feel myself maturing – just growing up to the point where I can look at different things about life in a whole new light. At times I like to sit in the baby's room. I feel so warm and happy inside. I feel real womanly, I guess. Like a flower that's almost in full bloom in spring. Maybe it's just in anticipation of getting something that you've wanted in the back of your mind for a long time, then being able to have made and share that with someone you love very much.

Ms. Santa's statement is a wonderful example of the paradigm shift described earlier – the sense of looking at the world with new eyes and of unfolding and evolving in the maternal role.

Change was perceived as a threat in some cases. As Ms. Hayes's due date was approaching, she confided in her diary that she anticipated postpartum depression; she saw herself "somewhat falling apart and not too willing to do anything." She continued, "I got a rush of semi-panic at the overwhelming responsibility and change that is going to occur in my life." Another woman, Ms. Penn, who thought of children as "monsters," anticipated motherhood as a threat to the peace and quiet of her house. It was difficult for her to accept the fact that children create noise and disorder, and that preserving a quiet home was an unrealistic expectation. A few other women in the sample were unable to envision significant changes in their lifestyle or, in effect, found it problematic to concede the possibility of change.

Maladaptive cognitions or attitudes about motherhood regarding role change, and expectations of motherhood and oneself as a mother, like those described, have been associated with higher maternal prenatal trait anxiety (Hart & McMahon, 2006). Both prenatal state and trait anxiety were found to be related to maternal childbearing attitudes, such as worries about responsibility involved in childcare, self-confidence in caring for a child, identifying pregnancy as positive and fulfilling, and attitudes about children (Hart & McMahon, 2006).

Variation in the intensity of ambivalence about change, and in the nature of the ambivalence, cannot be equated simply with the degree of readiness of the gravida to nurture the forthcoming child. Variation in identifying with a motherhood role also can be the result of varying propensities for abstract thinking and fantasizing, or of differences in the availability of appropriate opportunities for observation.

3.2.2 Dreams About Pregnancy and Motherhood

Pregnancy can act as a catalyst to awaken unconscious fantasies, and revive long-inhibited conflictual and unresolved issues. The unconscious fantasies can be elaborated on in nighttime dreams and in conscious daydreams, and in imaginary thoughts about the mother's current and future life (Raphael-Leff, 1986). In these dreams, the mother's identity may often be fused with that of her mother and alternately with that of the embryo/fetus. Logic and causality often are suspended in fantasies. The dream often characterizes and idealizes the mother's wishes and hopes, or serves as a window to her emotional disequilibrium when fear is her prevailing emotion. For example, a woman with positive expectations may idealize the creative act and the fetus emanating from it, while a woman who is predominantly fearful may evade thoughts of the fetus, may feel invaded and sapped, and may resent all sensations and discomforts reminding her of the child within. Likewise, labor and birth may be regarded as a powerful, exciting process in which a woman exhibits trust in her bodily performance and anticipation of a new union with the infant, or labor and birth may be perceived as potentially humiliating and painful, and something to be avoided as much as possible through anesthesia and technological intervention. In accordance with her opinion of labor and birth, the mother either does what she knows is best and assumes rational control through preparation, or she feels vulnerable and defenseless under the weight of maternal obligation to a role that threatens her self-esteem and competence. Normal mothering may be a composite of both orientations, with variations in the predominant mode for different women (Raphael-Leff, 1986).

The women's reported dream content tended to parallel their actual concerns. Women's recordings of dreams peaked in the few days that followed an interview with the researcher. The dreams often focused on concerns or conflicts that had been raised in the interviews. Dreaming is discussed at some length, because the emotive content was more vivid than that reported in interview conversations. Five categories of dreams commonly occurred.

1. Reliving childhood
2. School dreams
3. Motherhood-career conflict
4. Confidence in maternal skills
5. Food dreams and infant intactness

3.2.2.1   Reliving Childhood

One woman relived her childhood in her dreams. In an interview, Ms. Uman said that she was having "a lot of dreams…that relate to people and experiences in my past." It surprised her that she dreamed about people she had not "seen in 10, 15 years." In one dream, in which she was fighting with her older brother, she was pregnant and was helping her brothers put up a fence to keep out deer.

> [My older brother] changes more quickly than I do, and nags me about being slow, lazy, and unhelpful. While trying to maintain my good humor, I tease back only to have him nag me some more…. I break down, cover my ears, and scream that I can't take any more of his yelling and criticism. I run away, ears still covered, convinced that I'm going crazy.

Ms. Uman saw, by way of association, that she was experiencing feelings of anger and frustration like those formerly engendered by her relationship with her older brother. Just as before she had fears of failing, perhaps with regard to mothering skills this time. Ms. Uman's concerns seemed to be associated with the physical limitations of late pregnancy. It appeared from the interviews that she had worked through this sibling rivalry and had reached a state of reconciliation with her brother. She felt that this had helped her to prepare for motherhood, especially in terms of understanding her child. In response to the question "Do you sometimes think that your child will have feelings like your brother had toward you?" Ms. Uman said:

> I think that to a certain degree jealousy can be expected at any level…. I think it can be overcome and you can reach a point where everybody understands that he has a part in your life;… you reach a point where there's a great amount of mutual respect and family love that can override this jealousy that sometimes shows up…. I think, too, that the child has to understand that he can feel jealous at times, and he shouldn't be ashamed or afraid of feeling jealous. He can learn that it's just a normal reaction, but that it hasn't changed anything at any level.

In this instance, Ms. Uman appeared to have relived a conflict, satisfactorily resolved it, and achieved a state of readiness to assist her child in resolving similar conflicts.

3.2.2.2   School Dreams

Several women had what were termed "school dreams," in which they saw themselves back in school, often in dormitories. The gravidas usually interpreted these dreams as a wish to return to the prepregnant state. Ms. Carre had many dreams in which she experienced frustration at the difficulty of looking back in time. In one dream, she found herself in a strange city looking for a school friend; she became lost and confused, but eventually reached her destination. Loss and confusion in this case may have indicated the presence of conflict about becoming a mother. Ms. Oaks saw herself back in her old university dormitory with her baby. The students were much younger than she and unfamiliar, but the housemother was the same person. Ms. Oaks recognized the incongruity of the setting, as well as the implied search for an understanding companion. She offered the following interpretation of her dream.

> Coming to college and to [the dorm] was my first extended separation from home and family, but by the same token it afforded me the first taste of freedom and self-responsibility and self-sufficiency, independence, etc. Returning for one last stay could be viewed in several ways. First, the relinquishing of the kind of freedom that I associated with college life… that now I had assumed the responsibility for a child,…giving up of some of that freedom I had grown accustomed to. And second, it was as if I returned there to pick up…collect, the kind of familial responsibility that my parents had partially relinquished when they brought me to college and no longer could assume the…responsibilities of feeding, clothing, overseeing my daily life. I found the cyclical nature of this dream very interesting and after I spent a little time trying to analyze it, I had quite a contented feeling about what the dream represented to me.

In this case, motherhood was recognized as a developmental step equal in significance to the "first extended separation" from the family. The dream also showed the extent to which Ms. Oaks identified with her parents' roles. The "contented feeling" appeared to stem from her success in working through the problem of the loss of freedom in favor of gaining a new independence, as well as responsibility for charting the future course of her life.

In another school dream, Ms. Acton found herself pregnant in the dormitory of a large university, but no one seemed to notice that she was pregnant. She made friends primarily with the male residents, who were very friendly. One suggested that she lose weight (her pregnancy) so that she would be more attractive. He also reminded her that she was married and, therefore, unavailable. Ms. Acton associated this dream with the conflict between herself and her husband over her fatigue and over being less socially and sexually active during pregnancy. She felt that her husband was not understanding, which upset her.

> I felt inadequate because I could not please Bob. We hadn't had sex in quite awhile and we could have had more fun that evening had I not been tired. I felt that at that point he'd be better off without me and vice versa.

In the dream, Ms. Acton felt "glad" that no one realized that she was pregnant, and she offered the following interpretation:

> [I want]…to be an individual again. No responsibilities to anyone but myself,… At the end [of the dream] it became apparent that although that guy didn't know I was pregnant, he… knew I was married…. I still had that written all over my face. There was no escaping the situation. I just had to face up to my responsibilities.

The dream contained the dual themes of the loss of an old lifestyle and the impossibility of retrieving it. Ms. Acton recognized and accepted these eventualities, and acknowledged the responsibility inherent in parenthood.

3.2.2.3 Motherhood-Career Conflict

A preoccupation with the problem of combining motherhood with school or a career often was expressed in dreams. Such dreams tended to reveal a considerable amount of anxiety. Ms. Fair dreamed that she was in her parents' house when her brother returned the family car with a flat tire.

> For some reason this was very serious, and it incapacitated the car. I got very upset and was yelling…. I felt like there was a terrible crisis and was very upset and tense over the situation.

Ms. Fair interpreted the dream as follows:

> Sometimes I get scared about the prospect of finishing school, taking care of a new baby and the trailer. I want to get through school badly. And I was very upset when we couldn't have a car so that I could do my public health nursing. I don't know if I was creating an excuse to get out of going to school, but I acknowledge the desire is still there – or that I am just afraid something is going to keep me from finishing,… and I couldn't figure out why the flat tire was such a disaster.

Two conflicts seemed apparent in the dream – one between her career in nursing and her responsibilities for the baby, and the other between returning and not returning to school. The deflated tire could have signified a wish to return to the prepregnant state where such intense conflicts and their resultant anxiety were absent, and it also hints at an acceptable excuse for missing school. In her interview, Ms. Fair acknowledged feeling especially divided between motherhood and finishing school; it was difficult for her to cope with this conflict because she viewed motherhood as a "full-time job."

Ms. Hayes dreamed of returning to teach kindergarten after her baby was 1 year old. In her dream, she was left with all the "messy" things by the other teachers, plus some unexpected feelings.

> The other two teachers had gotten rid of the sand table while I was out with the flu because of the smell. After looking around, in the dream, I decided to wait until the baby was at least two to go back to work.

Regarding an interpretation of her dream, Ms. Hayes said: "It was probably a response to the feeling of being tied down and changing identity – which I don't want to become an end, but a portion of my life."

In this dream, there was the sense of a fear of losing ground in her profession while she was busy with her child. Clearly, Ms. Hayes did not anticipate fulfillment solely through motherhood, and was anxious about "picking up my life after" the baby was born.

Ms. Jabon had a "career anxiety" dream in which she thought she would be unable to get a college-level teaching job because she had not completed her master's degree in dance, and had not attended classes since "hurting" herself in the third trimester of pregnancy. "Others" got jobs and one dancer, in particular, "seemed very unpregnant and professional in orientation." Of her associations, Ms. Jabon said:

> I've been bothered by not finishing up my degree before the arrival of the baby. Hurting myself seems related to my hurting myself teaching the other day. Mark [a friend] and the successful dance friends looking on [in the dream] seem [connected] to some resentment and jealousy – that is, their careers are going fine; they're not pregnant.

Ms. Jabon equated being pregnant with being unprofessional. Indeed, a dancer might face special difficulties in combining her profession with motherhood. The "resentment and jealousy" probably symbolized the painful sense of loss that was not compensated for by the reward of the baby.

In surmising the meaning of these remarks, it is important to point out that women established in a career, or in the process of establishing one, either compromised their careers temporarily or expected to remain active in their careers after childbirth. In no case was a career totally relinquished. Motherhood was added to career responsibilities, and provisions for child care were anticipated. For several women, the loss of career seemed to be equated with the loss of self; in these cases, replacement was not easily found or was impossible to find.

3.2.2.4 Confidence in Maternal Skills

Many women dreamed about their babies, not symbolically, but as real infants or toddlers. The concerns of these dreams often involved their ability to mother. Ms. Carre, for example, dreamed about a 2-year-old boy who was "sitting in his large toy car and rolling out into the street."

> I called to him to stop and turn around, but he either didn't hear me or just ignored me. Fortunately, he didn't go too far out into [the] street and came back in the next driveway. When he got back to the garage, I picked him off of the car and scolded him thoroughly for going out into such a busy street. His ride-um car was then taken away and he was confined to the inside of the garage.

Ms. Carre expressed a fear of failure in mothering in this dream, as well as a lack of confidence in the child's ability to thrive. The frequency of dream themes involving misfortune and infant anomalies has been acknowledged by other researchers (Gillman, 1968; Sherwen, 1981), but in Ms. Carre's dream potential misfortune was associated with concerns about maternal adequacy.

In a similar dream Ms. Zeff was pregnant, but "still at home with my parents."

> My father had decided we would leave the new house we had been in for six years and go back to our old one. I remember being so disappointed. I had had the baby on the day we moved and I drove to our old house and hid the baby in a neighbor's garden. For protection I had wrapped him in paper bags. I went back to help move, spent the night in the house and seemed to forget about the baby. The next day I remembered, and panicked because I thought the squirrels may have gotten him. I rushed back to the garden and he was all bundled up and all right. I was very, very relieved.

Ms. Zeff's diary entries showed considerable ambivalence about the coming child and resistance to the change in her lifestyle; she sometimes felt that "kids are too much trouble." In her dream, she felt ambivalent toward the child and guilty because of the ambivalence; she wished to return to the "old house," her parents' home, or perhaps to her premarital state.

Ms. Santa dreamed that she had just had a baby girl.

> After being home a few weeks it seemed that Judith wasn't eating much and slept all the time. Tom wanted to take her to the hospital, but I didn't want to. I knew my baby was all right – she had to be. Then for some reason I guess I had to go back to work. I was very upset at leaving my baby at home. Then one night when I came home I found a note; Tom had taken Judith to the hospital. How could he? There wasn't anything wrong with my baby! Quickly I drove to the hospital to find my husband waiting to see what the deal was. Finally the doctor came out and all he said is, 'You have a very lazy baby.'

Ms. Santa's associations revealed that she worried about her skills in perceiving needs and giving adequate care to an infant. Signs of possessiveness also existed. In another dream, she continued to express concern about adequately nurturing her baby.

> [I found myself standing] in front of my spider plant [which in reality I am proud of – it grows and grows and just looks good!], but in this dream… it curled up and died. I wasn't sad…, rather… I was very mad at the plant. I couldn't figure out why it had died, or how it could just up and die on me. Then there was my baby sitting there next to the plant. She began to coo and just look at the plant. Almost instantly the plant perked right up to its normal self [sic]. I picked up my baby and gave her a big hug just before I woke up.

In this dream, the spider plant (perhaps symbolizing the baby) died despite Ms. Santa's care. The stimulus for her anxiety may have been a recent and sudden tragedy in her family that left her with the unanswerable question "Why?" Her wish was that her baby would flourish despite her (undefined) shortcomings.

Ms. Tell, who was an emotionally disturbed woman, occasionally dreamed about her baby. She found these dreams so painful that she could not bear to record them. At the investigator's request, however, she recorded the following diary entry.

> I…was troubled with many of the emotional problems in my dreams that I…had as a child and teenager – very shy, quite depressed, lonely, often crying and fat. The baby didn't play much of a part in my dreams, but when it was in the dreams I always was mistreating it, didn't know how to take care of it, or, if the baby hadn't arrived yet, I was ashamed to be pregnant.

Ms. Tell had many nightmares about death and dying during her pregnancy. She summarized the nightmares in her dream record.

> … handicapped children were always in my dreams. Often children in wheelchairs were in the basement of my grade school. Often children were sick and hurt.

Several nightmares involved reliving her childhood.

> In all my dreams my husband and I always ran into a person I went to grade school with, who…teased and hurt me because I was such a fat ugly kid; … these [dreams] frightened me very much, brought back many bad memories, and made me worry too much of my own misgivings. I woke in the mornings very disturbed, and often crying. I decided to write this outline of the dreams that have occurred so far, and forget any future dream.

Again and again Ms. Tell appeared in her dreams as the handicapped, the sick and hurt, or the fat and ugly child. Dreaming did not help her resolve past or present conflicts as it did for other women. Caplan (1959) expressed a concern that dreams which are predominantly about older children may leave the mother unprepared for the reality of caring for a small infant.

Although there was wide variation in the gravity or morbidness of the women's dreams, dream material commonly illustrated the women's fear of being unsuccessful as mothers. The themes of women's dreams pertained to anxieties, fears, anger, grief, and rejection, as noted by others (Trad, 1991), and women may be ambivalent about expressing these feelings since they may be considered socially unacceptable or inappropriate for new mothers (Trad, 1991). The anxieties associated with fears may well be due to the dramatic changes and transformations women experience, particularly regarding their self-image (Leifer, 1977; Trad, 1991). The intensity of the women's fears is presumed to be influenced by the mother's past experience of mothering, her current life events, her support system, and following the birth by her actual experience of motherhood (Raphael-Leff, 1986).

3.2.2.5 Food Dreams and Infant Intactness

Many women had dreams about food, picnics, and feasts – each being a frequently recurring dream theme. Food was viewed as the equivalent of the baby or the fruit of the womb. It also could have meant nourishment for the baby either in terms of milk, or metaphorically, in terms of love. Ms. Banor reported the following food dream.

> … Milk was squirting from my breast while I was lying in bed and it got on my husband and the wall and bed linen. [The dream] only occurred once. Maybe I dreamed about this because I plan to breastfeed.

It is reasonable to interpret this dream as Ms. Banor's identification with motherhood or with breastfeeding. It also seems plausible to view the squirting of milk on objects and her husband as an act of aggression, because elsewhere in her diary Ms. Banor complained that her husband did not seem to understand her need to be reassured during pregnancy.

Ms. Fair dreamed that one night she made fruit salad "with watermelon balls, cantaloupe balls, grapes, cherries, strawberries, etc."

> It took a lot of time, but I made it well … as we started eating the salad we found that Lily [her sister] had not taken the time to pit the cherries or pull all the stems off the grapes. It made the salad very distasteful … and I was really mad because I had taken a lot of time in preparing the earlier salad, and she must have just thrown this one together, and people were laughing because it was so bad and we had said we made it together.

Because food often represents the baby, Ms. Fair may have been expressing concern that although the baby was made carefully, someone else could be responsible for its injury or deformity. On the basis of past experience, Ms. Fair distrusted doctors and had wondered whether they would act quickly enough if an emergency developed during labor. In describing an association, Ms. Fair said that her sister "is going to stay with us after the baby comes."

> Maybe I'm scared she [her sister] won't do the housecleaning or something and people will think that I keep a messy house when they come to visit and see the baby… . Maybe I'm afraid of having someone else in charge [who] won't do things the way I like them done.

Ms. Fair seemed to be concerned about subordination, helplessness, and failure.

Ms. Inis dreamed that she drove to her father's house with the baby, but failed to bring food with her. She searched the cupboards of the house and found only gourmet foods. She offered the following interpretation of the dream.

> The dream indicates to me that I'm worried about providing everything the baby needs....
> I don't feel this way really, and don't think I would ever forget food.

Ms. Inis saw her concern about not giving enough food (love) to her child as fleeting because on the whole she was confident in her ability to mother.

In one of Ms. Uman's dreams, she and her husband stopped by a fresh fruit and vegetable stand run by a former boyfriend. She asked for two potatoes, but noticed "the ends are sliced off diagonally. We notice one of the potatoes is rotten. Therefore, I ask for some tomatoes and am given two shaped like eggplants."

In a discussion about her dream, Ms. Uman could not understand her request for well-formed "eggplants" or the meaning of the cut potatoes; however, these items may have reflected her fear of bearing a deformed child. Interpreting the rotten potatoes as symbolic of a deformed baby seemed reasonable, because Ms. Uman had a subsequent "baby dream" in which her concerns were even more explicit. In the latter dream she had "finally given birth to twins." "The babies were strangely shaped with huge circular heads and small triangular bodies. I'm given one to hold and it flops around like a fish. I'm upset because I can't support its head." In offering an interpretation of the dream, she said:

> I have some feelings of awkwardness and fear I can't physically hold the babies. Some revulsion, too, as to the appearance of the babies.... The physical appearance of the babies is probably related to my fear of some abnormality plus the uncertainty of the actual appearance of my baby. Not being able to hold the baby relates to my inexperience in handling babies.

The doubt about being able to care for her infant successfully is quite explicit in this example.

Another woman, Ms. Xana dreamed that she "spoiled a jar of fish."

> My...sister found out and told on me. The previous night I felt bad about not using the top leaf of lettuce, which I think had something to do with why I dreamed about the spoiled fish.

The analogy of the spoiled fish with a deformed baby is clear. Moreover, Ms. Xana had a phobia about needles and medical instruments and lacked trust in the medical staff. She had been born by cesarean section herself, and her breast had been cut during the delivery procedure.

In summary, the content of dreams often presented a mixture of past experiences and present perceived tasks. The women borrowed from their past experiences and from accounts of their own births to formulate an image of their future experiences and roles. Fantasy and dreaming helped them to prepare for what was ahead. In this way, the trials of childbirth and the skills of mothering were rehearsed.

Concerns about creating, producing, and rearing a child often are expressed in dreams about the intactness of the baby. The baby's wholeness and wholesomeness are seen as a test of mothering skills, and of devotion and endurance in the face of novel and complex responsibilities. The women's dream content suggested that enduring was equated with giving or the ability to give; one example was the gravida's frequently voiced concern about managing labor without the aid of medications and anesthetics. Having the strength to sustain herself through prolonged labor, plus managing labor successfully, often was perceived as a measure of the gravida's ability to "give" to the coming child.

The magnitude of the life change that pregnant women confronted and the immensity of the responsibility to be assumed were predominant dream motifs. Self-evaluation of one's ability to meet the developmental challenges of pregnancy, parturition, and parenthood also was prominent.

3.2.2.6   Life Experience

The woman's ability to fantasize and think about being a mother depended to a large extent on her life experiences. If she had been well nurtured, then she had a good role model on which to build her own motherhood identity, as Ballou (1978) and Breen (1975) have indicated. Those women who wished to emulate their own mothers because they had been good mothers demonstrated the advantage of a good role model. They were able to elaborate on their concept of motherhood with several concrete examples. For example, in response to the question "What kind of mother do you want to be?", Ms. Cole answered:

> I guess I could compare it to my own mother. She was always there whenever I needed her, …. The best kind of mother you could be … [would be to be] loving and understanding and caring, and sharing more than anything.

Even when the women had good role models, it was common for them to wish to differ from the role models in some ways – for example, to be more even tempered with their own child. Although they might not have wished to model their mothers exactly, the gravidas were influenced by early experiences of feeling loved and cherished.

Several women feared that they would follow in the footsteps of a "poor mother" and repeat past mistakes. They had a sense of uneasiness about the inevitability of a repetition of behaviors. In talking about this feeling, Ms. Lash said:

> Anytime that I say something – it sounds terrible – but sounds like my mother. I catch myself in the middle of a sentence, and I know where it came from.

Ms. Bode expressed great difficulty imagining herself as a mother and also feared a reversion to the "poor mother. When I was younger, like everybody, I'm sure I looked at my mother and said, 'Well, I am not going to be like my mother,' but, ah, I probably will."

Mothers, mother substitutes, and other women were seen as rich sources of information. They served as confidantes – people with whom to share feelings and ideas that gave perspective. Many women said that despite their husbands' empathy, there were certain limits beyond which they could not convey their feelings about being pregnant and their anticipation of motherhood. Readiness to share feelings with the same sex can be looked upon as a measure of identification with other women, especially other mothers. Regarding this need to share feelings with other women, Ms. Banor confided in her diary.

> One change in my life, moving here in December from [Pennsylvania] made me miss the advantage of a lot of close female relationships that would understand the emotional needs of pregnancy more than a man. I visited my friends the week of graduation and so many of our interests, hopes, and fears were congruent in relation to my pregnancy that I knew how much I needed them. But I haven't had time to develop those types of deep female relationships here yet.... I wish I could share all these little thoughts about being pregnant with my mom.

Ms. Banor sometimes felt hurt because she thought that her husband failed to understand her psychological needs during pregnancy. Later, as she approached her due date, a friend appeared in her life. Her sense of relief at being able to share feelings was expressed in this diary entry.

> I have been helping a friend teach vacation Bible school. This is helping the time move fast. She's due in July too, so we have lots of feelings to share.

3.3   Conflict Resolution

Several excerpts have alluded to the fact that every woman brings some doubts and conflicts to pregnancy, and that they need not be considered abnormal or equivalent to a lack of preparation. Most women, especially in a first pregnancy, wonder whether they will be able to nurture their baby properly. Primigravidas tend to underestimate the resiliency of the newborn and worry about handling such a fragile being. It is not at all unusual for the professional woman to have doubts about balancing motherhood and career goals. Overall, if a woman's doubts are not obsessive or prevailing, then these conflicts can be worked through during pregnancy and she will reach a reasonable state of preparedness and confidence.

Some women expressed few doubts and seemed to rely on their intuition. Characteristic responses reflecting this attitude included the following comments: "I'll do just whatever feels right." "If problems crop up, we will do what is comfortable and hope that the baby turns out OK." "I'll take each day as it comes, and try to work everything out."

Ms. Ely's problems, on the other hand, were quite different. She saw herself as too selfish to nurture effectively, but thought that she would manage to be a good mother.

> Sometimes I get really scared, you know, that I am not going to be able to [give]. I'm worried that I am too selfish and I worry about too much of my own desires and ambitions, ... and it's going to interfere with my child's feelings of security and everything. But I think for the most part I feel pretty...capable. I think I'll be a pretty good mother... 'cause I want to be.

Ms. Jabon understood the enormity of the adjustment to motherhood and worried about being able to give enough. Nevertheless, she thought that she was empathic and realistic, and believed that she would gain confidence in her capacity to nurture her child.

I hope that I won't be too self-centered to be able to adjust to it. Sometimes, if I have to get up very early in the morning or if the cats get us up, or something happens and I am very grumpy getting out of bed I think, 'Oh dear, maybe this will be very traumatic for me to have this creature that is going to be totally dependent.' On the other hand, I know that I like people and have always had a soft spot for children, so I feel confident...in that... I am 'people-oriented' or 'children-oriented.' I also know that...I am set in my ways...and this is going to be a real adjustment.

Ms. Aaron was more anxious about her mothering skills than about labor and delivery. She obsessed about possibly doing the wrong thing, and about being a poor mother.

I've had lots of thoughts on the subject.... You wake up at night and you worry that maybe...you will be sick and you won't know... [what to do]. So I worry...that I won't be able to cope. My husband's had more experience with young children than I have...with baby-size children. So sometimes I feel that he can manage a little better than I can.

Ms. Aaron identified the recent, unexpected loss of a depressed parent as a possible basis for her fears.

Ms. Tell was a very troubled woman (and thus an extreme case) who had no confidence in herself as a mother. She was convinced that she would damage the baby. She said that she had "all doubts, as many doubts as there can be."

I know I will probably ruin that kid's life. I know that I'm not going to be a good mother. I'm going to try too hard. I think that I'm too sensitive to be a good mother...[and that the child will be] a spoiled, rotten, overprotected kid who can't handle himself outside the house – like me.

A statement as negative as this was extremely rare and was considered ominous. Indeed, Ms. Tell and Ms. Aaron made little progress toward acceptable maternal role identification as they neared term.

The conflict generated by attempts of some professional women to combine their careers and motherhood was entirely alleviated by women who simply defined themselves solely in terms of wife and mother. Those who wished to sustain their careers worked through the conflict by reorganizing their priorities and adjusting their timetables. They carefully made provisions for substitute mothers when they were unable to be home, or arranged alternative schedules with their husbands. Ms. Uman felt reasonably positive about managing both school and her baby.

The only thing is that I'm hoping that I'll be able to work out a closer to part-time schedule, perhaps a teaching assistantship and teach and have my classes say in the afternoon and have the morning with the baby so that I don't feel that I'm completely neglecting the kid.

Ms. Lash, an actress, saw no problem in combining her interests with motherhood.

See, what I want to do with drama is go into children's dramatics, and I would like to begin my own children's dramatics group. Working with kids...as the actors...doing impromptu things. I guess I feel that taking the baby along to something like that is not going to mess it up in any way. In fact I think it would probably be...interesting to see how that could figure in with playmaking sorts of things with children.

Ms. Yuth, who was pragmatic and flexible, was able to "play it by ear" and design a program for her unique family circumstance. She planned to work out an "arrangement" with her husband.

> I kind of want to go back to school. I don't spend that many hours in school where I'd be away from home that long a time. And my husband will be home every other day just about, so he can watch the baby.

In some cases, professional women were well aware of the need to use the 9 months of pregnancy to work toward the resolution of motherhood-career conflicts. In describing the "big change" that the baby would effect in her life, Ms. Jabon said:

> I think that the transition [is] from being a performer to being more strictly, I'd say, a dance educator, preparing to adjust to that, because in the past I have been able to be in a situation to take class every day, and teach, and rehearse at night, ... [and] we have gone to New York a couple of times to perform.... So performing has given me a lot of rewards, and a lot of ego gratification, and I enjoy performing. I realize that it's unrealistic to expect that I am going to be able to do everything, or that I would really want to be out of the house every night...plus out all day. I think that occasionally feelings of ambivalence would arise.

Although the transition was indeed difficult, Ms. Jabon was adaptable as demonstrated by the way in which she scaled down her aspirations and reorganized her priorities.

Ms. Quins at first found it extremely difficult to arrange to do her graduate research and care for her baby at the same time. She was under enormous pressure from her academic department, and her advisor lacked understanding of her situation.

> It's just that I have to go to Washington, D.C., for a week or two, like every month, to do my dissertation research. I've no one to take care of the child. How can I do that? I've tried to work out a compromise that we would go to London because my husband's family is in London, and they could babysit.

Ms. Quins did, in fact, go to London and was euphoric about having persevered and about achieving such a satisfactory resolution.

Some women continued to feel uncomfortable about integrating career goals with motherhood; they worried about being trapped at home or felt guilty about continuing their careers. Sometimes this concern continued into the third trimester. Ms. Fair wanted to combine school and motherhood. Although aware of the conflict, she was confused about how to resolve it. She wanted to breast feed and bottle feed at the same time; she wanted to be a full-time mother and a full-time student.

> Well I consider a baby a 24-hour-a-day job. And then I want to breastfeed at least for the first month. I know when school starts that we're going to have a lot of conflict there but I've always wanted to breast feed, so we're going to start that way anyway, and then if it doesn't work out we'll put him on a bottle and a formula. So that'll take time, and we're using cloth diapers so that's going to take time....I'm really excited about it. I think it's a full-time job. So that's...what we're planning on.

Ms. Dann also acknowledged conflict about going to school and about working. When asked, "How do you feel about going to school and working while you have the baby?" she replied:

> There's conflict there, a conflict of interest, interest of trying to be a good parent and at the
> same time leaving the child and everything. I feel that going to school would be a lot easier
> with the child than working…. I'm sure the baby will be distracting, but at least you're
> there. But once you're working…it's [the legal profession] a rather demanding career if
> I pursue it at all. I feel kind of guilty…like maybe the baby will suffer, but I'll work it out.
> I just feel like a little love is better than none. It's better that I love my child and have a life
> of my own, than despise the child and stay home with it.

Ms. Dann had great difficulty resolving her motherhood-career conflict.

For women in the study, conflict appeared to be most acute when the need to be a mother and the need to identify oneself as a career woman both were felt intensely. If one need or the other could be adjusted, the conflict was more amenable to reconciliation. Sustained motherhood-career conflict raised the possibility of feelings of inadequacy regarding mothering. In these cases, there was either an unwillingness to relinquish a source of "ego gratification" provided through career mastery, or a lack of perceived rewards for the effort that was to be expended as a mother.

3.4   Maternal–Fetal Attachment Representation and Maternal Role Evolution

Attachment behavior is associated with acceptance, nurturance, and protection of the child. The foregoing discussion of expectations, fantasies, dreams, and planning for motherhood suggests that the development of maternal attachment to the infant is part of an overall process that begins well before birth. The assessment of maternal attachment is part of the Identification with a Maternal Role questionnaire scale and Interview Schedule. Attachment is measured with items inquiring about maternal anticipation of enjoyment and looking forward to caring for the baby, feelings of love for the fetus-baby, and enjoyment of closeness to children.

An emerging body of literature reveals interrelationships among past childhood attachment representations and future infant attachment, adult couple attachment, maternal–fetal attachment, and maternal–infant attachment. Fonagy et al. (1991) were among the first to use a prospective design to measure attachment representations (adult depictions, during pregnancy, of childhood attachment relationships) and find a relationship with subsequent infant patterns of attachment to the mother at 1 year. Slade et al. (2005) replicated these results. Huth-Bocks (2003) found that the most important predictors of secure infant attachment were the mother's own childhood attachment experiences and their representations of the infant-to-be during pregnancy. The predictiveness of the mother's past attachment relationships to her current attachment responses and of her infant's attachment behavior was replicated by others using similar attachment measures (Frank, Tuber, Slade, & Garrod, 1994; Priel & Besser, 2001; Steele, Steele, & Fonagy, 1996). In addition, other researchers found a correlation between maternal–fetal attachment and postnatal maternal–infant attachment (Muller, 1996). Siddiqui and Hagglof (2000) similarly found an association between maternal–fetal attachment and postnatal maternal involvement with the infant, as did von Klitzing et al. (1996), who found high continuity between pre-and postnatal couple relationships, and between attachment representations (depictions) of the parents and the early relationship with their infant. Other researchers (Wilson et al., 2008), using the Adult Attachment Questionnaire measuring partner attachment, found that prenatal attachment anxiety (lack of confidence in partner's love) and attachment avoidance (anxiety about closeness to others) significantly predicted emotional responses to the newborn infant. At 2 weeks postpartum more avoidant women reported feeling less close to their newborns than less avoidant women. Prenatal and postnatal neuroendocrine measures of oxytocin provide further validity to self-report and interview measures of maternal attachment or bonding. Oxytocin is secreted during uterine contraction and milk ejection and plays a role in the initiation of maternal behavior (Insel & Young, 2001). Feldman, Weller, Zagory-Sharon, and Levine (2007) report that plasma oxytocin levels at early pregnancy and the postpartum period were related to maternal bonding behaviors, including vocalization, positive affect, and attachment-related thoughts.

During pregnancy, fetal movement can act as a projective stimulus from which mothers elaborate, attributing abstract human characteristics to the infant within, and which may enhance maternal–fetal attachment. Researchers have reported a relationship between gestational age and maternal–fetal attachment, and a progressive increase in maternal–fetal attachment throughout the course of pregnancy (Alhusen, 2008; Tsartsara & Johnson, 2006). There is evidence that parents' working models of their infants develop prior to birth and remain relatively stable into early infancy (Zeanah, Keener, Stewart, & Anders, 1985). Stable parental perceptions of infant temperament have been documented by Zeanah et al. (1985), in which parents vividly attributed abstract personality traits to their infants. Additional evidence of the importance of parents' prenatal mental representations of their infant also is demonstrated by the stability in mothers' perceptions of their infants' activity level, regularity of behavior, and quality of mood from late pregnancy to 6 months postpartum. Parents' prenatal mental representations of their infant also were related to infants' behavior at 6 months. These important findings in maternal prenatal and postpartum perceptions have important relevance for maternal–infant relationships.

There also is evidence that mothers' characteristics and experiences – that is, their descriptions of their own early childhood relationships – predicted the quality of attachment relationships with their children (Fonagy et al., 1991; Main, Gabbe, Richardson, & Strong, 1985; Ricks, 1985). Main et al. (1985) specifically assessed such aspects as the value parents placed on their past relationships, namely whether they felt there was undeserved mistreatment, their forgiveness of their parents, and the coherence of their descriptions.

In addition to the studies, other researchers have presented evidence in support of the significance of prenatal attachment to maternal development (Arbeit, 1976; Chojnacke, 1976; Cranley, 1981; Leifer, 1977). Behaviors that indicate attachment include recognition of the individuality and attributes of the fetus/child, imaginative role rehearsal, thoughts about giving of oneself to the child, and fantasy about interactions with the child. As such, maternal attachment often is embodied in the process of envisioning motherhood, although it may be recognized by a few distinctive, overt behaviors as well. In research investigating prenatal attachment, expressions of attachment included the selection of names and pet names, evaluation of feeding methods, talking to the fetus, and touching and stroking fetal parts through the abdomen. One patient, for example, named her fetus "Thumper" after quickening began. Ms. Katen expressed the need to feel closer to her infant through breastfeeding.

In contrast to the conception of maternal–fetal attachment as consisting of maternal–fetal behaviors and interactions, Condon and Corkindale (1997) developed an instrument measuring maternal affective experiences such as closeness, tenderness, positive feelings about the fetus, a desire to know it, and mental representations of the future baby, as well as the intensity of preoccupation with the fetus (i.e., the time that is devoted to thinking about, talking to, and dreaming of the unborn baby). An example of such a response is provided by Ms. Katen's terse statement of the need to feel close to her baby. "If I have milk and can breastfeed and the baby's healthy with that, that would be really good. I can see getting very close to the baby at that time." Numerous other examples of maternal–fetal responses are presented throughout this chapter.

Condon and Corkindale (1997) and others (Ard, 2000; Cranley, 1984; Colpin, De Munter, Nys, Vandemeulebroecke, 1998; Muller, 1992; Wachter, 2002) showed relationships between maternal–fetal attachment and marital satisfaction or social support from a partner. Condon and Corkindale (1997) also found that lower maternal–fetal attachment was associated with higher maternal prenatal anxiety and depression. Hart and McMahon (2006) similarly found relationships for state and trait anxiety, depression, and the quality of maternal–fetal attachment. While Lindgren (2001, 2003) likewise reported that women with lower depression had higher maternal–fetal attachment, he determined that those with lower maternal–fetal attachment reported fewer positive health practices. Monk reported that maternal attachment security ratings during pregnancy made a unique contribution to postpartum depression, beyond that contributed by depression during pregnancy (Monk, Leight, & Fang, 2008).

The development of attachment has been regarded as a transition during which the mother gains a sense of the child (Ballou, 1978). This transition is associated with increased feelings of maternal competence and effectiveness. Toward the end of the third trimester, attachment culminates in a readiness and eagerness to get through the pregnancy and to have and hold the baby. This attitude was consistently expressed.

3.5 Summary

Identification with a motherhood role is the goal of the paradigm shift or developmental step from the woman-without-child to the woman-with-child. This step is taken by degrees and is a process of unfolding.

A developmental step has been described as taking two steps forward and one step backward, because it is natural to have doubts and conflicts about a role change.

Role change profoundly affects the sense of self, and in the interim between roles the woman often is uncertain about where she stands (Trad, 1991). The challenges of pregnancy are associated with ambivalence, uncertainty, and even resentment (Trad, 1991). Progress in identifying a motherhood role evolves, accelerates, and is unceasing during the pregnancy, a process recognized by both Leifer (1977) and Trad (1991). Shereshefsky, Plotsky, and Lockman (1973) also found that progress in the process of adaptation was made over time. They found that psychological preparation for childbirth and motherhood involved both clarification of and confidence in the image of oneself as a mother. By the third trimester, accommodation to the reality of the anticipated birth generally had occurred.

Setbacks in the process leading to motherhood identification can result from low self-esteem, excessive narcissism, lack of a good role model, and motherhood-career conflict. Barriers to role formulation can cause extreme anxiety, making it difficult for the young mother to prepare for motherhood and to accept the trials inherent in labor, which in turn can lead to prolonged labor and delivery as discussed in Chapter 1.

Women who have severe doubts about motherhood tend to find it difficult to contemplate their new role. They may resist the role change and find it hard to "try on the new role." They also may find it hard to think about themselves as mothers, or about changes in their lifestyles. Life changes may be perceived as threatening, with little fulfillment anticipated. A poor relationship with the child may be envisioned in which the child does not thrive. The gravida may be plagued with obsessive thoughts about a "monster" child, or about damaging the child. Persistent doubts about maternal adequacy may prevail. In addition, children may be seen as too much trouble and as an encroachment on life plans. Hostility toward the fetus may be expressed, and little mention may be made of liking or enjoying children. Such women do not demonstrate a state of "readiness" to make the developmental step. They are less prepared for motherhood and have not progressed in identifying a motherhood role.

The articulation of a philosophy of motherhood is indicative of progress in role identification, but it is not sufficient in itself. The ultimate task is to find ways to express this philosophy in terms of real and concrete situations. To accomplish this, the woman often rehearses or pictures herself in the new role. She imagines herself as a mother with her new infant, dreams about the infant, and tries to discover the characteristics that a good mother should possess. A good mother is seen as loving, warm, available, relaxed, empathic, and communicative. This ideal mother answers questions, gives room for independent growth, and sets reasonable limits. Many primigravidas question their capacity to give enough to the coming child. The gravida tries to anticipate changes in her lifestyle, and assesses the significance of what she will be giving up or compromising compared to what she will gain. Deutsch (1945) articulated this dilemma almost 40 years ago, referring to it as "I or the child." The dilemma is resolved as the mother progresses toward a concept of "I and the child." The gravida comes to accept the loss of a former part of herself, realizing that the new role with its potential and its obligations will have compensations; that is, the perceived losses are balanced by clearly perceived rewards. Several women in the study were conscious of making a developmental step.

Paradoxically, all growth, from birth to death, involves loss and gain. The process of growth means acquiring and learning new tools of adaptation appropriate to different situations. Preparing for a role change at any stage of life depends on readiness and eagerness for information. During the adaptation to motherhood, significant others, particularly a woman's mother, are sought out and their roles "tried on" and tested as Rubin (1967a, 1967b) has documented. The pregnant woman often turns to her mother, not primarily because she needs a confidante, but because her mother is a source of information and experience and can serve as a role model. Observing other mothers and children and attending birthing classes also can serve as sources of information. Group interaction in prenatal classes can be a confirming experience that enhances the identification process.

Our research findings and those of others (Leifer, 1977; Shereshefsky et al., 1973) indicate that the questions "Who am I?" and "What will I be?" are paramount in pregnancy, as they are in adolescence when critical decisions about the future are encountered. In continuing and repeated attempts to contemplate the unknown, the gravida asks herself "What kind of a mother should I, can I, will I be?" Other authors have documented the mother's continued search, and struggle, to formulate and find gratification in a motherhood role (Chodorow, 1978; Rich, 1976; Trad, 1991). Gratification is more readily anticipated if the mother-to-be likes and enjoys children; therefore, the course of events is primarily dependent upon the mother's attitude toward children.

Both the interview data and correlational project data indicate that progress in identifying with a motherhood role is a critical task of pregnancy, and is consistent with the recognized task of generativity in adulthood. Adult maternal representations and maternal–fetal attachment are part of this process and are predictive of postnatal maternal–infant attachment and infant attachment responses to the mother. Lederman (1989) reported predictive correlations of prenatal maternal identification with a motherhood role to postpartum confidence in maternal role and satisfaction with motherhood, which is further discussed in Chapter 11.

References

Alhusen, J. L. (2008). A literature update on maternal-fetal attachment. *Journal of Obstetric, Gynecologic, and Neonatal Nursing*, *37*, 315–328.

Arbeit, S. A. (1976). A study of women during their first pregnancy (Master's thesis, Yale University, 1975). *Dissertation Abstracts International, 36*, 6367B-6368B. (University Microfilms No. 76-12, 745).

Ard, L. D. C. (2000). Adolescent prenatal attachment, psychosocial development, and parental bonding: Is there a relationship? *Dissertation Abstracts International: Section B: The Sciences & Engineering, 60*(10-B), 5049.

Baker, A. A. (1966). *Psychiatric disorders in obstetrics*. Philadelphia, PA: F.A. Davis.

Ballou, J. (1978). *The psychology of pregnancy*. Lexington, MA: Lexington Books.

Breen, D. (1975). *The birth of a first child*. London: Tavistock.

Caplan, G. (1959). *Concepts of mental health and consultation*. Washington, DC: Superintendent of Documents, U.S. Government Printing Office.

Chodorow, N. (1978). *The reproduction of mothering*. Berkeley, CA: University of California Press.

Chojnacke, S. (1976). Preparation for motherhood: A comparison of high risk and low risk pregnant women. Unpublished Master's thesis, University of Wisconsin-Madison.

Colpin, H., De Munter, A., Nys, K., & Vandemeulebroecke, L. (1998). Prenatal attachment in future parents of twins. *Early Development & Parenting, 7*, 223–227.

Condon, J. T., & Corkindale, C. (1997). The correlates of antenatal attachment in pregnant women. *British Journal of Medical Psychology, 70*, 359–372.

Cranley, M. S. (1981). Roots of attachment: The relationship of parents with their unborn. *Birth Defects: Original Article Series, 17*, 59–83.

Cranley, M. S. (1984). Social support as a factor in the development of parents' attachment to their unborn. *Birth Defects: Original Article Series, 20*, 99–124.

Deave, T. (2005). Associations between child development and women's attitudes to pregnancy and motherhood. *Journal of Reproductive and Infant Psychology, 23*, 63–75.

Deutsch, F. M., Ruble, D. N., Fleming, A., Brooks-Gunn, J., & Stangor, C. (1986, April). Becoming a mother: Information-seeking and self-definitional processes. Paper presented at the meeting of the Eastern Psychological Association, New York, NY.

Deutsch, F. M., Ruble, D. N., Fleming, A., Brooks-Gunn, J., & Stangor, C. (1988). Information-seeking and maternal self-definition during the transition to motherhood. *Journal of Personality and Social Psychology, 55*, 420–431.

Deutsch, H. (1945). *The psychology of women* (Vol. 2). New York: Grune & Stratton.

Feldman, R., Weller, A., Zagory-Sharon, O., & Levine, A. (2007). Evidence for a neuroendocrinological foundation of human affiliation. *Psychological Science, 18*, 114–135.

Flapan, M. (1969). A paradigm for the analysis of childbearing motivations of women prior to birth of the first child. *American Journal of Orthopsychiatry, 39*, 402–417.

Fonagy, P., Steele, H., & Steele, M. (1991). Maternal representations of attachment during pregnancy predict the organization of infant-mother attachment at one year of age. *Child Development, 62*, 891–905.

Frank, M. A., Tuber, S. B., Slade, A., & Garrod, E. (1994). Mothers' fantasy representations and infant security attachment: A Rorschach study of first pregnancy. *Psychoanalytic Psychology, 11*, 475–490.

Gillman, R. D. (1968, July). The dreams of pregnant women and maternal adaptation. *American Journal of Orthopsychiatry, 38*, 688–692.

Grossman, F. K., Eichler, L. S., & Winickoff, S. A. (1980). *Pregnancy, birth, and parenthood*. San Francisco, CA: Jossey-Bass.

Haedt, A., & Keel, P. (2007). Maternal attachment, depression, and body dissatisfaction in pregnant women. *Journal of Reproductive and Infant Psychology, 25*, 285–295.

Hart, R., & McMahon, C. A. (2006). Mood state and psychological adjustment to pregnancy. *Archives of Women's Mental Health, 9*, 329–337.

Huth-Bocks, A. C. (2003). Mother-infant attachment: The impact of maternal representations during pregnancy, maternal risk factors, and social support. *Dissertation Abstracts International: Section B: The Sciences & Engineering, 63*(9-B), 4374.

Insel, T. R., & Young, L. J. (2001). The neurobiology of attachment. *Nature Reviews Neuroscience, 2*, 129–136.

Lederman, R. (1988, April). Prenatal prediction of maternal postpartum adaptation. Paper presented at the Sixteenth Annual Meeting of the American Society for Psychosomatic Obstetrics and Gynecology, St. Helena, CA.

Lederman, R. (1989, June). Prediction of postpartum adaptation from maternal prenatal adaptation scales. Presentation at second International Nursing Research Conference on Social Support, Seoul, Korea.

Lederman, R. (1996). *Psychosocial adaptation in pregnancy: Assessment of seven dimensions of maternal development* (2nd ed.) New York, Springer.

Lederman, R., Harrison, J., & Worsham, S. (1992). Psychosocial predictors of low birth weight in a multicultural, high risk population. In K. Wijma & B. von Schoultz (Eds.), *Reproductive life: Advance in research in psychosomatic obstetrics and gynecology*. Carforth, UK: The Parthenon.

Lederman, R., Lederman, E., Work, B. A., Jr., & McCann, D. S. (1979). Relationship of psychological factors in pregnancy to progress in labor. *Nursing Research, 28*, 94–97.

Lederman, R., Lederman, E., Work, B. A., Jr., & McCann, D. (1985). Anxiety and epinephrine in multiparous labor: Relationship to duration of labor and fetal heart rate pattern. *American Journal of Obstetrics and Gynecology, 153*, 870–877.

Lederman, R. P. (1996) *Psychosocial Adaptation in Pregnancy: Assessment of Seven Dimensions of Maternal Development.* (2nd ed.). New York : Springer.

Lederman, R. P., Weis, K., Brandon, J., Hills, B., & Mian, T. (2002, April). Relationship of maternal prenatal adaptation and family functioning to pregnancy outcomes. Poster presentation at the Annual Meeting of the Society of Behavioral Medicine, Washington, DC.

Leifer, M. (1977). Psychological changes accompanying pregnancy and motherhood. *Genetic Psychology Monographs, 95*, 55–96.

Lindgren, K. (2001). Relationships among maternal-fetal attachment, prenatal depression, and health practices in pregnancy. *Research in Nursing and Health, 24*, 203–217.

Lindgren, K. (2003). A comparison of pregnancy health practices of women in inner-city and small urban communities. *Journal of Obstetric, Gynecologic, and Neonatal Nursing, 32*, 313–321.

Main, D. M., Gabbe, S. G., Richardson, D., & Strong, S. (1985). Can preterm deliveries be prevented? *American Journal Obstetrics and Gynecology, 151*, 892–898.

Monk, C., Leight, K. L., & Fang, Y. (2008). The relationship between women's attachment style and perinatal mood disturbance: implications for treatment and screening. *Archives of Women's Mental Health, 9*, 117–129.

Muller, M. E. (1992). A critical review of prenatal attachment research. *Scholarly Inquiry for Nursing Practice, 6*, 2.

Muller, M. E. (1996). Prenatal and postnatal attachment: A modest correlation. *Journal of Obstetric, Gynecologic, and Neonatal Nursing, 25*, 161–166.

Oakley, A. (1980). *Women confined: Towards a sociology of childbirth.* New York: Schocken.

Pohlman, E. H. (1969). *The psychology of birth planning.* Cambridge, MA: Shenkman.

Priel, B., & Besser, A. (2001). Bridging the gap between attachment and object relations theories: A study of the transition to motherhood. *British Journal of Medical Psychology, 74*, 85–100.

Raphael-Leff, J. (1986). Facilitators and regulators: Conscious and unconscious processes in pregnancy and early motherhood. *British Journal of Medical Psychology, 59*, 43–55.

Rees, B. L. (1980). Measuring identification with the mothering role. *Research in Nursing and Health, 3*, 49–56.

Rich, A. (1976). *Of woman born: Motherhood as institution.* New York: Norton.

Ricks, M. H. (1985). The social transmission of parental behavior: Attachment versus generations. In I. Bretheron & E. Waters (Eds.), *Growing points in attachment theory and research. SCRD Monographs, 48*, serial no. 209, Chicago, IL: University of Chicago Press.

Rubin, R. (1984). *Maternal identity and the maternal experience.* New York: Springer.

Rubin, R. (1967a). Attainment of the maternal role. Part I: Process. *Nursing Research, 16*, 237–245.

Rubin, R. (1967b). Attainment of the maternal role. Part II: Models and referents. *Nursing Research, 16*, 342–346.

Ruble, D. N. (1983). The development of social-comparison processes and their role in achievement-related self-socialization. In E. T. Higgins, D. N. Ruble, & W. W. Hartup (Eds.), *Social cognition and social development: A sociocultural perspective* (pp. 134–157), New York: Cambridge University Press.

Ruble, D. N. (1987). The acquisition of self-knowledge: A self-socialization perspective. In N. Eisenberg (Ed.), *Contemporary topics in developmental psychology*, (pp. 243–270), New York: Wiley.

Shereshefsky, P. M., Plotsky, H., & Lockman, R. F. (1973). Pregnancy adaptation. In P. M. Shereshefsky & L. J. Yarrow (Eds.), *Psychological aspects of a first pregnancy and early postnatal adaptation.* New York: Raven.

Shereshefsky, P. M., & Yarrow, L. J. (Eds.). (1973). *Psychological aspects of a first pregnancy and early postnatal adaptation.* New York: Raven.

Sherwen, L. N. (1981). Fantasies during the third trimester of pregnancy. *Maternal Child Nursing Journal, 6,* 398–401.

Siddiqui, A., & Hagglof, B. (2000). Does maternal prenatal attachment predict postnatal mother-infant interaction. *Early Human Development, 59,* 13–25.

Slade, A., Grienenberger, J., Bernbach, E., Levy, D., & Locker, A. (2005). Maternal reflective functioning, attachment, and the transmission gap: A preliminary study. *Attachment and Human Development, 7,* 283–298.

Steele, H., Steele, M., & Fonagy, P. (1996). Associations among attachment classifications of mothers, fathers, and their infants. *Child Development, 67,* 541–555.

Trad, P. (1991). Adaptation to developmental transformations during various phases of motherhood. *Journal of the American Academy of Psychoanalysis, 19,* 403–421.

Tsartsara, E., & Johnson, M. P. (2006). The impact of miscarriage on women's pregnancy-specific anxiety and feelings of prenatal maternal-fetal attachment during the course of a subsequent pregnancy: An exploratory follow-up study. *Journal of Psychosomatic Obstetrics and Gynecology, 27,* 173–182.

Wachter, M. P. K. (2002). Psychological distress and dyadic satisfaction as predictors of maternal-fetal attachment. *Dissertation Abstracts International: Section B: The Sciences & Engineering, 63*(4-B), 2080.

Wenner, N. K., Cohen, M. B., Weigert, E. V., Kvarnes, R. G., Ohaneson, E. M., & Fearing, J. M. (1969). Emotional problems in pregnancy. *Psychiatry, 32,* 389–410.

Wilson, C. L., Rholes, W. S., Simpson, J. A., & Tran, S. (2008). Labor, delivery, and early parenthood: An attachment theory perspective. *Personality and Social Psychology Bulletin, 33,* 505–518.

von Klitzing, K., Amsler, F., Schleske, G., Simoni, H., & Burgin, D. (1996). Effect of psychological factors in pregnancy on the development of parent-child relations. 2. Transition from prenatal to postnatal phase. *Gynakologisch-Geburtshilfliche Rundschau, 36,* 149–155.

Zeanah, C. H., Keener, M. A., Stewart, L., & Anders, T. F. (1985). Prenatal perception of infant personality: A preliminary investigation. *Journal of the American Academy of Child Psychiatry, 24,* 503–505.

Chapter 4
Relationship with Mother

The significance of the pregnant woman's relationship with her mother has been emphasized in the literature as an important factor in adaptation to pregnancy and motherhood (Ballou, 1978; Deutsch, 1945; Tulman & Fawcett, 2003, Uddenberg, 1974; Wenner et al., 1969). A positive relationship with the mother also predicted successful adaptation to pregnancy (Lewis, 1989). In our initial multidisciplinary research project presented in Chapter 1, the quality of the pregnant woman's relationship with her mother was related not only to psychosocial conflicts in pregnancy, but also to physiological measures of progress in labor (Lederman, Lederman, Work, & McCann, 1978, 1979). In another project (Lederman, 1989). Relationship with Mother was predictive of postpartum adaptation scales of Confidence in a Motherhood Role and Satisfaction with Motherhood and Infant Care Tasks. These studies also demonstrated that the relationship with the mother appeared to influence the gravida's identification with and adaptation to a motherhood role. It previously was noted that a woman's ability to identify her motherhood role depended on the availability of good models and on her early experience of mothering. The research results revealed the importance of the pregnant woman's past and current relationship with her mother.

Four components have been found to be important in the gravida's relationship with her mother:

1. The availability of the grandmother – that is, the gravida's mother – to the gravida both in the past and during pregnancy, i.e., being available when needed.
2. The grandmother's reactions to the pregnancy, especially her acceptance of the grandchild, and her acknowledgment of her daughter as a mother.
3. The grandmother's respect for her daughter's autonomy, as demonstrated by relating to the gravida as a mature adult rather than as a child.
4. The grandmother's willingness to reminisce with her daughter about her own childbearing and childrearing experiences.

The gravida's contribution to the relationship also was appraised. Her ability to empathize with her mother's trials in parenthood, and with the changes inherent in her mother's transition to the role of grandparent was found to be particularly important. Each of these aspects of the mother–daughter relationship is discussed in the following sections.

R. Lederman and K. Weis, *Psychosocial Adaptation to Pregnancy*,
DOI 10.1007/978-1-4419-0288-7_4, © Springer Science+Business Media, LLC 2009

4.1 Availability of the Mother

4.1.1 Infancy and Childhood

Henry (1973) has asserted that the availability of parents is a precondition of a child's availability to him or herself, the parents, and others. "An infant will become a self only if he or she is urged on by love." To become a self and human, "the primal requirement is the availability of another person" (pp. 287–288). Henry was referring specifically to active emotional availability – to the giving of love when needed – versus attention only to basic physical necessities such as food, cleanliness, and shelter. The converse of active emotional availability is detachment, indifference, and a passiveness. These findings are well borne out in research on prenatal maternal attachment and maternal reflective representations in pregnancy (Fonagy, Steele, & Steele, 1991; Huth-Bocks, 2003; Slade, Grienenberger, Bernbach, Levy, & Locker, 2005).

In the context of our research, the availability of the mother during childhood means that the mother is perceived as having been loving, present, and interested. Ms. Cole, for example, said that her mother "always had time for us," Ms. Raaf commented that her mother "didn't shove us away," Ms. Yuth said that her mother "was with us all the time," and Ms. Ely stated that "she turned to her mother" when she had problems. These women felt that they had the basic role models and coping resources to form positive relationships with their own children. Although all women expressed the wish to have loving, close relationships with their children and to be available when needed, Henry's (1973) work and that of other researchers (Fonagy et al., 1991; Huth-Bocks, 2003; Slade et al., 2005) suggest that the probability of the gravida's emotional attachment to her baby was directly related to the grandmother's past availability to her daughter during childhood. Our project data support the thesis that a warm, secure, loving mother serves as a model from which a young woman patterns her own maternal behavior.

In talking about the past, some women who participated in the study related negative perceptions of the early interactions between themselves and their mothers. Ms. Tell stated that she had been "alone most of the time," Ms. Carre that her "mother did not seem interested," Ms. Fair that she "could not talk" to her mother, and Ms. Katen that she "was not close" to her mother. Ms. Gale felt that her stepmother gave her attention, but at the same time played what she called "the silence game"; as a result, Ms. Gale turned to her sister with her problems. Ms. Gale recognized that she was relating to her husband in a similar manner and said that she had tried to overcome the pattern.

> I've caught myself a couple of times, when I'm really moody, using silence as a tool to manipulate him. But I'm really glad that I realized it, and then I really made an effort to talk about it because I realized that if I didn't talk about it, I probably would show it in other ways.... And I felt less moody, and I think that he started understanding that I was having conflict with his priorities and that [talking] helped.

This excerpt illustrates how early patterns of interaction can carry over into adult and marital relationships, and has been referred to as "intergenerational patterns of attachment" (Obegi, Morrison, & Shaver, 2004; Steele & Steele, 2005). According to some researchers (Shereshefsky & Lockman, 1973; Shereshefsky, Plotsky, & Lockman, 1973; Wolkind & Zajicek, 1981), attempts to overcome the perception of a detached relationship are difficult. Such attempts have been described as requiring a persistent and concerted effort, and the assistance of a supportive person often is helpful (Wenner et al., 1969).

4.1.2   Availability During Pregnancy

Even if the woman's mother had not been available to her during childhood and this fact had led to considerable hostile feelings, the research project data demonstrated that the woman still could perceive her mother as being available during pregnancy. The relevant question was whether availability during pregnancy could influence adaptation to pregnancy and identification with a motherhood role. Deutsch, Ruble, Fleming, Brooks-Gunn, and Stangor (1988) showed that the woman's self-definition of her maternal role was strongly correlated with the relationship to her mother during pregnancy.

Availability of the mother, in the context of having an influence on maternal role development and pregnancy adaptation, means that the mother was perceived as interested in her daughter, and emotionally supportive of her; accessibility in the relationship was between two adults, not between mother and child. If the mother had been aloof in the past but was currently interested and supportive, it was assumed that the two women had reconciled and developed a better attachment relationship. As a result of reconciliation, the woman 's mother recognized her daughter's developmental tasks in learning to become a mother, and the expectant woman recognized her mother's need to adjust to a grandmother role. Pregnancy and childbirth provided an opportunity for the mother–daughter relationship to evolve to a higher level. As could be expected, the evolution of the relationship was facilitated if the mother and daughter lived in close proximity to one another.

Many mothers offered assistance to their pregnant daughters and were happy with the prospect of having a grandchild, but these circumstances did not necessarily indicate a close mother–daughter relationship. When the daughter welcomed her mother's help without ambivalence and when she felt that she could learn from her mother, the mother was considered available and supportive. For example, Ms. Uman's mother had been assisting her by purchasing items for the baby.

> She's [mother's] been very practical telling me that you don't need 30,000 little baby dresses or romper sets. You can get by with a minimum amount. And the other thing is they [grandparents] tend to just tell us not to worry, that the baby is not as fragile as he looks, that he'll manage okay, to take everything with a grain of salt.

In this case, the grandmother was not only supportive, but also a source of welcome information. Other examples of daughters' receptivity to their mothers' support and interest included Ms. Carre, whose mother was the main person to help her after delivery because she could not count on her husband for such assistance, and Ms. Dann, who welcomed her mother's help and advice when needed, saying, "I'll just do whatever I feel is right. If I don't know, if I'm just completely at a loss, I'll probably call my mother."

Ms. Yuth respected her mother's wisdom in mothering. Feeling that she had a good resource, she had no reservations about accepting her mother's advice.

> She tells me…what's the best type of bottle, you know, and stuff to use…. I think my mom knows. She raised seven kids. She's pretty well aware of what not to use.

Ms. Fair felt that her mother had changed and become more open when discussing sexual matters. Ms. Katen anticipated a closer emotional relationship with her mother during pregnancy.

> I think I'm going to become closer with my mother than I was in the past… It's been her ambition to be a grandmother for a long time, and I can see that where we've argued in the past about…school…and my…friends or the life that I'm leading, I'm becoming more appealing to her, and so I can see getting to know her better.

In both cases, pregnancy stimulated openness that had not existed in the past. With the common bond of motherhood and mutual availability, women often described a closeness that appeared to facilitate the development and adaptation of both individuals.Several women in the study reported that their mothers were critical of them, and it became apparent that the women had a great desire to receive their mothers' support during pregnancy. Some women became hurt and resentful when their mothers were not encouraging and reassuring. Ms. Meta felt that her mother was unsupportive and critical of childbirth preparation classes. In addition, Ms. Meta's mother failed to listen to her and predicted the worst for her.

> My mother thinks I'm crazy for this reason…for having my husband in the delivery room. She keeps saying, 'Are you sure that you want to go through with it?' Definitely there will be pain, she says, and it's going to be a hard time.

Upon hearing of the decision to breastfeed, Ms. Meta's mother referred to her daughter as "an animal." She forewarned her daughter of postpartum depression, saying "you will have that for sure. Everybody does."

Childbirth preparation, natural childbirth, the husband's participation in labor and delivery, breast feeding, and hospital rooming-in were common targets of grandmothers' criticism when it occurred. Ms. Zeff felt that her "mother was distant and clung to a rigid, ethical code." Ms. Hayes refused to discuss anything with her mother, and she did not want her mother to come visit after the baby was born because she saw her as "cold" and "a very guilt-inflicting person."

> She's just a really foul person. She can't help herself, but I have a hard time coping with her. I just resent her terribly…. I've crazy about my mother-in-law. She's just great. And she's going to come out when the baby is born, and my mother isn't cause we don't want to cope with her then.

Although Ms. Hayes rejected her own mother as a role model, she attempted to use her mother-in-law as a substitute.

> She has an amazing knack of letting you do what you want…. Her upbringing was different, and she's very nonjudgmental and [not] guilt- inflicting.

Many women who rejected their mothers, or who simply had not used them as role models, tried to find substitutes. Ms. Inis's mother died when she was young, and she had a stepmother with whom she had a good relationship. She still had memories of being loved by her biological mother.

> I had bronchitis really bad every year and she would stay up with me, and I would sit on her lap, and she'd sing and stuff like that. I really liked that.

In addition to retaining an extremely positive memory of having been mothered, Ms. Inis found herself observing friends who were mothers and talking with her husband about childrearing. Since the completion of this study, Ms. Inis has been presented in the news media as a significant personal contributor to Parents Anonymous. The poignant memory of her deceased mother, the availability of a stepmother, and her personal observations of other women in the maternal role appear to have contributed to Ms. Inis's positive attitude and effective coping behavior.

Clearly, pregnancy stimulates a need to identify with other women, preferably one's own mother. If the mother is available, then the daughter feels free to explore the meanings of pregnancy, labor, and delivery with her, and is more likely to do so given the novel experience of a first pregnancy. If the mother is supportive, the daughter gains self-confidence. Shereshefsky and Lockman (1973) have reported that it is through gains in self-confidence that the adaptation to motherhood is facilitated; confidence helps the mother-to-be define her new role.

If the mother is unavailable because of emotional or geographic distance, divorce, or death, then the daughter often feels a painful void. She senses that she is being deprived of an essential figure who can act as a sounding board and give support when she has doubts about her emerging role as a mother. She often seeks to find another woman who can serve as a role model – a stepmother, mother-in-law, sister, aunt, or friend. But often this objective is difficult and unattainable. Cohen (1979) expressed concern about the gravida's added adaptive challenge in such circumstances.

Ms. Penn illustrates the struggle outlined. Ms. Penn's mother divorced her father, left the family for another man and his five children, and "relinquished everything." Even though Ms. Penn was about 7 years old when her mother left, she claimed that she could not remember anything about her natural mother. "I don't know if I have blocked it out of my mind – just totally put it out." Ms. Penn asserted that her stepmother had taken the place of her natural mother.

> She's [the stepmother] my mother as far as I am concerned. When I refer to my mother, that's who I mean. She was there during the upheaval and growing up; and she was the one that was at my wedding and helped plan my wedding; and she's the one who is going to come when the baby is born. I told her, I want you to come. I'm sure it meant a lot to her. She's great!

Nevertheless, Ms. Penn had difficulty in fantasizing about herself as a mother and about the coming child. She was preoccupied with concerns about discipline, worried that her child would interfere with her life, and tended to see other people's children as "brats." It is possible that she had, in fact, blocked out her resentment at having been abandoned by her natural mother. Her emotional reaction to her pregnancy may have reflected resentment at not having her own mother available to lend support and to help her identify her role in childbirth and childrearing. Ms. Penn denied any such void in her life and denied the pain from her childhood abandonment; yet, her hostility to other people's children may have been a displacement of her jealousy of the five children raised by her natural mother. The resentment, although denied, may have reactivated early feelings of abandonment. Ms. Penn's fear of abandonment, stimulated by the lack of an available mother, took the form of distrusting others. Equally important was the fact that Ms. Penn's stepmother could not serve as a completely satisfactory substitute, because she had no experience with infants and small children; she came into the home when the children were half-grown.

Ms. Gale's mother died of a heart attack when she was a preschooler. It was mentioned earlier that she saw her stepmother as loving, but rather manipulative; therefore, she did not wish to emulate her in all ways. Ms. Gale felt a great need to search for the memory of her real mother.

> When I first got pregnant, about the second or third month, I started thinking about my mother a lot, my own mother – trying to remember things about her. I tried to find a picture of her – I had a photo album and I looked for it and couldn't find the one picture that I had of her.... I asked my father how she died because I couldn't remember what she died from and I thought that I might need to know that.

Despite the repression of this painful childhood event, she persisted in her search for information about her mother by talking to her father and by desperately trying to recapture the memory of her mother's death.

Ms. Gale was able to express the void felt when her mother was not available due to death. During her postpartum hospitalization she thought that she had phlebitis and was very frightened. She said:

> I was afraid that I was going to die.... And then I really missed my mother. I wished that I had known her better and [I] thought about her... My mother died when I was about five years old, and I talked to my father about it this past Fall because I knew that we were going to have the baby. I was thinking about my mother's pregnancy and whether maybe there was something related...to our birth. He said, "No," but she did have some kind of heart condition and that was one reason they had waited so long to have another child after my brother because they thought it would damage her heart. The doctor she had at the time said, 'No, it wouldn't,' that her heart condition was O.K.... I think that I have always had a little bit of fear that I would die after having the baby.

These excerpts show how the need for the women to know their own mothers intensified during pregnancy. Sometimes it was felt that crucial questions could be answered satisfactorily only by the woman's own mother – that a mother substitute could not fully satisfy the need.

Not all women searched for a substitute in the absence of their mother, nor did all seek a new role model when the model presented by their mother was unacceptable. Ms. Aaron, for example, hesitated to emulate her own mother. She perceived herself as being very different from her mother, "like night and day almost."

> We both worry about things a lot, but she takes things very, very hard.... Usually things don't bother me, you know, if something goes wrong. She is a more methodical person than I am. I tend to be a slap-dash, happy-go-lucky kind of person. She is very set in her pattern of living... She angers more easily than I do. She is more emotional in every way than I am outwardly.

Ms. Aaron felt that she would act differently than her mother in several respects, but gave no indication of how she defined a more positive role. The lack of role definition in the days before delivery led to anxiety attacks that were expressed as insomnia.

> When I wake up in the middle of the night they [the doubts] are very strong, and I often have an urge to wake up my husband and ask him if he thinks I'll really be able to manage this. In the daytime when I am up and rational, not thinking about it so much, they don't bother me in particular… but…at night when I am lying in bed and can't get to sleep, that's when I worry about it the most.

A gravida may not actively seek alternative role models because she doubts her ability to be a parent and questions whether her goals are attainable. Failure to "try on" new roles may also be due to the unavailability of acceptable models (Rubin, 1967a, 1967b).

Ms. Tell described her childhood as very lonely, and her mother as disinterested and indifferent. Ms. Tell did make some attempt at reparation, but was unsuccessful. She suffered from a deep sense of worthlessness and had sought psychiatric help in the past. While being interviewed during the third trimester of her pregnancy, she turned to the principal investigator for guidance. Ms. Tell's paranoia prevented her from following through on suggestions, because she feared that if her uncontrollable rages and destructive tendencies were discovered her baby might be taken away. As a result, she relinquished initial attempts at finding someone from whom she could learn to be a mother. Unable to find assistance or a mother substitute, Ms. Tell struggled with repetitive self-doubts. She made no progress in reconciling with her mother; that is, she did not become more tolerant or accepting of her mother's behavior. She also failed to identify a viable motherhood role for herself – a role different from the one she had experienced with her own mother. At the end of her pregnancy, Ms. Tell stated "I know I will ruin that child's life." Such a statement seemed ominous and foreboding. She was the only participant in the study to voice such strong doubts. Ms. Tell's case represents an extreme example of the way in which fears can be stimulated by a poor relationship with an unavailable mother.

Ms. Aaron's and Ms. Tell's comments demonstrate how a young mother adapts to roles that conflict with long-standing patterns of interaction with others. The incorporation of undesirable and unwanted behavior patterns was seen as hard to renegotiate, especially when an exemplar was not consistently available. Occasionally, these women did try to learn from someone else such as a grandmother, but finding a substitute was rare at this late stage.

Another woman, Ms. Meta, did not wish to be like her mother in any way. In answer to the question "In what ways do you think that you would like to be similar or different from your own mother?" Ms. Meta replied:

> Different in most respects. I would like to be different…. It's hard to think of any ways I would like to be like her. All I can think of are the things that I don't want to do that she did. I can't think of anything.

Ms. Meta had deliberately chosen a career that enabled her to compensate for the deprivation of love she felt during childhood and to identify a more desirable mothering role. She worked as a special education teacher and appeared adept at her job. She was determined not to allow what happened to her in childhood to repeat itself in her children's lives. Ms. Meta had tried, tested, and formulated a mothering role; this role was reinforced by mothering models in her place of work and was rewarded by positive experiences with the children she taught. Consequently, she entered pregnancy already having worked through several developmental tasks, and she felt confident about mothering her own child. In contrast to another woman's comment, "I needed the whole nine months to gear up for this," Ms. Meta said, "One month of pregnancy would have been enough for me."

4.2   Reactions to Pregnancy

An important component of the gravida's relationship to her mother is the grandmother's response to the pregnancy. This response includes her acceptance of the grandchild and her acknowledgment of the daughter as a mother. Often, the daughter wishes to share with her mother the excitement over the coming child.

Most grandmothers were happy and excited. Ms. Carre's parents were typical in this regard.

> Here they have all these children, married, for years and years and years, and no grandchildren around. My poor mother. She is knitting little sweaters for every little kid in the church… so she is very happy.

Although many grandmothers were happy, this reaction did not always indicate that they were supportive. For example, Ms. Aaron's mother was delighted about the coming child.

> [My mother] has had more fun making things and buying things for this baby; it's really kind of funny. It's just like…her own child because she knows it's not and she's not expecting it to be, but she's just so excited about having a new baby in the family. And it's the first grandchild so she's very excited.

In reminiscing about her daughter's birth, however, this grandmother painted a frightening picture of labor and described Ms. Aaron as a "very ugly baby with a pointed head and black hair all over her body." Thus, it is possible for the grandmother to be excited about the coming grandchild and yet offer limited emotional support to her daughter.

Other grandmothers also were perceived as excited, but as nonsupportive or interfering. Ms. Hayes' mother, for instance, was "thrilled." "She's wanted to be a grandmother since I got out of diapers. And she can't wait to show the pictures to all her friends and be a grandmother." At the same time, however, Ms. Hayes was not moved by her mother's excitement. She was not eager to send photographs of her newborn to her mother, because she feared allowing the grandmother any control over the child.

Some grandmothers did not seem especially excited about the coming grandchild. Ms. Tell stated that it was "just an everyday thing" to her mother; she speculated that her mother felt this way because she already had three grandchildren. Ms. Zeff stated that her mother did not have "too much to say about it at all." Ms. Gale was ambivalent when her stepmother failed to show excitement about the pregnancy.

> My mother [stepmother] was great with us as kids, but she doesn't seem to really like little children that much. I don't think that she really likes little babies and little toddlers.

The grandmother's excitement about her coming grandchild does not necessarily mean that she accepts her daughter as a mother, even though she may accept the grandchild. If the grandmother is not enthusiastic, then the daughter begins to doubt her self-worth and the acceptance of her child by others (Rubin, 1975).

4.3 Respect for Autonomy

A third component that was assessed in considering the mother–daughter relationship was the grandmother's respect for the autonomy of her daughter. When a grandmother respects her daughter's autonomy, a relationship of mutual respect exists between the two in which they relate to one another as adults.

On the other hand, if a grandmother tends to be critical, interfering, or controlling, she probably still sees her daughter as a child. A grandmother's inability to respect the independence of her daughter may be caused by a failure to "let go" of the image of her daughter as a child. This problem frequently occurs when several maturing events follow in rapid succession, such as leaving home, going to school, getting married, and becoming pregnant. A critical attitude on the part of a grandmother also may reflect her own sense of past inadequacy as a mother. If she feels that she was not appreciated as a mother, then she may view the coming grandchild as a second chance at mothering. In this case, the grandmother identifies with her daughter as a mother rather than crystallizing her own grandmother role. In other words, she is seeking a vicarious mothering experience as opposed to a grandmothering experience. The grandmother may even suggest that if her advice is not followed the baby will get sick.

In the study sample, several grandmothers found it difficult to see their daughters as autonomous even when the women asserted themselves. Ms. Vale felt that her mother was domineering. Ms. Faber resented being treated as a child. She was ambivalent about her mother coming to help after the birth of the baby.

> I really don't like living with my mother anymore. We get along great for short periods of time, but otherwise she treats me like a little kid and drives me crazy.... If she's there... maybe she would want to take over.

Ms. Dunn felt that she and her husband were being treated as children by her parents. She wished that her parents could "realize what we're going through 'cause we're two young people who want to be independent." She went on to say:

> I'm sure they were young once and wanted to be independent and make some choices, but, instead, they're taking everything we do as a personal insult.

Ms. Dunn also was worried about other relatives (particularly her mother) who were not encouraging autonomy. She made an eloquent plea for the need to be allowed room to grow.

[They are] beginning to act as if it [the coming child] is theirs already just because they are related. This is very difficult for me to accept because both my husband and myself want to…devote ourselves to the child and too much interference is bound to drive us from our families rather than toward them. We need room to breathe and we are not being given that room. People are already making plans for us telling us where and when we will go on vacation and what we will do with the baby – and this is suffocating us.

On the other hand, several women said that their mothers had always encouraged them to be independent. Ms. Fair, a nursing student, felt that her parents were supportive but did not interfere.

They show a lot of interest, but they don't push in any way. I think they know that I know most of the alternatives, having just gone through obstetrics and pediatrics, so they are just interested in what we decided. And my Mom will ask me why, …but they don't ever pressure us one way or the other.

Similarly, Ms. Xana felt that her parents "would really help out" and would not interfere.

[Mother] told me, 'Betty, I don't think that you're going to want anybody to be there.' She went through the same thing, and her mother-in-law took care of us for about a month after…. She just really wanted to be on her own I think.

Ms. Santa, whose mother discussed her own delivery with her, said it was a discussion between adults.

I feel more adult to be able to talk about things like this you know…. When you experience it, you can relate to what they are saying because you're feeling the same things and doing the same things.

The sense here is of Ms. Santa's identification with her mother, as well as her verification of the processes of pregnancy and delivery, which aided in self-definition. In talking with her parents about her childhood, Ms. Uman said that she felt that "it was a very happy time for them." She reported feeling "somewhat excited" by these talks.

It is special too because they never told me about these things before. It is as if I gained another dimension for them too so that they can finally confide in me at a different level than they used to be able to. So I guess I'm finally beginning to feel like an adult to them, too.

Such increasing respect and encouragement for autonomy from others facilitates rational decision making by the mother-to-be and promotes self-confidence in the role of parent.

4.4 Willingness to Reminisce

The fourth component found to be important to a woman was reminiscing with her mother. If there was a high degree of mutuality and closeness between daughter and mother, there seemed to be a spontaneous need to share the daughter's early childhood experiences and the grandmother's account of her childbirth experience. Such information enables the gravida to anticipate labor and delivery and to prepare for the event (Levy & McGee, 1975). This sharing of information with the grandmother was enjoyable for many women, although face-to-face contact appeared to be necessary. Using a telephone did not encourage much reminiscing when mother and daughter were geographically separated. Leifer (1980) reported that good communication between mother and daughter tended to increase the gravida's ego strength and confidence in herself.

In recalling events of her childhood with her mother, Ms. Lash said: "I think that it's neat that she remembers that sort of thing. I think that babyhood is neat. I really do. I think that I ought to be remembered."

Ms. Uman felt "adult" when her parents shared the events of her childhood with her. She discovered that her parents were able to discuss the past more openly than before.

> They bring up little episodes about how I was the worst one to toilet train or to feed – little things. I guess that they're much more free and open now than they used to be.... They're tending to relive a little bit, too, that portion of their lives.

Ms. Yuth said that she liked to listen to her mother reminisce. In retrospect, her mother seemed remarkably tolerant.

> I like to hear what we all did when we were little because some of it you can remember, and some of it you can't.... She would laugh because one day she'd given me a bath, and the phone rang and I was out of the bathtub, and I was just roaming around behind her, and I turned around and grabbed a roll of toilet paper – nothing on – I walked right out of the door with it. I guess the mailman found me and he knew who I belonged to, so he brought me back home, and he held me up and he says, 'Does this belong to you?,' and she just laughed. She'd laugh about a lot of things unless we got really bad.

Other women also reported feeling "good" when mischievous episodes were recalled. Such reminiscing suggested that the gravida was loved unconditionally in spite of pranks and punishments. When Ms. Katen's mother talked about the past, she perceived that her mother "was really glad to have me.... And she was very proud."

There were, however, quite a few instances in which no reminiscing occurred. In Ms. Zeff's case, her father, rather than her mother, reminisced. In a few cases, reminiscing was not a positive experience. Ms. Meta reported feeling neutral when her mother reminisced. She derived little satisfaction from listening to her mother recall past events. Earlier, it was noted that Ms. Meta's mother, when discussing her own childbirth experience, predicted that her daughter would become depressed.

> [Mother] had a very difficult time after the baby was born – as far as being depressed. I definitely will have that my mother says. Be prepared for a depression and feelings that you don't want the baby because the baby cries all the time.

Several women remarked that while reminiscing, their parents had become more "open" and "free" and "close." This suggested that a closer link between the generations had been established. In remembering her own experiences as a mother, the pregnant woman's mother can convey a sense of love to her daughter, as well as inform her of what lies ahead in labor and motherhood tasks. The perception of unconditional love goes a long way in sustaining a healthy sense of worth.

When unconditional love exists, the daughter knows that her parents will be supportive even if she makes mistakes; furthermore, she senses that her children also will sustain their love for her even if they have misgivings.

4.5 Empathy with the Mother

If mutuality characterizes a mother–daughter relationship, then the daughter also is supportive of her mother. It is an indication of the gravida's maturity if she can accept her mother as a human being with limitations. Mutuality is based on empathy. A mature woman usually empathizes with her mother's experiences in parenting and if she is able to do this, she also will establish an empathic relationship with her husband, her children, and others.

Ms. Acton seemed to be tolerant of her mother's excitability. Ms. Jabon was tolerant of the fact that her mother still lived in a traditional way. Ms. Yuth sympathized with her mother's discipline problems. Ms. Oaks appreciated her mother's increased insight. Her mother, who was a good role model, had been "pressured by other people's doubts" in the past. "It's something that she had identified as a mistake and feels bad about now.... I agree with her there."

Ms. Aaron understood her mother's problems in communicating with her father. "He kept problems bottled up, which was very hard on my mother. She tried to pull them out, and it was like pulling teeth sometimes."

Despite ambivalent feelings toward their mothers, some women still struggled toward reconciliation. Ms. Lash wanted to name her child after her mother; she wanted to do this because her mother "is having a hard time now." Ms. Lash felt that her mother had become more tolerant.

Ms. Faber was rather hesitant about the arrival of her mother after the birth, because her mother tended to interfere. However, Ms. Faber decided to welcome her mother because she thought it might be a good idea to share the excitement of the new baby.

> But I thought with the excitement of the baby, maybe I just would want to share that with somebody; maybe that would be my mom.... I'm thinking about it now from more of a psychological standpoint than a practical standpoint, because I think I'll be able to manage by myself.

Ms. Faber seemed very caring toward her mother.

> I'm always felt kind of more protective of my mother, I think, than she has of me. She's a very small woman, and she had [a serious childhood disease]. She's crippled; I'm just a generally stronger person than she is.

Although Ms. Gale struggled to recapture the memory of her deceased natural mother, she demonstrated a great deal of understanding and compassion for her stepmother. In attempting to comprehend the source of her stepmother's style of manipulation, Ms. Gale realized that her stepmother didn't have a very good relationship with her own mother. "I think the things she used with us as children were things that she had learned to use all her life."

Reconciliation is more readily achieved when both parties are cognizant and tolerant of differences. Ms. Hayes failed to achieve a satisfactory reconciliation with her mother when her mother did not reciprocate. Ms. Hayes reached a certain level of understanding, but remained disturbed by the relationship with her mother.

> [Mother] can't help herself, but I have a hard time coping with her. I just resent her terribly.... I am at the point where I understand her, but I just wish that I could totally get over the anger and just kind of feel sorry for her and not let it bother me.

Ms. Hayes did, however, substitute her mother-in-law as a role model. She showed considerable insight into her mother-in-law's problem of coming to terms with grandparenting.

> When she first found out that I was pregnant, she was a little worried about the money. She was not sure that she wanted to be a grandmother either. She's 50 and she plays tennis and she is real perky. She plays with 35-year-old women, and she won't tell them how old she is or won't throw the ball to her.... In fact his [her husband's] whole family had been in family therapy with this psychiatric social worker, and he said that he would like for her to go and see [the therapist] so that she could get over some of these hurt feelings of not wanting to be a grand- mother, even though it's normal. And she did. She's really a good person, and she's anxious to understand and to make a good relationship.

In other cases, the daughter's intolerance may have impeded renegotiation of a relationship. Ms. Zeff was extremely intolerant of her mother's traditional attitudes, especially her mother's belief that it was impossible to combine a career and children. Ms. Zeff's mother disapproved of her daughter continuing her studies at the university following the birth.

> I'm going to graduate...and yet still do the housework and take care of the kids. And she's never worked...she's terribly spoiled. She thinks that we're supposed to be spoiled like she is. Nowadays nobody can afford to do that.... I think her ideas are ridiculous, so they don't bother me at all.

Ms. Meta resisted her mother's controlling behavior.

> I won't conform to her view at all. I mean I'll just explain to her that this is the way I want to do it. It doesn't bother me, upset me in any way. I feel that they're wrong; that that's probably why things were so bad for my sister because she didn't do things the way she [the sister] wanted to.

Ms. Meta and Ms. Zeff reported that the lack of harmony between themselves and their mothers did not disturb them. Each appeared to have taken and maintained an independent stand. They may have been denying the need to have their mothers close, or they may have found support elsewhere. For instance, Ballou (1978) has found that support from the husband can assuage conflict between the mother and daughter. Nevertheless, Ms. Hayes was constantly irritated by the disharmony with her mother, despite a supportive husband. Compared to Ms. Meta and Ms. Zeff, Ms. Hayes probably had not reached a sufficient level of maturity to come to terms with what appeared to have been a controlling and guilt-inducing mother.

4.6   Summary

If a pregnant woman's mother is available to her and their relationship is mutual – adult to adult – the mother probably will be enthusiastic, supportive, and reassuring during pregnancy and childbirth. The gravida's mother is likely to serve as a constructive role model so that the gravida can spontaneously emulate her in establishing her new identification as a mother. On the other hand, if hostility characterizes the mother–daughter relationship, the daughter may make an effort to heal the rift. Reconciliation is more difficult to achieve if the gravida's mother is unavailable, critical, or unsupportive. In these cases, the daughter tends to shun her mother's advice and companionship, and often does not want to be like her mother or sees herself as dissimilar. Such a perception of the mother–daughter relationship has been associated with a persistent negative attitude toward pregnancy (Nilsson, Uddenberg, & Almgren, 1971). If the daughter is unable to see her mother as good, either during the antepartum or the postpartum period, then according to Breen (1975), she also may experience greater difficulty in adjusting to parenthood.

A tolerant daughter often is responding to a tolerant mother, and a tolerant mother inspires confidence in her daughter, even if she occasionally fails in her mothering skills. Although she may continue to attempt reconciliation, an intolerant daughter may be defending her self-esteem against a critical mother. If this attempt at reconciliation fails, the daughter will try to find a substitute role model. One major drawback associated with a substitute is the lack of reminiscing occurring between the mother and daughter, which serves an important function in the formation of the daughter's self-definition and maternal role identification. If the gravida is hindered in the process of dispelling doubt and achieving self-confidence, she may feel less prepared for childbirth and may subsequently experience increased anxiety in the days before delivery. Drawbacks associated with these substitute relationships have been demonstrated empirically (Lederman et al., 1979).

As noted, the relationship of the gravida to her mother was found to correlate with the gravida's identification of a motherhood role, and with fears related to labor and delivery. A poor relationship with the mother was associated with poorer contractile activity in labor (as were all the prenatal dimensions) and tended to prolong labor. The data, in short, suggest that these unresolved mother–daughter conflicts confront the gravida during childbirth. Further, in terms of increased or decreased anxiety and conflict, there appears to be little change in the relationship over the three trimesters of pregnancy (Lederman, Harrison, Worsham, & Erchinger, 1991; Tulman and Fawcett, 2003).

References

Ballou, J. (1978). *The psychology of pregnancy*. Lexington, MA: Lexington Books.
Breen, D. (1975). *The birth of a first child*. London: Tavistock Publications.
Cohen, R. L. (1979). Maladaptation to pregnancy. *Seminars in Perinatology, 3*, 15–24.
Deutsch, H. (1945). *The psychology of women* (Vol. 2). New York: Grune & Stratton.

Deutsch, F. M., Ruble, D. N., Fleming, A., Brooks-Gunn, J., & Stangor, C. (1988). Information-seeking and maternal self-definition during the transition to motherhood. *Journal of Personality and Social Psychology, 55*, 420–431.

Fonagy, P., Steele, H., & Steele, M. (1991). Maternal representations of attachment during pregnancy predict the organization of infant-mother attachment at one year of age. *Child Development, 62*, 891–905.

Henry, J. (1973). *Pathways to madness*. New York: Random House.

Huth-Bocks, A. C. (2003). Mother–infant attachment: The impact of maternal representations during pregnancy, maternal risk factors, and social support. *Dissertation Abstracts International: Section B: The Sciences & Engineering, 63*(9-B), 4374.

Lederman, R. (1989). Prediction of postpartum adaptation from maternal prenatal adaptation scales. *International Nursing Research Conference on Social Support*, Seoul, Korea.

Lederman, R., Harrison, J., Worsham, S., & Erchinger, P. (1991). *Progressive prenatal personality changes: Patterns of maternal development, anxiety, and depression*. American Society of Psychosomatic Obstetrics and Gynecology Meeting, Houston, Texas.

Lederman, R., Lederman, E., Work, B. A., Jr., & McCann, D. S. (1978). The relationship of maternal anxiety, plasma, catecholamines, and plasma cortisol to progress in labor. *American Journal of Obstetrics and Gynecology, 132*, 495–500.

Lederman, R., Lederman, E., Work, B. A., Jr., & McCann, D. S. (1979). Relationship of psychological factors in pregnancy to progress in labor. *Nursing Research, 28*, 94–97.

Leifer, H. (1980). *Psychological effects of motherhood: A study of first pregnancy*. New York: Praeger.

Levy, J. M., & McGee, R. K. (1975). Childbirth as a crisis. *Journal of Personality and Social Psychology, 31*, 171–179.

Lewis, J. M. (1989). The Birth of the Family: An Empirical Inquiry. New York, Brunner/Mazel.

Nilsson, A., Uddenberg, N., & Almgren, P. E. (1971). Parental relations and identification in women with special regard to paranatal emotional adjustment. *Acta Psychiatrica Scandinavica, 47*, 57–78.

Obegi, J. H., Morrison, T. L., & Shaver, P. R. (2004). Exploring intergenerational transmission of attachment style in young female adults and their mothers. *Journal of Social and Personal Relationships, 21*, 625–638.

Rubin, R. (1967a). Attainment of the maternal role. Part I. Processes. *Nursing Research, 16*, 237–245.

Rubin, R. (1967b). Attainment of the maternal role. Part II. Models and referents. *Nursing Research, 16*, 342–346.

Rubin, R. (1975). Maternal tasks in pregnancy. *Maternal-Child Health Nursing Journal, 4*, 143–153.

Shereshefsky, P. M., & Lockman, R. F. (1973). Background variables. In P. M. Shereshefsky and L. J. Yarrow (Eds.). *Psychological aspects of a first pregnancy and early postnatal adaptation*. New York: Raven Press.

Shereshefsky, P. M., Plotsky, H., & Lockman, R. F. (1973). Pregnancy adaptation. In P. M. Shereshefsky and L. J. Yarrow (Eds.), *Psychological aspects of a first pregnancy and early postnatal adaptation*. New York: Raven Press.

Slade, A., Grienenberger, J., Bernbach, E., Levy, D., & Locker, A. (2005). Maternal reflective functioning, attachment, and the transmission gap: A preliminary study. *Attachment and Human Development, 7*, 283–298.

Steele, S., & Steele, M. (2005). Understanding and resolving emotional conflict: The London parent–child project. In K. E. Grossmann, K. Grossmann, & E. Waters (Eds.), *Attachment from infancy to adulthood: The major longitudinal studies* (pp. 137–164). New York, Guilford.

Tulman, L., & Fawcett, J. (2003). *Women's health during and after pregnancy: A theory-based study of adaptation to change*. New York: Springer.

Uddenberg, N. (1974). Reproductive adaptation in mother and daughter: A study of personality development and adaptation to motherhood. *Acta Psychiatrica Scandinavica*, Supplement, 254, 1–115.

Wenner, N. K., Cohen, M. B., Weigert, E. V., Kvarnes, R. G., Ohaneson, E. M., & Fearing, J. M. (1969). Emotional problems in pregnancy. *Psychiatry, 32*, 389–410.

Wolkind, S., & Zajicek, E. (1981). *Pregnancy: A psychological and social study*. New York: Grune & Stratton.4   Relationship with Mother.

Chapter 5
Relationship with Husband or Partner

The marital relationship has been reported as the most significant dimension affecting the course of pregnancy (Wenner et al., 1969). This finding is not always borne out (Shereshefsky & Yarrow, 1973), but the results of studies on the importance of the marital/partner relationship to postpartal adjustment are compelling (Lederman, 2008a; Melges, 1968; Russel, 1974; Shereshefsky & Yarrow, 1973; Tomlinson, 1987a, b). Even when partner support and support of others are both present, partner support tends to make the greater contribution to maternal well-being during pregnancy (Brown, 1986), and it has been associated with earlier prenatal care and more prenatal care visits (Lederman, Weis, Brandon, Hills, & Mian, 2002; Zambrana, Dunkel-Shetter, & Scrimshaw, 1991).

In our initial research project, a poor marital relationship was associated with earlier admission to the labor unit, administration of sedatives and tranquilizers in early labor to quell anxiety, and subsequent prolonged duration of labor (Lederman, Lederman, Work, & McCann, 1979). In the second research project cited in Chapter 1, regression analyses showed that relationship with husband was a significant predictor of gestational age at first prenatal visit and of the length of gestation (Lederman, et al., 2002). Other researchers have found that family and marital dysfunction were significant determinants of preterm birth (Dole et al., 2004) and lower infant birthweight (Abell, Baker, Clover, & Ramsey, 1991; Keeley et al., 2004; Ramsey, Abell, & Baker, 1986). A poor relationship with the husband is also associated with depression during pregnancy and is predictive of maternal postpartum depression (Centers for Disease Control and Prevention: Morbidity and Mortality Weekly Report, 2008; Dimitrovsky, Perez-Hirshberg, & Itzkowitz, 1987; Graff, Dyck, & Schallow, 1991). In addition, and importantly, mothers' and fathers' prenatal and postnatal aggressive marital conflict predicted attachment measures of infant withdrawal at 6 months (Crockenberg, Leerkes, & Lekka, 2007).

There is ample evidence that the transition to parenthood is a drain on the emotional, physical, and material resources of many parents (Pacey, 2004), and that for most couples there is a decline from pregnancy to postpartum in marital quality and satisfaction (Gottman & Notarius, 2002; Lawrence, Rothman, Cobb, Rothman, & Bradbury, 2008; Schultz, Cowan, & Cowan, 2006). Lawrence et al. (2008) also found that couples with planned pregnancies had higher marital satisfaction scores, and that planning of pregnancy slowed the husbands' decline in marital satisfaction

R. Lederman and K. Weis, *Psychosocial Adaptation to Pregnancy*,
DOI 10.1007/978-1-4419-0288-7_5, © Springer Science+Business Media, LLC 2009

postpartally. Both maternal and paternal happiness about pregnancy also are associated with birthweight, and differentiated low- and high-risk birth weight groups (Keeley et al., 2004).

In evaluating the quality of the gravida's relationship with her husband, it was important to learn whether a state of "mutuality" existed between the expectant couple. Did they support one another and trust one another? Did they, in other words, have an interdependent and egalitarian relationship at the time when the woman found herself pregnant? An interdependent relationship implies that the partners are neither dominant nor submissive. Such a relationship is associated with few emotional and physical symptoms (Grossman, Eichler, & Winickoff, 1980). According to Wenner et al. (1969), an interdependent relationship provides a favorable framework for completing preparation for motherhood. It also appears that active support and involvement during pregnancy are associated with lower levels of anxiety, and, for expectant fathers, represent the best means of coping with the stress of pregnancy (Teichman & Lahav, 1987). Couples who report high prenatal relationship quality (relationship satisfaction, communication, and interpersonal processes) also are more likely to remain involved in co-parenting (versus paternal disengagement) postpartally (Florsheim & Smith, 2005). How positively or negatively partners engage with one another tends to predict the quality of parenting and the parent–child relationship, and is referred to as the "spillover theory" (Krishnakumar & Buehler, 2000). Research also shows some degree of consistency between how a husband relates to his wife and how he behaves toward his child, suggesting that the interpersonal skills needed to relate to a partner are closely related to skills needed to become a competent parent (Margolin, Gordis, & John, 2001; McHale, Keursten-Hogan, Lauretti, & Rasmussen, 2000). These interpersonal skills include the capacity to focus on another's needs for the sake of that person's well-being, to remain warmly engaged under stressful conditions, and to maintain a balance between providing guidance and caring, and facilitating autonomy (Edwards et al., 1994a, b; Grossman & Grossman, 2000). The "spill over" theory and findings on relationship quality and interpersonal skills have some analogy to attachment theory and family systems theory (Cowan & Cowan, 2002; Grych, 2002; Lerner, Rothbaum, Boulos, & Castellino, 2002; Slade, Grienenberger, Bernbach, Levy, & Locker, 2005). These theories posit that couples need to work together to create a relational context for child rearing (Heineke & Guthrie, 1992).

A distinction can be made between interdependency and excessive dependency on the part of either the wife or the husband. Interdependency implies a two-way relationship between two reasonably autonomous adults. In this type of relationship, there is an overlapping area of interchange between the two self-defined persons, in which sharing and the satisfaction of dependency occur. In the case of excessive dependency, one person needs the other for survival and identification, or to fill needs that she or he is not able to confront and satisfy. Excessive dependency also is associated with low autonomy and low self-esteem (Wenner et al., 1969). Conversely, maternal efforts to maintain psychological independence from their partner is associated with "avoidant" maternal behaviors; that is, feeling less comfortable with closeness in emotional intimacy, and tending to be less invested in their relationships. In addition to avoidant attachment, another attachment dimension, "anxious attachment," is characterized by maternal worry about being rejected or abandoned (Wilson, Rholes, Simpson, & Tran, 2007).

To understand the nature of the marital bond under the impact of pregnancy, four areas were evaluated:

1. The husband's concern for his wife's needs as an expectant mother with regard to:

   (a) Empathy (understanding, tolerance, supportiveness)
   (b) Cooperativeness
   (c) Availability (sharing and communication)
   (d) Trustworthiness (reliability)

2. The wife's concern for her husband's needs as an expectant father.
3. The effects of the pregnancy on the marital bond with regard to the degree of:

   (a) Closeness
   (b) Conflicts

4. The husband's adjustment to his new role, specifically his identification of a fatherhood role.

In addition to maternal accounts, we review factors in the literature found to be pertinent to the transition to fatherhood.

Assessment of the impact of pregnancy on the marital relationship is an assessment of change in the marital bond. This aspect of the relationship was addressed in interviews with the following questions: "Are there any differences in your relationship to your husband now that you are pregnant? If so, how has pregnancy changed your relationship?" It should be pointed out that information concerning marital relationships can be difficult to glean from interviews. If marital problems existed, some women felt a need to deny them during pregnancy. Therefore, attention was focused on behavioral descriptions of the husband–wife relationship, as well as on their initial responses. In addition, responses to questions were further explored. For example, if a woman stated that her husband was supportive, she was asked in what ways he was supportive.

5.1   The Husband's Concern for His Expectant Wife's Needs

5.1.1   Empathy

5.1.1.1   Empathic Partners

First, it was determined whether the husband was empathic, supportive, and understanding, and whether he provided strength and dignity in response to his wife's doubts and feelings of vulnerability and dependency, or whether he exhibited negative behavior.

Some husbands clearly demonstrated empathy with their wives. Ms. Hayes felt that her husband would help her a great deal in labor because he understood her.

> I think when you have anxiety or when you have pain, if somebody is there who understands it, who's right with you and knows how you feel, [it's better]. And he does understand me so well; I can say what I have to say and share it with him. I really feel that I will be sharing it [labor]; he won't be distant. He won't feel the physical sensation as I will, but I can almost imagine that he will feel the intensity of it with me.

Ms. Uman anticipated feeling a little "panicky" with her newborn, but she said:

> My husband keeps reassuring me things will work out and I'll get used to it once I get over the first fears of, Is the baby okay? Did I do something wrong?

The ability to listen is complementary to empathy. Quite a few husbands in the research sample were able to listen effectively. Mr. Quins, for example, was attentive and interested when his wife discussed labor with him.

> He always listens. After [childbirth] class, we'll talk about it the most. He asks me a lot of questions about it. He wants to make sure he knows.... Right now, he's not very confident.

Several gravidas reported that their husbands were tolerant of their mood swings, and that their husbands understood that increased emotional lability was characteristic of pregnancy.

Ms. Santa indicated that her husband made an effort to comprehend her changing moods.

> Sometimes it seems it's harder for me to explain what I feel because I'm pregnant and he's not. Sometimes I feel real moody and ugly because I've got this bulge in front of me, and I'll get upset over it. He is really good. He tries to understand and kind of pampers me along.

Ms. Eaden wanted her husband to be with her in labor, saying "He cares about me" and "knows me."

> I think he'll understand if I feel all of a sudden, 'Don't even touch me. Get away from me.' He'll understand; he won't be offended. It's important to me to share the experience with him.

Ms. Uman reported that she had been subject to "fits" – feeling fine one day and bad the next. She stated that this condition became much more pronounced in the third trimester than it had been earlier. In general, she felt that she had become less sociable, but that her husband responded very well.

> He's been that way the whole nine months. He understands at times I'm going to have to be moody, and puts up with it. Of course he's always put up with me, so!

The gravidas often felt that their husbands were accepting of their changed body size. Ms. Katen said:

> [My husband is] amazed at what actually happens to the female body, and what happens in the birth process. He's been very supportive, telling me I still have my figure.

Most women reported that their husbands adapted to the decreased sex drive resulting from pregnancy. (Only two women reported no decrease in the desire to have intercourse during the last trimester.) Ms. Raaf said intercourse had been "fine" throughout her pregnancy, but that during the last couple of weeks it had become "more difficult."

> Sometimes I just don't want sex at all, but Mike never forces me. We just talk about [it] and everything works out and then the next time I am ready for it again.

Supportive husbands had a calming effect on their wives and, as Cohen (1966) notes, the husbands' sensitivity to needs eased the gravidas' sense of vulnerability. Ms. Aaron wanted her husband to be with her in labor.

> ... first of all he gives a fabulous backrub. He'll be a great help with that because I do get severe backaches. He will be able to help me relax. I don't think he'll get flustered like I will.... I think he'll help to keep me calm.

Her husband's patience, optimism, and confidence were encouraging to Ms. Aaron.

> He's a very confident person. He's sure that everything is going to be just fine; that's very reassuring to me.

Ms. Inis also reported that her husband's gentleness, even temper, and caring would help her in labor.

> He'll stick with it and stay calm. He doesn't get all hassled about things. I'm sure he'll just keep it all under control. In fact...he saved me from some robbers one day in my dream. I look at him as my stabilizer.

This perception of the husband as a stabilizer was commonly reported by the women during pregnancy. It was for this reason that Ms. Carre wanted her husband to be with her in labor. "He's the person I'm used to being around most of the time. He's a very calm sort. I tend to get in a panic; he doesn't. I feel better when he's there." This role of the husband was sought after by the women and appreciated whether or not a woman tended toward dependency. Fridh, Kopare, Gaston-Johansson, and Norvell (1988) found that expectant fathers' positive feelings toward pregnancy appeared to be an important element in decreasing their partners' feelings of apprehension. Furthermore, the authors extrapolated that when fathers are more supportive of their partners during pregnancy, the women may subsequently experience less pain during labor.

5.1.1.2   Unempathic Partners

Some husbands were perceived as nonsupportive for a variety of reasons. Sometimes they felt threatened by the pregnancy and the prospect of becoming a father, and sometimes they were overly concerned with their careers. New emphasis on fathers' participation in the pregnancy process can place additional stress on a young husband. He may feel inadequate in the eyes of his wife when compared to the obstetrician, whom he may view as heroic. He may also feel incapable of being with his wife in the labor room, and may not want to attend childbirth preparation classes (DeGarmo & Davidson, 1978). Occasionally, the wife may have misperceived her husband's character because of her own dependency needs.

Ms. Dann did not wish to have her husband with her in labor because he had no understanding, no empathy, and he could not help her to relax or to be calm.

> The things I can imagine William saying would probably upset me because he's never been sick and has never had pain. He's the type that feels like 'Well, it can't be that bad. Everybody does it. As many women as have had babies, you know, it can't be that bad or women wouldn't have babies.' I mean he would give me a lecture on pain in the labor room. That's not what I would need. I get 100 lectures a week. I can imagine myself wanting to kill him, you know.

Ms. Dann expressed a great deal of overt anger at her husband's lack of understanding. Nevertheless, her husband was extremely supportive in labor, although he had not been supportive during the pregnancy and was not supportive during the postpartum period.

Ms. Vale said that she would not feel comfortable with her husband present during labor, and she was unsure about whether he would be supportive in a crisis.

> I hope he's got a good stomach. I'm not sure whether he does or not. If he doesn't, fine, he doesn't have to be there. I think he doesn't feel as subjective [as I do]. He'll really hate it if I'm having a hard time, but that's not his main concern right now.

Mr. Vale's "main concern" was for his unborn child, whom he anticipated with excitement, but this exhilaration did not include being with his wife during labor.

Ms. Allen's husband, a physician, tended to minimize his wife's concerns. Ms. Allen did not feel that the continuing presence of her husband in labor or delivery would be sufficient to quell her concerns of being alone in pain. Although he was supportive and encouraging at times, she remained doubtful of his attitude as labor approached.

Many husbands found their wives' dramatic mood swings difficult to understand at first. Most tried to come to terms with this difference in moods, but a few could not tolerate the changes in their wife's behavior. Ms. Bode said that her husband expected her to be stoic and to refrain from expressing her feelings openly. Sometimes he listened with sensitivity, especially when she was depressed. She had made the decision not to let herself "be inhibited emotionally" while in labor, even though she would be embarrassed if she lost her temper. Her husband did not "worry about labor." She said:

> He doesn't anticipate it the same way I do....it's going to happen to me; it's not going to happen to him. He's going to stand there and watch, and if he can help, he's going to help.

Ms. Bode's perception of her husband's behavior seemed equivocal; he was both empathic and nonempathic. He did not, in fact, lend his support during labor and was not with his wife. Her seeming confusion may have been an expression of doubt about the extent of her husband's concern for her.

Ms. Yuth's husband helped her relax "better than anyone," but he was less tolerant of her mood swings, indicating that "it upset him a lot."

He would call me fat belly and all this. He was teasing. At first it would hurt a little bit, but now I've gotten used to it. Because I've grown out so much, I wonder if he's going to like me like this for nine months. I wonder if he might resent the bigness.

Similarly, Ms. Inis felt that she was not as attractive to her husband as before, even though he was supportive in some ways.

He just doesn't think that a pregnant woman's body is sexually appealing. So we do have sex still, but I don't think as often. I don't think he's into it.

Ms. Dann reported becoming enraged because of the way that she felt her husband rejected her. She said:.[I approached him]…affectionately, and [he] just said something like,

'So the big, fat pregnant woman wants a little affection, huh? And I just blew up…. I told him that was the most terrible thing he could ever say.

In a somewhat reversed situation, Ms. Santa wrote in her diary that her husband, who was generally supportive, felt rejected when she was reluctant to have intercourse with him.

It seems like the biggest problem facing us as far as just husband and wife is our sexual relationship. I just don't seem interested and haven't been in a few months. I don't know why it's so far from my mind. Sometimes I know my husband feels hurt and rejected. He can't understand how I can change so, and I can't explain why when I don't know [myself].

In another situation, Ms. Cole said that her husband experienced a lower sex drive during her pregnancy. She stated that he did not care whether she wanted intercourse, and that her husband was tired of sex and tired "all the time." Subsequently, she discovered that he was having an affair during her pregnancy.

Ms. Carre reported feeling sad because her husband was not available to her. He was hardly ever home and did not keep her company. Despite his behavior, she preferred him over anyone else during labor because he remained "cool." She wanted her baby to be a girl.

… I need someone to keep me company. And you can't expect your sons to sit home and keep Mom company. My husband certainly doesn't sit home and keep me company. He sleeps in the morning and works in his lab at night, so I see him for dinner and that's it. I knew before I married him. So I can't complain.

Ms. Carre's husband was not supportive, seemed very involved with his work, and did not easily manage to change his priorities.

Ms. Meta complained that her husband joked about labor, sometimes unkindly.

He said,'We'll probably be there [in the labor room] 24–28 hours, so I'll just be laying there.' He said that he'll bring a deck of cards because some friends of his were playing cards all night. What if he gets tired? Will they have a bed in there for him to sleep? And will they serve him meals?

In her diary record, Ms. Meta recounted a dream in which she was swimming in a pool and knew she was "just as pregnant as now," but her stomach was flat. In her associations she said that her husband, although happy and excited about being a father, was frightened of labor and delivery; she thought that he made unsympathetic jokes about labor because he was so nervous.

From the foregoing excerpts, it is evident that husbands also experience anxiety and stress during pregnancy and childbirth and see the process as a developmental challenge (Berry, 1988; Glazer, 1989; Wilson, et al., 2007). Conflict is expressed by the husband when the gravida reveals her anxiety, vulnerability and dependency; spouse behaviors that indicate avoidance and distance are then frequently observed. Wilson et al. (2007) noted that women who scored higher in anxiety perceived less support from their partners than mothers scoring lower in anxiety. This finding was borne out by husbands' responses as well. Men whose partners were more anxious also reported providing less support relative to men who had less anxious partners.

In a few instances, it appeared that the wife's conflict was greater than her husband's, and that his readiness to confront the tasks of pregnancy was greater than was hers. Ms. Penn wanted to preserve an emotional distance and was afraid that her husband would show her more affection as labor and delivery approached. He had been "really great" from the time that he had learned of her pregnancy.

> He's probably looking forward to it more than I am, if that's possible. It seemed he was more accepting, or became more accepting earlier than I did. I seemed not to believe it for a longer time. I can't say that he's any more loving because he's always been a very affectionate person, and I would hate to think of him getting any more affectionate.

Ms. Penn's need for distance may have been an expression of her greater ambivalence about the coming child; for this reason, her husband's excitement may have been threatening to her. Conversely, her lack of appreciation for her husband's need to express himself may have been threatening to him. Interestingly, May (1978) notes analogous distancing behavior in the father when he is ambivalent and when he expresses a lack of readiness for pregnancy. On the other hand, Wilson et al. (2007) noted that men partnered with women having a strong prenatal desire for children reported giving greater support, regardless of the women's anxiety levels.

There also is the possibility that when the gravida's conflicts and needs are inordinate, a reasonable level of support from the husband may not be enough. For example, because of her very excessive need for reassurance, Ms. Tell misperceived her husband's overall feeling when he was silent. Her behavior illustrates, in the extreme, a phenomenon that often occurs. (Brown, 1987). Ms. Tell experienced rages over her husband's "lack of concern about everything." In talking about this, she said:

> I guess it's just his insensitivity. I get supersensitive, and I see that he's so insensitive, I get super-mad at him. He's super-intelligent.... He's so mathematical and science-oriented that nothing can get past that. I've never seen any emotion in him.

Her husband was, however, was more caring and supportive in labor than had been expected. Throughout all her criticisms and protests, he gently reassured her and offered physical aid for her discomfort.

In summary, empathic husbands were perceived by their wives as good listeners and as providers of physical support and emotional reassurance. They generally were accepting of their wives' mood swings and anxiety, their altered body shape, and their lowered interest in sex. In addition, empathic husbands were valued sources of stability and confidence under stress. Nonempathic husbands were described by their wives as distant or disinterested. These men sometimes mocked their wives' pregnant bodies, were less tolerant of emotional lability and an increased need for affection and reassurance, and were unreliable as sources of support in labor. A few women misperceived or did not welcome expressions of empathy and concern from their husbands.

5.1.2   Increased Cooperativeness and Flexibility

In general, the more empathic the husband, the more he cooperated with the limitations imposed by the pregnancy. This attitude especially was evident as the wife became tired, increasingly vulnerable, and awkward. Many women reported that their husbands were much more protective and thoughtful, and pampered them more than ever during the pregnancy. These women enjoyed this extra attention. Ms. Dann felt that her husband tended to worry about her more.

> Any time I have to spend by myself, he worried about me. That's one thing that's changed. Normally he wouldn't worry so much about my being home alone. He makes sure that I have a phone number if he goes somewhere.

Ms. Raaf's husband cooked dinner when she was tired.

> And he helped me bake Christmas cookies. I told him as long as I can move around, it doesn't bother me, but when I have to stand in one spot and keep beating that cooking mix, I'd start feeling sick. He says, 'Well then, I'll do that.'

Ms. Lash felt proud of her husband's ability to reorganize his priorities.

> I was concerned initially that he would become like his father and be separate from the family; work would be the all important thing, especially as Gerald is deeply involved in natural resources. But I don't think that's going to be the case. He's very willing to put that aside if I need him. He does feel the family is more important.

Ms. Penn felt that her husband was nurturing and said that "things were better" when he was with her.

> When I'm sick he comes in with the wet wash cloth and wipes my face, or helps me back into bed in those situations when you just feel like you're going to die any minute.

Some husbands afforded their wives no special treatment during their pregnancy. Ms. Bode noticed no change in her husband's behavior toward her. He was "thrilled" about the coming child, but was no more protective than usual and did not treat her "with kid gloves." She said that his attitude toward her was matter of fact, just one of "do whatever you have to do."

Ms. Carre adjusted to her husband's involvement with his research and did not expect help at home with the baby. It was Ms. Carre's mother who would help her."He will do as little as he can get by with, but if I ask him to do something, yes, he'll do it. My mother will be helping me out at first."

Ms. Gale was upset by her husband's inability to change priorities and to find time to practice breathing exercises with her. She avoided responding to the question "Are there any differences in your relationship to your husband now that you are pregnant?" Instead she said:

> I guess we're starting to move into new roles and finding our way. We're both expecting a change in our relationship because of the baby.... The amount of time we can spend together will be altered when the baby is there, and we're going to have to divide our time among the three of us, instead of the two of us.

Ms. Gale preferred to talk about changes that she anticipated in her marital lifestyle, but perhaps because her husband resisted alterations in his timetable, it was anticipated that he might not be cooperative in helping with the practical details of life during his wife's third trimester, or after the child was born.

5.1.3 Availability

It was helpful for a woman if she could communicate easily with her husband about pregnancy and childbirth. When the husband was empathic, he was likely to be available and involved in his wife's pregnancy, as well as in labor and delivery. This differed from the more traditional situation in which the husband kept a safe distance from the whole childbirth sequence because he considered it to be "women's work." Women once were culturally conditioned to think that it was inappropriate to share labor and delivery with their husbands. Today, men's (in addition to friends and family) attendance during labor and the birthing experience is routine and expected (Capogna, Camorcia, & Stirparo, 2007; Trainor, 2002).

Husband's are better prepared to help their wives when they understand their own emotions (Pavill, 2002). Attending prenatal or childbirth classes promotes an understanding of the birthing process and an opportunity to confront one's fears. In doing so, the husband is then able to encourage and promote confidence in his wife during labor (Trainor, 2002). It is the husband's helpfulness that has been reported as the most useful behavior during labor (Nichols, 1993), and the mechanism necessary for the woman to find the inner strength necessary to make it through the difficult birthing experience (Keenan, 2000).

Several participants in the project reported speaking quite openly about childbirth and child care with their husbands. Ms. Dann's husband had attended all the childbirth preparation classes. She said that he had "his own game plan" to help her keep up with her breathing exercises and to ensure that she was relaxed.

> I've talked to him about the contractions I've had and what I've done about them, so he knows what to expect. He always asks me how I feel, and he always makes sure he's kept fully in touch.

It was common for couples in the sample to view pregnancy as a shared experience. Ms. Hayes spoke about this.

> He's just been incredible about helping and doing things in the house, and talking whenever I feel the need to, and being really interested in the whole thing.

Some husbands also accompanied their wives to the doctor. Ms. Acton explained that there was nothing about her pregnancy that she could not discuss with her husband."He's come to all the examinations with me, and if I hesitate to ask the doctor anything or talk about anything with the nurses, he would [do it]." Like most of the women, Ms. Jabon wanted her husband to be with her in labor, although he had resisted practicing the breathing exercises with her.

> I'm very close to him. I feel that the pregnancy has been a shared experience. He is really my best friend. Sometimes I feel he is almost too relaxed, although I know he's also nervous. Sometimes I want him to be more interested in rehearsing and practicing the breathing techniques. I can tell he doesn't find it all that fascinating to go through this rehearsal every night.

Ms. Eaden's husband, who did a great deal of reading, organized taped exercises for his wife to practice when he was not available, thereby arranging for her to practice in the morning without him. Then, they practiced together at night.

Insofar as the degree of sharing during pregnancy depends on the degree of communication, most women reported that they were "open and free" with their husbands. However, in answer to the question "How does your husband seem to react when you try to discuss labor?" several women said that they seldom discussed childbirth with their husbands, or that they seldom found a receptive climate to do so. Ms. Quins said that her husband did not like to talk about labor, although he enjoyed the childbirth education classes; she thought that his being Iranian may have contributed to his reluctance.

> I think he was affected by his mother's labors. A lot of Persian folk think you just have to suffer, and that's the end of it. I think he was affected by the movie we saw and the relaxation techniques. He has had times when he's been positive about it, and other times, I don't want to go; I'm not going.

Ms. Tell probably was too disturbed to promote more than a cursory discussion with her husband. After they attended classes, she said that she would tell him what she wanted him to do and how she wanted him to coach her, and he would simply answer "okay. ' They did not discuss labor.

Ms. Bode said that her husband discouraged talk by diminishing her concerns.

> I sometimes asked him questions, or told him thoughts I've had, but if they're dumb questions, he tells me so, or if they're something I shouldn't worry about, he'll say so.

Mr. Bode was not enthusiastic about being with his wife in labor and delivery. His wife quoted him as saying:

> I've seen enough that it's not a new thing for me. That bothered me. But now I've accepted that and can understand that it's not a new experience for him, but I still think he will be excited.

Mr. Bode had witnessed several animal deliveries. He neither practiced breathing exercises with his wife nor was he more protective or caring than before the pregnancy.

In one case, it was the husband who wished to share while the wife was somewhat unwilling. Ms. Penn reported that her husband was the one who brought up the topic of labor, not she. She characterized herself as the "slipshod one who puts things off," whereas he demonstrated a "positive attitude," saying about practice sessions, "Let's do it right now."

Some husbands did not enjoy the childbirth preparation classes and showed considerable resistance to practicing breathing exercises with their wives. Ms. Vale said that she and her husband never discussed labor, perhaps because Mr. Vale, who grew up in Ireland, had seen many childbirths; he "hated" the classes and was "bored" by them. The researchers interpreted such remarks as an attempt by Ms. Vale to defend her husband's lack of interest; as it turned out, he gave almost no support to his wife in labor.

Ms. Gale, who felt that her husband was too engrossed in his work to change his priorities easily, had hoped that as soon as his "qualifying exams were over" he would "throw himself" into the childbirth classes.

> Well, he didn't. He did while he was there in the classes, but at home it was not a priority for him, and it was a priority for me. I felt we ought to get everything out of the classes we could, and we weren't, so I was a little frustrated with that.

When Ms. Gale expressed her frustration to her husband, he agreed to practice breathing exercises with her.

Generally, the women discussed above either attempted to rationalize their husbands' noninvolvement or tried somehow to accept it. Ms. Cole, for example, described her husband as a private person who therefore was unavailable to her.

> He doesn't tell me how he feels, and he's really not sure how I feel. I don't know if it bothers him that much. He's worried about the financial situation more than anything. So they have their worries and we have ours.

In fact, Mr. Cole showed little empathy, care, or consideration for his wife. He never talked about helping her in labor and delivery, never attended classes, and never wanted to discuss childbirth.

A minority of gravidas, like Ms. Gale, reported difficulty in communicating their feelings to their husbands. Ms. Katen seemed to have a good relationship with her husband, but was reluctant to express her "ups and downs" with him because he seemed intolerant of her mood swings and fatigue. In addition, she found it difficult to talk to him about some of his habits that irritated her. She tended to keep certain feelings to herself, even though she was outspoken about women's rights and assertive in achieving her goals.

Ms. Dann was the most explicit of any woman about her problems with her husband. She complained that he did not listen to her and that he disregarded everything she said. Essentially, there was little discussion about anything and this fact, she said, drove her "up the wall." Most women in the study, however, tended not to admit to difficulty in communication because then they would have been admitting that difficulties and conflict existed in their marriages. Goldstein (1993) also noted that expectant mothers tended to respond in a socially desirable manner regarding spousal support. The sincere report of prenatal marital satisfaction posed a dilemma at a time when family unity, rather than disunity, was paramount. The level of father involvement during pregnancy is best determined through a balanced approach in which fathers, in discussions with their partners, choose levels of involvement that are consistent with their desires, skills, and perceived roles (Condon, 2006; Palkovitz, 1985). Findings reported on military wives in Chapter 9 reflect a direct relationship between the gravida's perceived flexibility of the husband within the family system and a decrease in her prenatal maternal adaptational conflict. In other words, the gravida's increased perception of the husband's flexibility within the family decreased her anxiety related to her and her baby's well-being and safety, her fear of helplessness and loss of control in labor, and her ability to identify with being a mother.

5.1.4   Trustworthiness and Reliability

The pregnant woman needs to know that she can trust her husband to lend support when necessary in labor and delivery. Moreover, the husband's reliability and the wife's ability to trust are likely to have an impact on the expectant woman's experience of labor. Regardless of the woman's true labor experience, the quality of support received during labor impacts the woman's memory of the experience as depersonalizing and degrading or as an experience that increases her self-esteem and self-confidence (Trainor, 2002). Most women in the sample said that they could count on their husbands to be with them in labor and delivery, helping them to maintain control. Ms. Raaf wanted her husband with her, not only because she had "a lot of trust" in him and his ability to handle an emergency if it arose, but also because "I want him to be able to experience it with me because it's his child too." Ms. Dann said:

> There's got to be someone there you know; for me, it has to be someone I'm really close to, someone I can feel secure enough with. He's got the strength and power to keep me hanging in there, and I think that will be very important. That's why I'd like to have him around for the whole thing, even if he falls asleep.

Ms. Meta was bothered when her husband occasionally joked about labor and delivery because she needed to see him as someone on whom she could rely. She described him as otherwise nurturing and resourceful.

> He makes me very comfortable. He's realistic about everything where I tend not to be. I'm confident that if I lose control, or something comes up, he'll be aware of everything going on. He'll be able to bring me back to the right breathing, or if I feel something's going wrong, or somebody's not telling me something, he can reassure me, or tell me the truth.

Both Ms. Dann and Ms. Meta thought of their husbands as rational, controlled people. The husbands thus had a calming, comforting effect on their wives.

Ms. Xana exemplified mature dependency in all the interviews, never indicating that she would be unable to cope without her husband. She particularly wanted her husband to be with her in labor because he would be supportive, and help in sustaining her.

> I know if I get out of hand, he's going to be there to say, Come on! He knows how I feel about medication. I think if he kept telling me to stick it out, maybe I could do it with him there. Just being alone would be harder.

In contrast, some gravidas found it inconceivable to go through labor and delivery without the presence of their husbands. Not only did Ms. Aaron rely heavily on her husband to help her maintain control, but she needed his support to bolster her vulnerable self-esteem.

> We've practiced so much at home…he is a strengthening force in my life. He rarely loses his calm, and he is a very encouraging person. I think that he will definitely be a help. If I had to have someone I didn't really know well, I think…I would worry more about making a spectacle of myself,… like we were talking about defecating; I think that would bother me more if he were not there.

Ms. Aaron also expressed the idea that if something bad happened to her, her husband could take over because he was so attached to the coming child. Because of Ms. Aaron's low self-esteem, this statement may have indicated a lack of confidence in her own ability to manage.

Some women displayed excessive dependency on their husbands' goodwill; that is, their self-esteem depended on their husbands' approval. Often, such women appeared to have an underlying lack of trust in their partners. Ms. Yuth worried that she would lose face with her husband if she lost her temper or misbehaved, and if she lost face, she might be abandoned. She told of a dream in which she had gone into labor and had looked everywhere for her husband, but was unable to find him.

> He had gone to work and I tried there, but no one could find him anywhere. It seemed as if he had vanished. The time kept growing closer. I finally left for the hospital with some friends while his boss kept trying to locate Dick. Finally they found him and he got there just in time to see his child born.

Ms. Yuth's dream expresses a fear of abandonment in labor and delivery. In another dream, she was washing the car and "all the paint fell off." She became so upset by this occurrence that she "left home because my husband would be mad and I thought he wouldn't like me any more." Her dream expressed both a fear of rejection and her evident insecurity about her marriage. Her fears were distinguishable from the more common concern of gravidas that the husband or someone else be available for transportation to the hospital when labor starts (DeGarmo & Davidson, 1978).

Occasionally, the woman's fear of abandonment was based on a realistic appraisal of the husband's immaturity and, consequently, of his inability to be supportive. Ms. Bode was uncertain whether her husband would be with her in labor, and she tried to persuade herself that he would be there.

> Before I was pregnant we sometimes talked about labor. He would tease me and say he didn't want to be with me. I never ask him whether he really wants to be there. I think he does – for my sake maybe, more than seeing the baby.

She explained that her husband had "certain, not chauvinistic, but role-type feelings," and that he felt "having a baby" means "he had helped make it," but that he was "not going to bring it into the world." In other words, delivery was not the man's job. In the end, he did not remain with her during labor and delivery.

Ms. Cole, who had complained that her husband was neither caring nor concerned about her, was aware that he might "chicken out" and not be available to her in labor and delivery.

> I would like Jim there. But every time I bring it up he says he's really not sure; it all depends on how he feels at the time.... It doesn't make that much difference, you know. I'm not going to force him if he doesn't want to because that's his decision.

Although Ms. Cole truly wanted someone's hand to hold, preferably her husband's, she did not think that he would be able to help her even if he did come to the labor unit with her.

> I think he'll be worse off than me. I think that it [the childbirth experience] is really going to break him down. He'll probably sit here and go through a carton of cigarettes. He's the type that'll get real nervous.

Ms. Ely, a lawyer and feminist, experienced some motherhood–career conflict. She wondered whether she was too self-centered and ambitious to mother her child adequately, and she was uncertain whether her husband would live up to his promises of "taking an equal share of the burden" for the child.

> You know, doing the diapers, especially right now because I know I won't be able to go out and be self-supporting instantaneously like I've always been before. It's been a big thing with me to be independent economically. That's one of the things I get upset about, that bothers me – I don't like being dependent.

Ms. Dann similarly was occupied with women's rights and the development of her career. She found herself in disagreement with her more traditional husband. This confrontation seemed to lead to a rather defensive stance on the part of her husband, who apparently felt threatened. Consequently, conflict, mutual hostility, and misperceptions of each other's positive attributes resulted. For example, Ms. Dann said that she had no confidence in her husband's ability to help her during labor.

> I don't discuss labor with him. I have mentioned to him that I don't think he'll be helpful to me, and he just kind of brushes it off. At first I told him that he wasn't going to be there. He said, 'Oh yeah? I'm going to be there!' From the very beginning he decided he was going to be there, and I just went along with it. It's the way they do it here anyway.

However, Ms. Dann's husband was supportive in labor, helped with back rubs, brought roses to his wife, and so on. The couple separated soon after childbirth due to disagreement over Ms. Dann's pursuit of a career outside the home.

Ms. Tell, who felt both angry and fearful toward her husband, expected no support from him during labor. Here, again, there was misperception. Mr. Tell was highly supportive during labor, even when his wife lost control to the point of hysteria.

Ms. Fair reported that her husband was extremely frightened of childbirth, although he had attended childbirth classes and presented an outward appearance of strength. Ms. Fair felt that he would be supportive as long as she maintained control, but his anxiety worked to reinforce her fears about herself and her husband.

> I hope to keep my husband sane! I can't really foresee any problem at all [with my labor]. He's just scared to death! He's scared about everything. If he drops out during the labor, I wouldn't be surprised at all. If I lost control, he would be upset, and he wouldn't be able to function at all. I think he is more worried for me than I am. He's really scared about the baby – if everything will come out right. He's more scared about that than I am, a lot more.

Nevertheless, Ms. Fair felt it necessary, with the advent of childbirth, to continue seeing her husband as strong and dependable. In contrast to the preceding statements, she stated that she wanted her husband to be with her in labor because he was "strong, both emotionally and physically," as well as empathic. In this case, Mr. Fair found it difficult to be supportive because childbirth triggered underlying fears of his own. On the other hand, Ms. Fair's denial (avoidance) of her husband's real feelings served to give credence and recognition to her own needs. Despite Mr. Fair's anxiety, childbirth was a positive experience for this couple because he was able to be supportive during his wife's labor.

At the extreme end of the interdependency–dependency spectrum were a few women like Ms. Dann and Ms. Ely, who could not accept even minimal dependency needs in themselves.

5.2 The Wife's Concern for Her Husband's Needs as an Expectant Father

During the interviews, the wife's degree of empathy and understanding of her husband's needs also was considered. The marital relationship is reciprocal when both partners respect each other's needs and limitations. If the woman's interactions with her husband are adult (that is, not like the early dependent relationship she had with her mother), she is not likely to see him as an all-protecting, nurturing figure. She is able to like him as well as love him. Liking implies respect, whereas loving may not necessarily have this component.

Many women in the sample were aware that their husbands needed to make emotional adjustments to the pregnancy, and to the idea of having a child. Ms. Gale thought that she and her husband had an equally important adjustment.

> We both are finding that there's more psychological and emotional switching to do than we expected. And it's the combination of needing to do that and having everything else to do too. We worry about work and school and things like that.

Ms. Uman said that she felt it was harder for her husband to adjust because he "can see the changes in me, but he can't feel them because he hasn't had the constant physical presence I've had."

Ms. Eaden saw herself as a "mother hen" in the way she worried about her husband because she understood that he would need support when she was in labor. Mr. Eaden was nervous and anxious about this experience, his wife said.

> He's basically a quiet person. Whether he'll be verbal enough with everything else going on, and encouraging me is one thing I think about. I don't think he realizes how much

> encouragement I may be going to need, and I'm sure I probably don't even know. But the
> fact that someone is there to help him if he needs help is important.

Ms. Lash also was sympathetic with her husband's struggle to crystallize a father-hood role for himself. Although it was easy for her to see herself as a mother, she was conscious that her husband was unsure of his fatherhood role.

> [He]...is still petrified about being a father; he still really doesn't know what he's going to
> do with the whole thing. Theoretically he knows, but when you put him on the spot, I don't
> know how he'll respond. I would be interested in finding out what fathers in general feel
> as they approach the birth of their baby. People center so much on the maternal side of it.
> I think people leave fathers out too much.

The desire on the part of many women to include their husbands in childbirth and childrearing is indicative of their interest in obtaining a greater degree of paternal involvement with their children (Palkovitz, 1987). The birth event is a crucial time for men's emerging sense of paternal identity and their growing relationship within the infant (Pruett, 1989). Ms. Inis said that the baby became more "real" for her husband as he encountered experiences revolving around the preparation for the newborn. She said that she wished he had been present at her baby showers: "I would just come home with the stuff and show it to him, but I think he should have been included there too."

While discussing the desire to share her labor and delivery, Ms. Eaden speculated that this desire was related to her strong need for her husband to formulate his fatherhood role. She thought that he would love the baby more if "he actually saw it being born." Ms. Raaf did not want her husband to be left out of "an amazing event." Ms. Aaron placed significant value on her husband's interest in the baby.

> My father was always very involved with us as children, and both my sister and I had a
> good relationship with my father. And I want Chris to have a good relationship with his
> children. A lot of fathers get left out, or choose to be left out of it, and I don't want that if
> I can avoid it.

Because Ms. Aaron was not confident in her own ability to nurture, she had a strong emotional stake in having her husband, who had no ambivalence about fatherhood, present for the birth event.

Many women expressed concern that their husbands were frustrated over various unmet needs. For instance, Ms. Xana worried because she interrupted her husband's sleep.

> I conk out in the middle of the day unless I've had a terrific sleep.... My husband and I
> have not been getting very good sleep. I toss and turn so much during the night, I keep him
> awake. And I think Oh, no. When the baby comes, we're not going to be able to sleep very
> well at all unless we [learn to] get better sleep now.

Sexuality was another concern for many couples. How each couple dealt with differences in sexual libido caused by pregnancy, was a particularly important indicator of their sensitivity and responsiveness to each other. In the third trimeseter, most gravidas experienced a decline in their desire to have intercourse because it was uncomfortable and awkward, or because they had a lowered sex drive (Condon, 2006; May, 1987). Some couples experimented with alternate positions, and if these attempts proved unsuccessful, the wives were concerned about depriving their husbands. Ms. Bode felt badly about her diminished interest in having sex with her husband.

> I have absolutely no sex drive, absolutely none. I haven't during most of the pregnancy, and I feel like it's hard on him. He wouldn't turn it down if I, ...but he's not at all pushy.

Several gravidas displayed consideration, tenderness, and understanding toward their husbands during pregnancy. Ms. Santa, understanding that her husband might feel rejected and even jealous of the pregnancy, wanted to include him in the childbirth experience. When the interviewer remarked to Ms. Xana in a postpartum meeting that she had coped extremely well, and that even during labor she had been considerate toward her husband, she said:

> I never did once feel irritable towards Tom. I knew he was busy trying to find out a lot of things. If he wasn't right there, I could just go into the breathing pattern. We were going to have our first baby and I just wanted to get through it staying in control. Tom was being so considerate, and that made me want to be considerate towards him.

Ms. Faber said that when she was at home and thought she was going into the first stages of labor, she did not tell her husband until she was positive.

> I had 12 hours sleep, but he was exhausted. I gave him a beer at lunch knowing he'd fall asleep immediately instead of watching TV. I told myself I'd let him sleep at least 4 hours or as long as I could. By about 4:30 my contractions had been consistently 5 minutes apart and extrapolated 40 seconds long for a couple of hours. I went to the A & P, cashed a check, got some milk, and filled the car with gas. I knew he would appreciate not having to bother with that for the next few days.

Ms. Jabon packed her husband's favorite food before she went to the hospital. Despite her husband's fervent desire to share the responsibility of child care, Ms. Jabon expected that after his initial involvement he would gradually slack off as he became absorbed with his career again, and she was quite prepared to tolerate the possibility of his decreasing involvement with the baby. Ms. Aaron expressed a sense of mutual support in her marriage, saying that her husband tended to be patient with her throughout the pregnancy.

> When he gets impatient it is almost always with himself, and that gives me something to do, to kind of calm him down. I think it [labor and delivery] will be a good sharing experience for both of us.

Rarely did women register "no concern" for their husbands. Nevertheless, some women expressed an inability to empathize with their husbands. This lack of empathy was manifested in different ways: resentment of the husband's habits or an apparent lack of concern for his welfare, oblivion to his needs, acts of omission, fears of abandonment, and excessive dependency.

Ms. Katen was one of the gravidas who seemed to be aware of a father's need to bond with and nurture his child. She said:

> It may be hard for Mick not to be able to feed it [the baby], and that would be an advantage of bottle feeding. Even if we did use a formula, the baby would be close in terms of being held and given milk rather than propped up.

Ms. Katen was ambivalent about her own motherhood role, however. She voiced considerable motherhood–career conflict and was not able to anticipate changes in her lifestyle. It seemed plausible, therefore, that she really favored bottle feeding more for her own benefit than for her husband's. She was resentful of her husband's intolerance of her mood swings and, at the same time, found it impossible to talk to him about certain habits of his that irritated her. She perceived herself as tolerant of him, yet some resentment appeared to hinder an accepting attitude. In a dream about labor, it was her dog, Sonny, who was with her. She said:

> He's [the dog is] my solace when I'm sad and shares in joy when I'm happy. He and I can read each other very well, and it's going to be a long separation. I hate to leave him even when we go on vacations where he can't come. I guess the dream might say I'd be more comfortable in labor with him around.

In her interpretation of this dream, Ms. Katen felt that her dog possessed the characteristics of sharing, loyalty, and understanding that a close friend possesses. However, she seldom referred to others close to her in such unequivocal terms. In addition, the designation "housewife" upset Ms. Katen. She viewed this as a devaluation of herself. Thus, she was sensitive to any disregard of what she thought was her just due. According to the investigators' assessment, Ms. Katen's husband was empathic and involved in the birth process.

Ms. Fair found her husband's messy habits annoying.

> He just doesn't care. He'll take his clothes off and two days later I'll have a pile of 90 clothes. So I have to go down to the laundromat and wash them all. Two days later there's another mound of clothing.

She claimed that she tried not to get frustrated, but it was obvious that she had not been successful, partly because she was unable to communicate the full impact of this problem to her husband. Her husband also was not receptive to such confrontation.

The foregoing excerpts indicate how reciprocity in the marital relationship was marred by perceptions of lack of concern and involvement, poor communication, and conflict about assuming a parenthood role.

5.3 Effects of the Pregnancy on the Marital Bond

5.3.1 Closeness and Intimacy

No marital bond remains static; it evolves continuously. One event that changes the nature of the marital bond is the addition of a child to the marriage. This change usually signifies a developmental challenge for both the husband and the wife. Adding the role of mother or father to one's identity can be a positive experience, and changes in partners' self-concepts can be linked to changes in the marital bond resulting from the newborn's presence (Cowan & Cowan, 1988; Wilson et al., 2007). Therefore, it was expected that the anticipation, and then the actual presence of the newborn, would add a new dimension to the way couples related to one another.

Many women said that they grew closer to their husbands during pregnancy. The feeling of increased closeness usually resulted from sharing the pregnancy, and from the maturity that came from the process of merging into their new roles together and discovering new aspects of one another. In a study examining changes in the marital relationship, Saunders and Robins (1987) found that despite increased discussion of relationship issues and possible increases in stress and conflict, spouses tended to feel greater love for one another and reported no decrease in marital satisfaction during pregnancy. This increased intimacy strengthened the marital bond. Women with such a positive marital relationship tend to adapt more easily to pregnancy (Lederman, 2008b; Westbrook, 1978). Lederman (2008b) found that the couple relationship, as measured by the Revised Dyadic Adjustment Scales (Busby, Crane, Larsen, & Christensen, 1995) significantly correlated with Acceptance of Pregnancy, and with several other prenatal adaptation scales: Relationship to Husband, Preparation for Labor, Fears about Labor, and Relationship with Mother. These results suggest that the quality of the marital or couple relationship has a significant bearing on adaptation to pregnancy. As an example of a positive marital relationship and its effect on pregnancy adaptation, Ms. Xana said that her relationship with her husband had "gotten better" and that they had become closer. Ms. Uman noticed that the pregnancy had brought her and her husband "much closer together." She said:

For one thing I'm discovering a lot of qualities that I didn't know he had before. The first four months were a very bad time for us, and during that whole time he was very understanding, very patient. I know I would have been the opposite. I'm beginning to realize he's a very steady, calm person. The effect this has had on me is to make me more steady and confident. We're just so much more close, I think, because we realize that we're sharing an experience together.

Ms. Raaf said: "We were close before, but something's added, not sexually, especially the last month, but there's something there. We've talked about and we don't understand it. There's a closeness that wasn't there before."

Ms. Yuth felt that her husband had become more responsible, caring, and considerate since she had become pregnant.

He'll do a lot more for me around the house. He won't let me carry things; he carried all my laundry back and forth because we live in a three-story house. And he'll go up and downstairs for things I need so I don't have to make the extra trips.

Ms. Hayes remarked on her husband's heightened sense of commitment.

It [the child] makes Doug's plans more important. His parents always gave him money; he never felt financial insecurity or needed to make it on his own, whereas my family didn't have anything, and I always knew I would have to take care of myself. Now this [the child] gives him a commitment to get going in law school and to get through. He's taking a real interest in the whole thing. His father has no interest in the kids. ... It gives us both more responsibility; we're more a family unit.

Ms. Eaden suffered some anxiety about the pregnancy disrupting their relationship, and was initially upset at the news that she was pregnant.

> We've had a good marriage. There's no reason why we didn't want children, but we were satisfied with our life the way it was. You think of how a baby is going to disrupt your nice, quiet, secure little twosome. We talked about it. I'd cry once in a while. I'd be upset because I thought we're selfish really. Once the baby started to move, then everything was okay.

With the awareness of fetal movement, Ms. Eaden resolved her doubts, managed to overcome her hesitance, and ultimately made an immediate and delighted contact with her new baby.

On occasion, as indicated earlier, a woman was alarmed at the growing closeness of her husband. Ms. Penn had a protective and comforting husband who took the initiative for coaching breathing exercises, and who was less ambivalent than she was about the coming child. She seemed alarmed at his growing affection and wished to maintain distance, evidently finding this situation threatening.

Most women, however, consciously looked for increased commitment on the part of their husbands and thought that it was occurring. Ms. Zeff, for example, said that her husband had accepted their marriage once she became pregnant. Nevertheless, she felt that her best support in labor was the delivery staff, not her husband. Ms. Vale said that she thought her husband had matured and had become "a little more responsible." He had never driven a car before and he took driving lessons, which she thought made him feel "really good." Some women, like Ms. Vale, needed to reassure themselves of their future welfare by envisioning their husbands in an appropriate light, because they had not been accepting of the pregnancy. It is significant that Porter and Demeuth (1979) and Lederman (2008b) reported a high correlation between the husband's acceptance of pregnancy and the health of the marital relationship.

As noted earlier, it was difficult to obtain information about whether the pregnancy tended to separate couples because acknowledging this separation would be tantamount to admitting that there were marital problems. Yet, it was particularly relevant that several women reported seeing no change in their marital relationships. Generally, it was assumed that if a husband did not show more concern and more empathy toward his wife, then either no progress was taking place toward a mature acceptance of the fatherhood role, or there was a deterioration of the marital relationship. Pregnancy and childbirth, with their potential turmoil, can strain a relationship already in jeopardy, and can be the decisive events that overturn a floundering marriage.

Ms. Meta could see no change with respect to her husband exhibiting "more affection and more concern, showing more interest, or being at home more," but she insisted that this did not make her envious or regretful. The lack of change in the way her husband related to her may have been the result of his fear and anxiety about the coming child, which he expressed indirectly, often unkindly, by joking about her pregnancy. In addition, Ms. Carre, who reported "no change," said that her husband also seemed ambivalent about the coming child and was seldom at home.

Several women alluded somewhat obliquely to their husbands feeling threatened by the pregnancy and the coming infant. Ms. Jabon expressed doubts about her husband's ability to accept responsibility. Ms. Dann reported that at times her husband seemed hostile, and then at other times he showed consideration. In this particular case, the reality was that the marriage was disintegrating. Although it was apparent that Ms. Cole and her husband also were growing apart during the pregnancy, this fact was volunteered only after the birth of their child, and then in written communication. Ms. Cole was not able to confront this reality directly during the third trimester.

5.3.2　Increased or Decreased Conflict in the Marital Bond

The generalization can be made that pregnancy and parenthood, as a rule, do not help resolve conflicts, and are not a remedy for marital problems (Robson & Mandel, 1985). It was difficult for the researchers to pinpoint areas of marital conflict because of most women's reticence concerning this subject. Ms. Vale, for instance, stated that she had "a really good marriage," but, in fact, she was extremely fearful of being abandoned because her marriage was insecure. Usually, it was not possible to know whether the couples in the project resolved their problems through argument, or whether they discussed their difficulties while maintaining an atmosphere of trust and relative ease. In addition, it could not be ascertained whether one partner gave in to the dictates of the other, or whether both discovered that mutual compromise was the solution.

In some cases, we could conclude that the marital bond was reasonably conflict-free when there seemed to be agreement on value systems, areas of responsibility, sex roles, and child care. Fishbein (1984) found that agreement between partners concerning particular roles appeared to be more important than what form the roles would assume. For example, if both partners agree to more traditional roles in which the husband is the breadwinner and the wife is a full-time mother, one would predict relatively low levels of marital conflict and anxiety. In one case, a marital bond characterized more by traditional values than by mutuality appeared reasonably stable, because both partners were satisfied with this state of affairs. Ms. Meta said that she and her husband both agreed that the wife should be a full-time mother. She felt that the experience of adjusting to pregnancy was more difficult for her than for her husband.

> My first concern was losing my job. I was very happy with it, and I didn't want to leave it. He was always saying, 'Well, you can go back later.' But then he would say he did want me to be a full-time mother, and I said that was something I wanted also.

Ms. Meta said she was ready to have a baby, was confident she would be good at mothering, and had few qualms about staying home.

Some women were able to identify conflicts in their marital relationships. Ms. Gale, who was somewhat dependent on her husband and who had been jealous when his attention turned elsewhere, felt that she gave more to the relationship than he did. She had feared being abandoned in labor and delivery, and was distressed that her husband appeared to place her needs low on his priority list. She was able to specifically identify areas of conflict in their relationship. "I think the focal points were conflict over priorities and my tiredness. And I think that I am starting to deal with both of those."

Ms. Gale tried to talk openly with her husband about her frustration over his detachment from the pregnancy, and he seemed to respond.

> He's taken the initiative a couple of times now in suggesting we do the exercises at home and things like that, which he hadn't done at all up to that point, not until after we talked about it.... So that made me feel one hundred percent better.

In another situation, the marital conflict was so open that the gravida's tension and resentment emerged in the interviews. Ms. Dann stated unequivocally that she and her husband agreed on virtually nothing. They simply had different views and different sets of values. Ms. Dann had to deal with resolving her own motherhood–career needs, and with the discovery that her wish to combine both conflicted. This difficult situation was exacerbated by her husband's rigid stance. Ms. Dann said that he was "like a rock; doesn't budge." She perceived herself as being more open-minded than her husband.

> He's dogmatic about his traditional theories. He kind of says, 'This is right, and this wrong.' I say, 'If you look at it this way, it's not so right, and if you look at it from that way, it's not so wrong.' We have all kinds of little conflicts because he expects me to know what he thinks is right and wrong according to his values and I don't have his values. That's why communication is such a problem.

Conflict was particularly evident concerning sex, and each partner expressed anger toward one another in this area. For example, when Ms. Dann approached her husband for affection he ridiculed her enlarged shape, and when she tried intercourse a few times in the last trimester and did not enjoy it, she said that she "saw no reason to go through it just so Bill could"; so she "just kind of dropped it." She elaborated:

> Maybe I'm extraordinarily selfish these days. I just said, I'm not going to bother, if I'm not getting anything out of it. Things haven't been that great, you know. I'm sure if I had more positive thoughts towards him right now, I'd even encourage it. There are different ways to have sex besides intercourse that could probably satisfy both of us, but I just haven't bothered.

Such mutual antagonism and devaluation seemed characteristic of this marriage, whereas several other women gave evidence of progress in conflict resolution, and of a growing closeness in the relationship during pregnancy. It is important to note that alienation within the sexual relationship can damage the woman's psyche causing conflict and alterations in her self-concept and identity at a time when she is struggling with an adaptation process (McCaffrey, Barnett, & Thomas, 2001).

5.4 Identification of a Fatherhood Role

If mutuality is viewed as the key defining characteristic of a healthy marital bond, then each partner's attitude toward the coming child is equally important. It was of interest, therefore, to determine whether the husband was able to establish a fatherhood role for himself, and whether he accepted that role with relatively little ambivalence and conflict.

Husbands prepared for fatherhood in many of the same ways as did their wives for motherhood: reading and planning, fantasizing and thinking about the baby and the subsequent changes in their lifestyle, attending classes, and talking to other fathers. Many husbands were aware that if they attended childbirth classes and were present during labor and delivery, they were more likely to become integrated into their roles as fathers. Thus, they could see themselves as major figures in the whole pregnancy–birth process. Although it does not follow that if a marriage bond is strong a man would necessarily wish or need to be a father, our data indicated that husbands who had difficulty accepting the responsibility of fatherhood also related poorly to their wives. Cohen (1966) reported a similar observation. More recently, McHale and Rotman (2007) found that husbands' negative outlooks regarding parenting prenatally predicted co-parental solidarity and cohesion postpartally. It could not be concluded that if a husband was excited about the coming child, he necessarily would be supportive of his pregnant wife. For instance, he could have perceived his wife merely as a vehicle for childbirth, an attitude more characteristic of a conservative, traditional view of a wife.

Most expectant fathers were happy and excited, and they proudly anticipated the arrival of the child. Although Mr. Aaron was extremely nervous about labor and the prospect of his wife's suffering, Ms. Aaron said: "He is very proud of the fact that I am going to have a baby. We both really want this baby. It is very important to us as a couple and as individuals." At first, Mr. Aaron appeared to be more involved in parenting than his wife, but ultimately he needed more nurturing and support in childbirth than she did.

Another husband, Mr. Quins, crystallized his fatherhood role before his wife, because she was occupied with her efforts to resolve her motherhood–career conflict. Ms. Quins reported that when she was having no dreams about the baby or labor, her husband had two dreams about the baby. She reported: "In both [dreams], the child could walk and talk right after it was born."

Ms. Wooly said she was depressed when she discovered that she was pregnant.

[But my husband] was so happy…. He was just ecstatic the day he found out. He's really taken an active interest in it [the pregnancy]. He always listens and talks to it [the baby].

Ms. Santa reported that her husband had thought a great deal about his fatherhood role.

He worried about whether he was ready to be a father, if he could be the right kind of father, if he was ready for the responsibility, if we'd be able to afford it. But now he looks at it a little bit different; it's more a matter of, 'I am going to be a father and I am going to have to adjust to a lot of things, but I can only do the best I can and do what I feel is right.'

Ms. Santa also felt that her husband was making progress with respect to recognizing the reality of the baby.

> The baby right now is so alive for me. It's really neat to watch him [her husband] progress because when I was first pregnant, he didn't think so much of it. But now that the baby moves so much, he really gets a kick out of it and both of us are waiting to have it on the outside.

The process of the father's coming to terms with the reality of the baby is similar to the process described in identification of a motherhood role (Sherwen, 1986).

Several women expressed confidence in their husbands' abilities to be good parents. Ms. Fair, for example, stated that her husband liked children and was "good with them." In her diary, she wrote:

> [My husband]... is so good with kids it's unbelievable; they really like him too. I can't wait until our baby's born and watch John play with him. He can handle any kid of any age it seems. I'm excited to see the two of them together. He isn't going to be the typical father because he isn't scared of handling babies, and he's just dying to see and hold and touch and bring up ours.

One clear indication of the husband's anticipation of fatherhood, and of mutuality in the marital bond, was the assertion of a considerable number of women that pregnancy and childbirth are shared experiences. Several examples demonstrated how mutuality and anticipation of parenthood coexisted. Ms. Acton said:

> [My husband]...seems to be the mainstay in the whole thing. He's been the most – well, more willing – to be pregnant with me, and he's just as excited about it as I am. He's been more sure of it than I have and that always helps. I think his being sure about my labor will help.

As previously noted, Mr. Acton accompanied his wife on all her prenatal visits. Ms. Penn recognized that her husband needed a clearly defined role in labor.

> He would like to be in the labor room with me if at all possible. Before the ...classes he felt that he would just be standing there watching, and he really didn't want to do that. But I think now he understands that he can have such a beneficial role to play in helping me that he wants to help me.

Ms. Katen described her husband as "A proud father. Really excited. He told everybody that we were pregnant before I did."

The idea of husband and wife sharing pregnancy and childbirth, and of the need for the husband to develop his fatherhood role, are complementary and contemporary views (DeGarmo & Davidson, 1978). The corollary of these ideas, documented in both professional and lay publications and discussions, is illustrated in Ms. Jabon's description of her husband's reactions.

> He is very nervous and excited. I think that he probably feels somewhat less anxiety than I do as far as what will happen after the baby is born and on the scene. He is probably more relaxed than I am, and I think that that has to do with sex roles and general expectations about whose major responsibility a baby really is. Although we both read Father Power and he is planning on being very active and very involved, I think our society fundamentally expects that and rewards the man for maybe taking a few days off, then returning to his career full time.

On the whole, those husbands who found it difficult to be empathic, under-standing, and concerned about their wives, and found it difficult to share and communicate with them, also seemed to be ambivalent and even resentful and fearful of fatherhood or of the coming child. Ms. Carre reported little sharing and said:

> [My husband]…knows nothing and wants to pretty much know nothing about children. He has this arm's length attitude toward them. This [having a child] is kind of like all my idea, a you-take-care-of-it kind of thing. I'm sure that will change when the child actually is here. But I think he assumes that I know what I am doing.

Mr. Carre appeared to take some interest in childbirth and childrearing as time went on, but his wife reported that he was absorbed in his career, which probably explained his detachment. She accepted the situation, although she continued to wish and hope that her husband would be more enthusiastic. Consequently, Ms. Carre stood almost alone in her new motherhood role. She seemed to be a reasonably self-assured person with a healthy sense of her own self-worth, and with a realistic appraisal of the changes that the new baby would bring to her life. For these reasons, the lack of support from her husband did not permeate or disrupt the process of preparation for motherhood.

Similarly, Ms. Cole, who wholeheartedly wanted her baby and who had confidence in her ability to mother, established a happy, healthy bond with her newborn even though her husband had disappointed her by having an extramarital affair. It is possible that Mr. Cole engaged in the affair partly because of fear and his inability to accept the responsibilities of fatherhood.

Ms. Lash needed to be supportive of her husband, who was frightened of being a father, and she showed concern and sympathy with his difficulties in coming to terms with his new role.

In contrast, Ms. Vale, who was beset with fears and anxieties, had low self-esteem, was unclear about what kind of mother she wanted to be, and lost control in labor and delivery when her husband behaved in a nonsupportive way. This marriage was weak with little sharing and closeness, although Ms. Vale felt it necessary to deny the equivocal nature of the marriage bond. Mr. Vale appeared excited about the idea of becoming a father, but not about the added responsibilities of fatherhood. At times he seemed jealous of the fetus. In addition, Mr. Vale was not able to tolerate his wife's interest in a musical career, and his intolerance further decreased her self-esteem. Ms. Vale seemed highly dependent on her husband's whims, and her dependence was accompanied by an underlying fear of abandonment. Both partners seemed excessively dependent. This marital relationship clearly represented an extreme case in which neither partner was able to develop an adult romantic attachment, appropriate coping mechanisms for parenthood and co-parenting, or a coherent representation of the infant and relationship to the coming infant (Slade et al., 2005; Wilson et al., 2007). Rather, they appeared anxiously and avoidantly attached and had feelings of jealousy of the baby (Wilson et al., 2007).

Clearly, analogies exist in the formulation of motherhood and fatherhood roles. May (1982a, b) found support for ongoing prenatal and neonatal paternal involvement throughout the birth process. Yet, preoccupation with a difficult career, as well as a lack of interest in children, could forestall or preclude identification with a fatherhood role. Progress in expectant fathers' role identification can be accomplished through reading, thinking about life changes, fantasizing about fatherhood, attending classes, and attending professionally led group discussions with other fathers and couples (Condon 2006; Schultz et al., 2006). Participation in such activities facilitates role integration, as well as continued involvement in the birth process and with the newborn.

5.5   The Transition to Fatherhood[1]

In this section we review the literature to identify factors associated with readiness for fatherhood, the stresses of fatherhood, and the significant contributions of fathers to pregnancy and to the father–infant relationship.

When compared with the substantial body of research examining maternal prenatal and postpartum adaptation, a dearth of research exists concerning paternal transition to parenthood (Bouchard, Boudreau, & Hebert, 2006; Clinton, 1987; Clinton & Kelber, 1993; Hanson & Bozett, 1986; Henderson & Brouse, 1991; Schultz et al., 2006). Fathers have been viewed primarily as a source of support for the mother, with little research devoted to the impact of fatherhood on the man's own development (Clinton & Kelber, 1993). However, research evidence has begun to accumulate which suggests that the transition to fatherhood is a significant developmental event in men's lives (Clinton, 1987; Condon, 2006; Hanson & Bozett, 1986). Reports are emerging on paternal development of attachment to the fetus, adjusting to becoming a family triad versus a dyad, conceptualization of self as a father and the changes inherent with parenthood, and the type of father to be (Condon, 2006).

5.5.1   Readiness for Fatherhood

In an investigation involving first-time fathers, May (1982a, b) identified four factors that the fathers believed were important to their readiness for parenthood: whether the man intended to become a father at some point in his life, his perception concerning the stability of the couple relationship, the couple's relative financial security, and a sense of having completed the childless period of his life. These findings imply that if a man has problems associated with one of these factors, he may be ambivalent about beginning a pregnancy. Usually, assuming the difficulties

[1] This section is prepared by Scott Worsham with Regina Lederman.

are not severe, the man will overcome his doubts and become involved in the pregnancy to a degree that is comfortable for him and his wife (Battles, 1988). However, if the man never intended to father children or perceives problems in more than one of these areas, he is unlikely to become involved in the pregnancy and his detachment will adversely affect both his fathering and the marital relationship (Battles, 1988; May, 1982a, b; Bronte-Tinkew, Ryan, Carrano, & Moore, 2007).

In a study by Fein (1976), men perceived four factors as important to their successful postpartum adjustment: the baby's health, negotiating processes and roles in the couple relationship, family support, and work support. Preparing for and participating in infant care enables men to share their experiences with their wives and to deal with changes in the marital relationship.

5.5.2   Stress Associated with Fatherhood

The changing roles of men and women, along with the increasing number of mothers who work outside the home, have increased the opportunities and pressures for men to assist their wives with child care. In past research, men have expressed a number of difficulties adjusting to pregnancy and parenthood, including the possibility of financial problems, adapting to new routines, loss of sleep, and conflicts between work hours and participation in child care (Hangsleben, 1980; Tiedje & Darling-Fisher, 1993; Wente & Crockenberg, 1976).

Although parenthood is a normal life event, the birth of a child alters the structure of the family system as boundaries, roles, and duties must be reorganized to accommodate a new family member (Battles, 1988; Condon, 2006; Hangsleben, 1980). Generally, because the mother immediately becomes the most involved in infant care, the couple's time for conversation and mutual nurturance decreases. To the degree that the mother's emotional energy is focused on the infant, the new father may experience a loss of emotional support, because wives often are the only source of emotional support for adult men (Battles, 1988; Cronenwett & Kunst-Wilson, 1981). Consequently, some of the difficulty associated with the transition to fatherhood is related to disruption of the existing couple relationship (Wente & Crockenberg, 1976) and the noted decline in marital satisfaction postpartally (Schultz et al., 2006; Lawrence, Rothman, Cobb, Rothman, & Bradbury, 2008).

5.5.3   Paternal–Infant Attachment

Until recently, paternal–infant bonding has received little research attention, but available evidence indicates that fathers bond with their infants in a way similar to maternal–infant bonding (Condon, 2006; Hanson & Bozett, 1986). For example, a characteristic increase in attachment occurs with quickening for the woman, and for the father when he observes and palpates fetal movement (Condon, 2006). Evidence also shows that how fathers later treated their infants reflects how they were treated by their wives (Florsheim & Smith, 2005). That is, the quality of the expectant mother's behavior (hostile or negative) toward her partner predicted paternal behavior at follow-up when the infant was 2 years old.

Results of a study by Greenberg and Morris (1974) suggest that fathers begin developing a bond with their newborns by the 3rd day following birth. The fathers exhibited traits such as absorption, preoccupation, and intense involvement with their infants, behaviors which these investigators termed "engrossment." Characteristics of engrossment include visual and tactile awareness of the newborn, awareness of the newborn's distinct features, perception of the infant as perfect, a strong attraction to the infant, a feeling of extreme elation, and an increased sense of self-esteem. Greenberg and Morris (1974) hypothesized that newborns have the capacity to release fathers' innate potential for engrossment. Early physical contact between a father and newborn may encourage engrossment, and aid the father in developing a continual close bond with his infant; in other words, extended early contact may be an important first step in the development of a strong paternal–infant bond.

Research indicates that fathers and mothers interact differently with their children, and that infants relate to each parent in different ways (Hanson & Bozett, 1986; Pruett, 1993; (Wilson et al., 2007). Infants seem to relate to their mothers as mainly an attachment figure, a source of security, while the father is seen not only as an attachment figure, but also as a playmate (Hanson & Bozett, 1986; Tomlinson, 1987a, b). When mothers are not present, fathers tend to play differently with their children, using fewer toys; men encourage their children's curiosity and persistence in solving problems, and do not become overly concerned with their children's failures (Pruett, 1993).

In at least two studies, early paternal involvement was found to have significant mitigating effects on the long-term vulnerability of premature infants, and another study suggests that, because of their use of gender-specific language, fathers are important in clarifying children's gender roles (Pruett, 1993). Moreover, the father–infant relationship appears to be essential in loosening the symbiotic relationship with the mother which, in turn, allows the child's ego boundaries to develop and expand continuously (Hangsleben, 1980). Father absence during a child's early years may cause adjustment problems for the child and be a contributing factor in faulty personality development (Hangsleben, 1980; Pruett, 1993).

5.5.4   Paternal Involvement in Child Care

Father–infant involvement is significantly related to the father's earlier intentions for pregnancy. Men who did not want the pregnancy are less likely to show warmth toward the infant following birth, while men who wanted the pregnancy sooner than it actually occurred were more likely to show nurturing behaviors toward their infants (Bronte-Tinkew et al., 2007).

Paternal involvement and closeness to their infant is related to their family of origin relationships (Beaton & Doherty, 2007). Fathers who were either very close to their parents or very distant during childhood had more positive attitudes about father involvement prior to the birth of their first child, and at 6 and 12 months postpartum; likewise fathers' closeness to their fathers also predicted postpartum co-parenting of their infants.

In general, fathers are more likely to engage in play activities with their children than to perform caretaking tasks such as feeding and changing diapers (Tiedje & Darling-Fisher, 1993; Tomlinson, 1987a, b). The findings of one study indicate that greater paternal involvement in child care activities is associated with greater paternal preparation for child care, greater marital cohesion, and lesser maternal ambivalence about paternal involvement (Tomlinson, 1987a, b). In another study, better educated fathers with shorter work hours participated more in child care (Tiedje & Darling-Fisher, 1993). However, paternal participation in child care activities appears to remain limited, despite the increase in dual-earner families (Hanson & Bozett, 1986; Tiedje & Darling-Fisher, 1993; Tomlinson, 1987a, b).

The benefits of fathers' participation in child care appears to extend beyond reducing the workload of mothers. A father who is involved in the daily physical care of his child, during a significant period before the child becomes 3 years old, is much less likely to sexually abuse his own or anyone else's child; the intimacy of child care appears to create a barrier against subsequent violation of that inti-macy (Pruett, 1993). Also, research throughout the United States, Australia, and Europe demonstrates that involved fathers are less prone to physical illness, have better self-esteem, have spouses who are more satisfied in their marriage, and have children who are better able to cope with the stresses of life (Pruett, 1993). Health care providers who understand the transition to parenthood from the perspective of both fathers and mothers are better able to provide support and counseling appro-priate to each couple's circumstances.

5.6   Summary

Mutuality and relational attachment were described as the defining characteristics of a healthy marital bond, and several examples were provided which demonstrated how this was manifested in responses to pregnancy, childbirth, and emerging parenthood.

Some factors that may have interfered with the consolidation of the marital bond included a fundamental lack of caring or empathy, and an inability to share, com-municate, and trust on the part of either the wife, the husband, or both. The marital bond also could have been threatened by a lack of maturity on the part of the wife, as demonstrated by overdependence, by insufficient concern for her husband, or by misunderstanding the support that he offered. Moreover, the marital bond may have been jeopardized by a lack of maturity on the part of the husband, as demonstrated by excessive anxiety about the responsibilities of being a father, by insufficient concern for his wife, or by anxiety about his role in labor. As Deutscher (1970) poignantly described, the marital partners must first learn to parent and nurture each other, and to assuage the fears and doubts that arise during pregnancy and preparations for parenthood. An important developmental shift that occurs in both partners in the transition to parenthood is the shift in their behavior towards each other, i.e., becoming parental partners in addition to marital partners (Saunders & Robins, 1987; Wilson et al., 2007). Pregnancy is then more likely to be perceived as satisfying (Gladieux, 1978).

Objective and accurate responses about the marital relationship may be difficult to obtain (Goldstein, 1993). This difficulty may, in part, account for the early disparity in the literature regarding the significance of the marital relationship. Therefore, methods of inquiry need to be in-depth and validated through further inquiry. If the couple is interviewed together, they should also be interviewed separately to decrease socially desirable responses. Of particular importance are: (1) assessments of change in the relationship, and (2) methods the couple uses to solve differences in sexual libido during pregnancy. Responses to these questions provide a strong indication of the degree of empathy, cooperation, and support in the relationship. Obtaining an accurate assessment of the partner or marital relationship is particularly important during pregnancy, not only for the significance in pregnancy adaptation, but also for anticipating postpartal maternal and family adaptation. Spousal issues, including marital problems and arguments, the assumption of household responsibilities, and issues pertaining to sex were considered among the most stressful events of pregnancy in a study by Arizmendi and Affonso (1987). An assessment of partner attachment, if individual partner attachment relational representations, and conceptions of parenthood and co-parenting may also be warranted, given the significance of the marital relationship to adaptation to both pregnancy and the postpartum, and it's reported predictiveness to preterm birth and low birthweight.

Success in establishing a fatherhood role was observed in husbands who were highly motivated to nurture a child, who were excited and proud in anticipating fatherhood, and who were reasonably confident about their fatherhood skills. These fathers tended to like children, to think about their fatherhood roles, and to share the pregnancy–childbirth experience with their wives. Establishing a fatherhood identification is a paramount developmental step for a man, in the same way that establishing a motherhood identification is important for a woman (Clinton, 1987; DeGarmo & Davidson, 1978; Glazer, 1989). This process of establishing a fatherhood role may temporarily reactivate the husband's conflicts with his own parents, intensify feelings of separation, heighten dependency needs, and rekindle feelings of sibling rivalry. The husband who can look at these temporary regressions honestly is more likely to effect attachment and bonding with his partner and newborn. Two husbands in the study, Mr. Aaron and Mr. Quins, established their parenthood roles more easily than did their wives.

In contrast, husbands who had difficulty establishing their fatherhood roles were ambivalent about the added responsibility that a child would bring, thought of children as interfering, showed little interest in their wives' pregnancy and childbirth, and tended not to think about fatherhood. Some traditional husbands were excited about the child, but either they wished to be left out of the childbirth and childrearing experience, or they felt resentful of the added responsibility and decreased freedom that caring for a child would bring to their lifestyle. Some husbands, like Mr. Gale and Mr. Carre, became irritated at any impingement on their timetables and resented interruptions of their sleep routines during their wives' pregnancies. Others, like Mr. Vale, demonstrated signs of jealousy of the fetus or of their pregnant wives. One husband, Mr. Fair, identified to such an extent with his pregnant wife that he suffered more fears and doubts about labor and delivery than she did. A few husbands left their wives alone during labor, or they withdrew from their wives in other ways: through an extramarital relationship, through engrossment in a career, or through viewing the wife merely as a child-bearing vehicle. Similar behaviors have been described by Hobbs (1965) and Liebenberg (1967).

In general, the experience of pregnancy and childbirth appears to mature husbands who are in various stages of readiness for parenthood, but does not rectify severe marital rifts (Robson & Mandel, 1985). Many husbands found the birth of their child to be both a dramatic growth experience and an expression of deep commitment to wife and child (Greenberg, 1985).

Literature is also emerging on the contributions that can be made by preventive intervention for mothers, fathers, and couples. Schultz et al. (2006) reported efficacy for a prenatal couple intervention that decreased the decline in marital satisfaction postpartally. Since coping skills and communication are important factors in interpersonal relationships and the adaptation to pregnancy (Condon, 2006; Dole et al., 2004; Facchinetti, Ottolini, Fazzio, Rigatelli, & Volpe, 2007; Martin & Baker, 2004), curricula have also been developed to enhance these skills (Gardner, Giese, & Parrott, 2004).

References

Abell, T. D., Baker, L. C., Clover, R. D., & Ramsey, C. N. (1991). The effects of family functioning on infant birthweight. *The Journal of Family Practice, 32*, 37–44.

Arizmendi, T., & Affonso, D. D. (1987). Stressful events related to pregnancy and postpartum. *Journal of Psychosomatic Research, 31*, 743–756.

Battles, R. S. (1988). Factors influencing men's transition into parenthood. *Neonatal Network*, 63–66.

Beaton, J. M., & Doherty, W. J. (2007). Fathers' family of origin relationships and attitudes about father involvement from pregnancy through first year postpartum. *Fathering, 5*, 236–245.

Berry, L. (1988). Realistic expectations of the labor coach. *Journal of Obstetric, Gynecologic, and Neonatal Nursing, 17*, 354–355.

Bouchard, G., Boudreau, J., & Hebert, R. (2006). Transition to parenthood and conjugal life. *Journal of Family Issues, 27*, 1512–1530.

Bronte-Tinkew, J., Ryan, S., Carrano, J., & Moore, K. A. (2007). Resident father's pregnancy intentions, prenatal behaviors, and links to involvement with infants. *Journal of Marriage and Family, 69*, 977–990.

Brown, M. A. (1986). Social support, stress, and health: A comparison of expectant mothers and fathers. *Nursing Research, 35*, 72–76.

Brown, M. A. (1987). How fathers and mothers perceive prenatal support. *The American Journal of Maternal Child Nursing, 12*, 414–418.

Busby, D. M., Crane, D. R., Larsen, J. H., & Christensen, C. (1995) A revision of the Dyadic Adjustment Scale for use with distressed and nondistressed couples: Construct hierarchy and multidimensional scales. *Journal of Marital and Family Therapy, 21*, 289–308.

Centers for Disease Control and Prevention: Morbidity and Mortality Weekly Report. (2008). Prevalence of self-reported postpartum depressive symptoms—17 states, 2004–2005. CDC: Atlanta, GA, *299*(19), 2268–2270.

Clinton, J. (1987). Physical and emotional responses of expectant fathers throughout pregnancy and the early postpartum period. *International Journal of Nursing Studies, 24*, 59–68.

Clinton, J. F., & Kelber, S. T. (1993) Stress and coping in fathers of newborns: Comparisons of planned versus unplanned pregnancy. *International Journal Nursing Study, 30*, 437–443.

Cohen, M. B. (1966). Personal identity and sexual identity. *Psychiatry, 29*, 1–14.

Cohen, R. L. (1988). Developmental tasks of pregnancy and transistion to parenthood: An approach to assessment. In R. L. Cohen (Ed.), *Psychiatric consultation in childbirth settings: Parent- and child-oriented approaches* (pp. 51–70). New York: Plenum Medical. Book Co.

Condon, J. (2006). What about Dad? Psychosocial and mental health issues for new fathers. *Australian Family Physician, 35*, 690–692.

Capogna, G., Camorcia, M., & Stirpara, S. (2007). Expectant father's experience during labor with or without epidural analgesia. *International Journal of Obstetric Anesthesia, 16*, 110–115.

Cowan, C., & Cowan, P. (1988). Changes in marriage during the transition to parenthood: Must we blame the baby? In G. Michaels & W. Goldberg (Eds.), *The transition to parenthood: Current theory and research*. New York: Cambridge University Press.

Cowan, P. A., & Cowan, C. P. (2002). Interventions as tests of family systems theories: Marital and family relationships in children's development and psychopathology. *Development and Psychopathology, 14*, 73–759.

Crockenberg, S. C., Leerkes, E. M., & Lekka, S. K. (2007). Pathways from marital aggression to infant emotional regulation. *Infant Behavior and Development, 30*, 97–113.

Cronenwett, L. R., & Kunst-Wilson, W. (1981). Stress, social support, and the transition to fatherhood. *Nursing Research, 30*, 196–201.

DeGarmo, E., & Davidson, K. (1978). Psychosocial effects of pregnancy on the mother, father, marriage, and family. *Current Practice in Obstetric and Gynecologic Nursing, 2*, 24–44.

Deutscher, M. (1970). Brief family therapy in the course of first pregnancy: A clinical note. *Contemporary Psychoanalysis, 7*, 21–35.

Dimitrovsky, L., Perez-Hirshberg, M., & Itskowitz, R. (1987). Depression during pregnancy: Quality of family relationships. *The Journal of Psychology, 12*, 213–218.

Dole, N., Savitz, D. A., Siega-Riz, A. M., Hertz-Piccioto, I.,McMahon, M. J., & Buekens, P. (2004). Psychosocial factors and preterm birth among African-American and White women in Central North Carolina. *American Journal of Public Health, 94*, 1358–1365.

Edwards, C. H., Cole, O. J., Oyemade, U. J., Knight, E. M., Johnson, A. A., Westney, O. E., et al. (1994a). Maternal stress and pregnancy outcomes in a prenatal clinic population. *Journal of Nutrition, 124*, 1006S–1021S.

Edwards, C. H., Knight, E. M., Johnson, A. A., Oyemade, U. J., Cole, O. J., Laryea, H., et al. (1994b). Multiple factors as mediators of the reduced incidence of low birth weight in an urban clinic population. *Journal of Nutrition, 124*, 927S–935S.

Facchinetti, F., Ottolini, F., Fazzio, M., Rigatelli, M., & Volpe, A. (2007) Psychosocial factors associated with preterm uterine contractions. *Psychothreapy and Psychosomatics, 76*, 391–394.

Fein, R. A. (1976). Men's entrance to parenthood. *The Family Coordinator, 25*, 341–347.

Fishbein, E. (1984). Expectant father's stress – Due to the mother's expectations? *Journal of Obstetric, Gynecologic, and Neonatal Nursing, 13*, 325–328.

Florsheim, P., & Smith, A. (2005). Expectant adolescent couples' relations and subsequent parenting behavior. *Infant Mental Health Journal, 26*, 533–548.

Fridh, G., Kopare, T., Gaston-Johansson, G., & Norvell, K. (1988). Factors associated with more intense labor pain. *Research in Nursing and Health, 11*, 117–124.

Gardner, S. P., Giese, K., & Parrott, S. M. (2004). Evaluation of connections: Relationships and marriage curriculum. *Family Relations, 53*, 521–527.

Gladieux, J. (1978). Pregnancy – The transition to parenthood: Satisfaction with the pregnancy experience as a function of sex role conceptions, marital relationship, and social network. In W. B. Miller & L. F. Neman (Eds.), *The first child and family formation* (pp. 275–295). Chapel Hill: Carolina Population Center, University of North Carolina.

Glazer, G. (1989). Anxiety and stressors of expectant fathers. *Western Journal of Nursing Research, 11*, 47–59.

Goldstein, L. H. (1993). Associations among maternal characteristics and resources during pregnancy and mother-infant interactions at 3-months postpartum. Paper presented at the Society for Research in Child Development, New Orleans, LA.

Gottman, J. M., & Notarius, C. G. (2002). Marital research in the 20th century and a research agenda for the 21st century. *Family Process, 41*, 159–197.

Graff, L. A., Dyck, D. G., & Schallow, J. R. (1991). Predicting postpartum depressive symptoms: A structural modeling analysis. *Perceptual and Motor Skills, 73*, 1137–1138.

Greenberg, M. (1985). *The birth of a father*. New York: Continuum.

Greenberg, M., & Morris, N. (1974). Engrossment: The newborn's impact upon the father. *American Journal of Orthopsychiatry, 44*, 520–531.

Grossman, F. K., Eichler, L. S., & Winickoff, S. A. (1980). *Pregnancy, birth and parenthood*. San Francisco: Jossey-Bass.

Grossman, K., & Grossman, K. E. (2000). Parents and toddlers at play. In P. M. Crittendon & A. H. Claussen (Eds.), *The organization of attachment relationships: Matuation, culture, and context* (pp. 13–37). New York, Cambridge University Press.

Grych, J. (2002). Marital relationship and parenting. In Borenstein (Ed.), *Handbook of parenting: Social conditions and applied parenting* (vol. 4, 2nd ed., pp. 203–225). Mahwah, NJ: Erlbaum.

Hangsleben, K. L. (1980). Transition to fatherhood: Literature review. *Issues in Health Care of Women, 2*, 81–97.

Hanson, S. M. H., & Bozett, F. W. (1986). The changing nature of fatherhood: The nurse and social policy. *Journal of Advanced Nursing, 11*, 719–727.

Heineke, C. M., & Guthrie, D. (1992). Prebirth marital interactions and postbirth marital development. *Infant Mental Health Journal, 17*, 140–151.

Henderson, A. D., & Brouse, A. J. (1991). The experiences of new fathers during the first 3 weeks of life. *Journal of Advanced Nursing, 16*, 293–298.

Hobbs, D. F. (1965). Parenthood as crisis: A third study. *Journal of Marriage and the Family, 27*, 367–372.

Johnson, M. P. and Baker, S. (2004) Implications of coping repertoire as predictors of men's stress, anxiety and depression following pregnancy, childbirth and miscarriage: a longitudinal study. *Journal of Psychosomatic Obstetrics and Gynecology, 25*, 87–98.

Keeley, R. D., Birchard, A., Dickinson, P., Steiner, J., Dickinson, L. M., Rymer, S., et al. (2004). Parental attitudes about a pregnancy predict birthweight in a low-income population. *Annals of Family Medicine, 2*, 145–149.

Keenan, P. (2000). Benefits of massage therapy and sue of a doula during labor and childbirth. *Alternate Therapies, 6*, 66–74.

Krishnakumar, A., & Buehler, C. (2000). Interparental conflict and parenting behaviors: A meta-analytic review. *Family Relations: Interdisciplinary Journal of Applied Family Studies, 40*, 435–441.

Lawrence, E., Rothman, A. D., Cobb, R. J., Rothman, M. T., & Bradbury, T. N. (2008). Marital satisfaction across the transition to parenthood. *Journal of Family Psychology, 22*, 46–51.

Lederman, R. P. (2008a). *Predictiveness of postpartum maternal psychosocial adaptation from prenatal ccales of adaptation, dyadic adjustment, and maternal attachment.* San Diego, CA: Society of Behavioral Medicine.

Lederman, R. P. (2008b). *Relationships among psychosocial adaptation, attachment, and dyadic adjustment.* San Diego, CA: Society of Behavioral Medicine.

Lederman, R., Lederman, E., Work, B. A. Jr., & McCann, D. S. (1979). Relationship of psychological factors in pregnancy to progress in labor. *Nursing Research, 28,* 94–97.

Lederman, R. P., Weis, K., Brandon, J., Hills, & Mian, T. (2002). *Relationship of maternal prenatal adaptation and family functioning to pregnancy outcomes.* Washington, DC: Society of Behavioral Medicine.

Lerner, R. M., Rothbaum, F., Boulos, S., & Castellino, D. R. (2002). Developmental systems perspective on parenting. In Borenstein (Ed.), *Handbook of parenting: Biology and etiology of parenting* (vol. 2, 2nd ed., pp. 315–344). Mahwah, NJ: Erlbaum.

Liebenberg, B. (1967). Expectant fathers. *American Journal of Orthopsychiatry, 37,* 358–359.

Margolin, G., Gordis, E. B., & John, R. S. (2001). Coparenting: A link between marital conflict and parenting in two-parent families. *Journal of Family Psychology, 15,* 3–21.

May, K. A. (1978). Active involvement of expectant fathers in pregnancy: Some further considerations. *Journal of Obstetric, Gynecologic and Neonatal Nursing, 7,* 7–12.

May, K. A. (1982a). Factors contributing to first-time fathers, readiness for fatherhood: An exploration study. *Family Relations, 31,* 353–361.

May, K. A. (1982b). Three phases of father involvement in pregnancy. *Nursing Research, 31,* 337–342.

May, K. A. (1987). Men's sexuality during the childbearing year: Implications of recent research findings. *Holistic Nursing Practitioner, 1,* 60–65.

McCaffrey, R., Barnett, S., & Thomas, D. J. (2001). Seeking satisfaction: Treating decreased libido in women. *Lifelines, 5,* 31–35.

McHale, J. P., Keursten-Hogan, R., Lauretti, A., & Rasmussen, J. L. (2000). Parental reports of coparenting and observed coparenting behavior during the toddler period. *Journal of Family Psychology, 14,* 220–236.

McHale, J. P., & Rotman, T. (2007). Is seeing believing? Expectant parents' outlooks on coparenting and later coparenting solidarity. *Infant Behavior and Development, 30,* 63–81.

Melges, F. T. (1968). Postpartum psychiatric syndromes. *Psychosomatic Medicine, 30,* 95–108.

Nichols, M. R. (1993). Paternal perspectives of the childbirth experience. *Maternal Child Nursing Journal, 21,* 99–108.

Pacey, S. (2004). Couples and the first baby: Responding to new parents' sexual and relationship problems. *Sexual and Relationship Therapy, 19,* 223–246.

Palkovitz, R. (1985). Fathers' birth attendance, early contact, and extended contact with their newborns: A critical review. *Child Development, 56,* 392–406.

Palkovitz, R. (1987). Fathers' motives for birth attendance. *The American Journal of Maternal Child Nursing, 16,* 123–129.

Pavill, B. C. (2002). Fathers & Breastfeeding. Consider these ways to get Dad involved. *AWHONN Lifelines, 6,* 324–331.

Porter, L. S., & Demeuth, B. R. (1979). The impact of marital adjustment on pregnancy acceptance. *Maternal-Child Nursing Journal, 8,* 103–109.

Pruett, K. D. (1989). The nurturing male: A longitudinal study of primary nurturing fathers. In S. H. Cath, A. Gurwitt, & L. Ginsberg (Eds.), *Fathers and their families* (pp. 389–405). Hillsdale, NJ: The Analytic.

Pruett, K. D. (1993). The paternal presence. *Families in Society, 74,* 46–50.

Ramsey, C., Abell, T., & Baker, L. (1986). The relationship between family functioning, life, events, family structure, and the outcome of pregnancy. *Journal of Family Practice, 22,* 521–527.

Robson, B., & Mandel, D. (1985). Marital adjustment and fatherhood. *Canadian Journal of Psychiatry, 30,* 169–172.

Russel, C. (1974). Transition to parenthood: Problems and gratifications. *Journal of Marriage and the Family, 36*, 294–301.

Saunders, R., & Robins, E. (1987). Changes in the marital relationship during the first pregnancy. *Health Care for Women International, 8*, 361–377.

Schultz, M. S., Cowan, C. P., & Cowan, P. A. (2006). Promoting healthy beginnings: A randomized controlled trial of a preventive intervention to preserve marital quality during the transition to parenthood. *Journal of Clinical and Consulting Psychology, 74*, 1–31.

Shereshefsky, P. M., & Yarrow, L. J. (Eds.). (1973). *Psychological aspects of a first pregnancy and early postnatal adaptation.* New York: Raven.

Sherwen, L. (1986). Third trimester fantasies of first-time expectant fathers. The American *Journal of Maternal Child Nursing, 15*, 153–170.

Slade, A., Grienenberger, J., Bernbach, E., Levy, D., & Locker, A. (2005). Maternal reflective functioning, attachment, and the transmission gap: A preliminary study. *Attachment and Human Development, 7*, 283–298.

Teichman, Y., & Lahav, Y. (1987). Expectant fathers: Emotional reactions, physical symptoms and coping styles. *British Journal of Medical Psychology, 60*, 225–232.

Tiedje, L. B., & Darling-Fisher, C. S. (1993). Factors that influence fathers' participation in child care. *Health Care for Women International, 14*, 99–107.

Tomlinson, P. S. (1987a). Father involvement with first-born infants: Interpersonal and situational factors. *Pediatric Nursing, 13*, 101–105.

Tomlinson, P. (1987b). Spousal differences in marital satisfaction during transition to parenthood. *Nursing Research, 36*, 239–243.

Trainor, C. L. (2002). Valuing labor support. *Lifelines, 6*, 387–389.

Wenner, N. K., Cohen, M. B., Weigert, E. V., Kvarnes, R. G., Ohaneson, E. M., & Fearing, J. M. (1969). Emotional problems in pregnancy. *Psychiatry, 32*, 389–410.

Wente, A. S., & Crockenberg, S. B. (1976). Transition to fatherhood: Lamaze preparation, adjustment difficulty and the husband–wife relationship. *The Family Coordinator, 25*, 351–357.

Westbrook, M. T. (1978). The reactions to childbearing and early maternal experience of women with differing marital relationships. *British Journal of Medical Psychology, 51*, 191–199.

Wilson, C. L., Rholes, W. S., Simpson, J. A., & Tran, S. (2007). Labor, delivery, and early parenthood: An attachment theory perspective. *Personality and Social Psychology Bulletin, 33*, 505–518.

Zambrana, R. E., Dunkel-Schetter, C., & Scrimshaw, S. (1991). Factors which influence use of prenatal care in low-income women in Los Angeles County. *Journal of Community Health, 16*, 283–295.

Chapter 6
Preparation for Labor

Preparation for labor by expectant women is preparation for work and stress. It is comparable to preparation for motherhood in the sense that the desire to be prepared is not sufficient. The gravida must take steps to reach a state of mental/ emotional and physical readiness, through both concrete actions and imaginary rehearsal. Preparation takes the form of "nesting behavior," attending childbirth preparation classes, reading books about labor, and specifics such as arranging transportation to the hospital. Preparation also entails confronting one's fears and anxieties and, in general, gearing up or "psyching up" for the ordeal of labor. This process of gearing up is closely related to the gravida's level of self-confidence and self-esteem, and to her personality style, her past experience with stress, and her manner of resolving conflicts about motherhood.

In this chapter, planning for labor is discussed under the following three behavioral dimensions:

1. Activity characterized by practical steps
2. Activity characterized by imaginary rehearsal or fantasizing
3. Dreaming about labor

Imaginary rehearsal or dreaming about labor is examined in terms of the following factors:

(a) Thinking versus avoidance of thinking about labor
(b) Congruence between fantasy and reality with respect to contractions, work and pain, and risks
(c) Doubts and fears
(d) Level of confidence
(e) Envisioning the challenges of labor for oneself and the fetus.

6.1 Planning for Labor: Practical Steps to Gather Information

Practical steps refer to the specific resources that the gravida utilized in order to become better prepared and informed about the processes of labor and self-help methods. Most women who participated in the study wanted to gather information about the labor process before delivery. By attending and participating in prenatal childbirth preparation classes, by sharing feelings, fears, and experiences with other women, and by using books, films, and various other resources for gathering information and further learning, the gravidas prepared themselves for the labor experience (Aaronson, Mural, & Pfoutz, 1988). Being informed about labor and delivery is generally considered helpful by women (Mackey, 1990).

6.1.1 Prenatal Classes

With few exceptions, the sample in our original project attended childbirth preparation classes. The two most common reasons given by the women for attending classes were to learn what to expect in labor and to share the experience of labor and delivery with their husbands. Ms. Inis explained that she attended childbirth classes with her husband.

> [I want]…to find out what's going on and be prepared for each stage with Sam. I just don't believe in doing this alone….. I don't have a real hang-up on the anesthetic, although I'd rather do it natural. But my main purpose is to have it [the baby] with knowledge and to have him [my husband] with me.

A good example of the way in which preparation helped a gravida overcome fear was the following response by Ms. Santa.

> I really liked them [the classes] and Tim did too. This is our first baby and we didn't know what to expect, and you hear so many bad things – about labor especially. Everybody says, 'Oh it's so painful and it's just terrible.' After going to childbirth classes, I'm not afraid at all. I know it's going to hurt. I feel really informed and I'm just eager.

Although attendance at childbirth preparation classes helped reduce anxiety about labor, many women commented afterward that labor was, in fact, more difficult than they were led to believe, a finding noted by others (Kuczynski & Thompson, 1985; Melzack, 1984; Stolte, 1987).

Ms. Lash, who was very anxious, said:

> [The classes]…are really helping me to put my mind at another place when my body is here. And they've…been helping me to relax…. I…feel better after I leave the class because I have been so relaxed… I can lie on my back during the class while I'm doing the breathing exercises and… it doesn't hurt like it hurts other times; I don't notice the pain.

Ms. Lash had strong feelings about not having anesthesia, fearing repetition of the trauma of feeling "trapped" which occurred when a dentist had used "gas." She felt that attending childbirth classes would help her go through labor and delivery without the use of anesthetics (Greenfield & Tepper, 1981).

Several women expected that the breathing techniques, in addition to knowledge about the processes of labor, would enable them to take a more active role in childbirth (Crowe & von Baeyer, 1989). Ms. Carre felt that parenthood and childbirth classes instructed one "…in how to control as much as you can of the labor process. Now obviously it's still going to be quite a trial, …but you at least know what's coming." On the whole, those women who said that they profited from classes felt that the classes answered many questions, made labor and delivery easier, and heightened their husbands' interest in the processes of pregnancy and childbirth (Delke, Minkoff, & Grunebaum, 1985).

In addition to childbirth education, recent educational and counseling support groups found added benefits to both adaptation to pregnancy and the postpartum (Schachman, Lee, & Lederman, 2004). Schachman et al. (2004) compared a traditional 3-h, 4-week childbirth education course with an experimental course in which the expectant mothers, who were military Air Force wives, received the same traditional course with one hour added to class each week that included content and counseling designed to facilitate maternal role adaptation. Using the Lederman Prenatal Self-Evaluation Questionnaire (Lederman, 1996), significant differences in results were found between the two groups both prenatally and postnatally. The experimental counseling group with added maternal role counseling content, compared to the traditional group, attained a significantly higher total prenatal questionnaire scale score, and higher scores on scales indicating they felt more prepared and less anxious about labor, and also less anxious about fears of pain, helplessness, and loss of control in labor, as well as concerns about the well-being of self and the fetus in labor. Likewise postpartally, the experimental group attained a higher total questionnaire scale score, and higher adaptation scale scores on satisfaction with labor and delivery, confidence in motherhood, satisfaction with motherhood, and support from family and friends. These results stand in contrast with those found by Hodnett and Fredericks (2003), but are supported by the pivotal study conducted by Norbeck, DeJoseph, and Smith (1996).

Childbirth classes may include content on risks associated with the birthing process which may heighten the gravida's fears. During the instructor's discussion of common complications in labor Ms. Uman felt that she was "learning too much" in her classes.

> [I]....got to the point where I know so much that I'm afraid of...failure in childbirth. In certain ways I am afraid I'll panic, even though I know what's going to be happening. The problem is that they present all the alternatives to you. This may happen, and that may happen, but not necessarily. You tend to think that they all are going to happen.

Nevertheless, Ms. Uman thought that the advantages of attending classes outweighed the disadvantages.

> I'm grateful in that I'm aware of everything. I think I'd hate to go in totally ignorant, and I'd hate to wonder what was happening to me. They say it is a lot better to know what is happening and try to cope with it.

A small minority of women favored clinic classes offered by the hospital. Ms. North was not certain why she decided against attending childbirth classes, except that her husband did not wish to attend. This attitude seemed to be connected with Ms. North's tendency to avoid all thoughts about labor. She had lost a baby due to a miscarriage and then suffered a septic infection because of it. As a result, she was terrified of labor and extraordinarily afraid of injury or death to her baby. In addition, she gave the impression of being passive and of simply allowing things to be done to her. She said that the breathing and relaxation classes she took at the hospital clinic "kind of helped."

Ms. Cole, who attended clinic classes at the hospital, thought that her mother might not have had as much pain in childbirth if she had attended preparatory classes. She said:

> [The classes]...teach you how to help yourself,...how to breathe with your contractions and how to...limber up before you go in, ... what you can do for backache and things like that.

Ms. Cole prided herself on not depending "on people too much for anything." Her reason for going to clinic classes was to learn how to take as much responsibility for labor as possible, and she was quite prepared to work actively in labor.

Ms. Zeff wished to attend childbirth classes, but failed to organize herself sufficiently to sign up for them. In the third trimester she was still not attending classes, and she placed the responsibility for this on instructors who did not call her back. In a retrospective study of patients in a large hospital who received minimal prenatal care, Joyce, Diffenbacher, Greene, and Sorokin (1984) found that both internal and external barriers to care exist. However, most women reported that internal barriers such as depression, denial, and fear kept them from obtaining prompt prenatal care more than did external barriers such as financial problems, lack of transportation, and lack of child care. Ms. Zeff rated low on the identification of a motherhood role scale and very high on fear of loss of self-esteem, fear of loss of control, and fears of injury and death scales. Her extreme anxiety evidently interfered with her preparation for labor.

6.1.2 Conversing with Other Women

More traditional sources of information about labor include talking to one's own mother, sister, relatives, friends, or even strangers (Aaronson et al., 1988). Ms. North, who did not attend childbirth classes, related how she had overheard her sister and sister-in-law talking about labor. Apparently they had normal deliveries, but Ms. North claimed that she did not listen to the two women attentively enough to remember what they said. Again, it appeared that Ms. North's anxiety about her fetus's well-being, following a previous spontaneous abortion, prevented her from integrating such information, and blocked further inquiry.

Another such case of selective blocking, but in a positive sense, was Ms. Meta. She did not identify with the negative experiences recounted by the women in her family, particularly her mother, presumably because they had not gone through childbirth training classes.

> I don't even listen to them when they...[mention] the problems they had in labor. My mother-in-law had a very difficult time, and it was... hard on her. She...really dramatized the whole situation. It was bad also for my mother; ....she went through a lot of pain.... It was just a whole different experience; it wasn't...the same thing that I am going to go through.

Ms. Meta made the clear assumption that she would have an easier time in labor and refused to consider the possibility of difficulties. At the same time, however, she wished that she did not have to go through labor.

Often the expectant mothers were upset by "horror" stories told to them by other women. Ms. Zeff related her mother's description of Ms. Zeff's own birth.

> I was a breech birth and…was going to be a C-section…. She told me about how she was in labor for 32 hours, and how she was screaming and beating on the bed, and how after a while they just couldn't control her anymore….. I gave her such a hard time and…this and that and the other. And my grandmother…said, I know you'll be glad when it's all over….. I wanted… [my] baby more than anything in the world, but after I had that first child, I said I would never do this again. It was so horrible. I just don't believe…it [labor] being that bad.

Ms. Zeff felt resentful about having such gory details of childbirth inflicted on her and thought that they were "uncalled for." Throughout her pregnancy, the rift between Ms. Zeff and her mother showed no sign of healing. Ms. Zeff expressed hostility toward her mother whom she perceived as a rather cold and stern woman, one who was generally nonsupportive and who did not help her to prepare for childbirth in any way. Other researchers have noted that when a mother conveyed such extreme childbirth evaluations, the gravida often felt less prepared for labor and delivery (Levy & McGee, 1975). Dissimilarity in the mother–daughter relationship also is associated with greater prenatal and postnatal adjustment difficulty (Nilsson, Uddenberg, & Almgren, 1971). However, it did not necessarily follow that mothers who described their difficult childbirths to their daughters were unavailable or punitive. Some mothers were happy that their daughters were better prepared and hoped that they would have a better experience than their own.

6.1.3   Books and Films

Most women read something related to childbirth, if only the pamphlets distributed by the clinic. All the childbirth education instructors with whom the women worked suggested a few standard books to read, and films were shown in class. The amount and kind of reading completed by each gravida depended greatly on her educational level and available time. Ms. Eaden was typical of the group in that she read in order to visualize and anticipate labor. She talked about her interest in reading books that would help her "to tell if you're really in labor." Ms. Eaden had read one such book early in her pregnancy and said that her husband wanted her to read it again and go to childbirth classes as well. She also felt that she would "get more out of it [reading the book] the second time." While speculating about labor, she said:

> It's hard to imagine what a contraction feels like…. Right now I'm thinking about when they [contractions] are going to start, what I'll be doing, if I'm going to be ready for it with my hair clean – and it won't be in the middle of the night or something.

Some participants' reading was wide ranging. Ms. Banor said that she read *Birth* and at least ten other books on childbirth until she became "bored" with the repetition.

And then I read a book on nursing by Karen Pryor, Nursing Your Baby. A couple of the books were more centered around the biological processes of the…fetus…. And two or three were just around different people's birth experiences….. Others, kind of like encyclopedias, told a little bit about everything. And then I read a couple [of books] by people whose philosophies give the foundation for childbirth without fear….

Ms. Banor was, in fact, well prepared for labor. Her husband, a social psychologist, seemed to have encouraged her in her reading. Another participant, Ms. Jabon, and her husband also read extensively and thoughtfully. She noted that in *Our Bodies, Ourselves*, it was suggested that the woman sit up during labor so that gravity could do some of the work.

I was asking about this, and he [the doctor] said something like 'Oh, my dear, surely you don't expect us to jack you up like a car and work on you that way, do you?' …. It irritated the hell out of me because I thought, Well, if hospitals were really designed for the welfare of women, that is exactly what they'd do – they'd jack you up and work on you as if you were a car. Instead of being [placed] for the ease of the physician, what would really be the concern is the ease of the patient and getting the baby out.

As Ms. Jabon's comment suggests, on occasion reading led to conflict with the medical staff.

A few women, like Ms. North, read nothing at all. Some tended to read excessively, perhaps to ward off anxiety. Ms. Katen's style of reading was a case in point. She was particularly afraid of losing self-esteem and control in labor, and of being coerced and interfered with; moreover, she worried considerably about her own health. She said:

[When I read about]…other people going through it….it was kind of scary to think that… such an intense thing…was going to happen…. Like I would read it, and then maybe a couple of days later go back and read it again because it had left a bad flavor in my mouth when I read it the first time.

Ms. Katen would read the same "scary passages" repeatedly, apparently to confront her feelings and achieve clarity. The result, in any case, was that she came to feel that she was well informed.

…. the best thing that I've got going for me is that I am well informed…. I have more of an idea than most all the women that I've ever spoken to about what to expect, and that John is somewhat informed and he is looking forward to being with me.

Similarly, Ms. Bode also did an extensive amount of reading, and even read a new medical obstetrics book. She tended to identify with women who had problems during pregnancy.

You read about birth defects…, even imagining harelip or something like that…. That's the main reason I want my pregnancy to be over, because it's been very pleasant…. When I first started reading it [an obstetric text…], I not only read the normal pregnancy parts, but I also read the problem pregnancy parts.

Ms. Bode admitted that such reading made her more anxious about the well-being of her baby, and she stopped reading on the advice of her sister. She was concerned about birth defects throughout her pregnancy.

In addition to attending classes and reading books, wives and husbands were encouraged by childbirth education instructors to practice breathing exercises.

Most women practiced with fair to moderate consistency, and many felt that they could have been more conscientious. A few women were well disciplined. Ms. Santa stated that she and her husband tried hard to do her natural childbirth exercises. She said: "We practice breathing together…every day, but sometimes we don't and that is not too good. Still, he looks forward to it." Ms. Eaden practiced alone or with her husband to a taped recording that her husband had made.

> My husband has really helped me out a lot in the sense that he has taped the exercises for me and recorded it. We have a whole program worked out, so I can do my part of the exercises without taking up his time, and then we can practice together at night. So I do them in the morning. It's so easy to hear his voice tell me what to do. If I taped it, it wouldn't have meant anything to me.

Some husbands put up considerable resistance to practicing exercises, and a few wives hardly practiced their exercises at all. After her baby was born, Ms. Carre admitted that she had not practiced.

> [I]…was not practicing up the way you're supposed to be…because I am notoriously bad on practicing anything. And I did not really practice my breathing…and when they'd say, 'Well, let's try a little accordion something or other,' I would say to my husband, 'Is that the five or the three?' He says, 'Haven't you ever read your book?' [I said] 'No.'

Ms. Carre had strong wishes to have her baby without labor and was not at all interested in preparing herself for "something unpleasant."

Ms. Gale, on the other hand, was overly meticulous about details. Describing how she and her husband practiced, she said:

> He's concentrating and I'm concentrating on getting it down to something that's comfortable for both of us. I think we've decided not to be too picky whether I'm breathing out exactly at the right second, but whether it's regular, whether I'm relaxed. The beginning was sort of like we were trying so hard to get every second exactly right, and we both realized that it was a little ridiculous because I was getting out of breath too, just concentrating on when I was supposed to be relaxing.

Ms. Gale harbored a fear of death during or after delivery. She knew that her fear was irrational and tried to work through it. She admitted in the postpartum interview that "on and off through the pregnancy" she had "worried about dying during labor." For the women in this project, extreme anxiety either precluded preparation or was associated with overpreparation.

The amount of reading done by the women did not always parallel the amount of exercises that they practiced, because they read primarily to gain knowledge and practiced in order to acquire coping skills. Practice was facilitated by the husband's interest, encouragement, and participation. It is noteworthy that when women in another research project had greater knowledge about childbirth, the father of the child attended delivery significantly more frequently (Rautava, Erkola, & Sillanpää, 1991); these women also had significantly fewer newborns that were small for gestational age. Attendance at childbirth education classes by women often appeared to diminish fears about pain, injury, and death, although this outcome depended on the instructor who taught classes. After completing classes, gravidas were sometimes overly concerned with managing and maintaining self-control during labor. Common childbirth themes, as reported by DiMatteo, Kahn, and Berry (1993), include women's reports of loss of control, and of unexpected pain and emotional reactions. In a Taiwanese population of expectant parents who were administered a childbirth expectations questionnaire the results showed five areas of expectations pertaining to the caregiving environment, labor pain, spousal support, control and participation, and medical and nursing support (Kao, Gau, Wu, Kuo, & Lee, 2004).

Lederman, Harrison, and Worsham (1995) and Lin and Cho (2008) found, as might be expected, that primigravidas reported greater anxiety and concerns about feeling prepared for labor than did multigravidas in every trimester of pregnancy. Lin and Chou (2008) replicated these findings.

6.1.4   Other Practical Steps

Preparation of a layette was a key activity in preparing for childbirth and the baby. Some women enthusiastically organized layettes, while others procrastinated. Differences in performing this task tended to indicate each gravida's preparedness for the newborn. Ms. Penn, for example, saw the obvious connection between her lagging practical preparations and her psychological state of readiness for having the child.

Most women considered the need for additional help at home after their baby's birth. A few gave no thought to how they would manage afterward. In one such instance, Ms. Tell showed a high degree of general anxiety, which thwarted constructive preparation of any kind.

6.2   Planning for Labor: Maternal Thought Processes

Planning refers to specific thought processes – fantasies, doubts, and fears – that the gravida confronts and her coping methods in meeting the challenges of labor.

6.2.1   Thinking Versus Avoidance of Thinking About Labor

Just as it is a developmental step for a woman to imagine herself as a mother and, as Rubin (1967a, 1967b) described, to "try on the role," it also is a developmental step for her to anticipate labor in fantasy. These steps are understandably difficult for the primigravida. There appears to be a relationship between the practical and psychological aspects of planning for labor. If a woman can project her imagination into the labor scene, she will be more likely to prepare herself for labor. The act of making practical arrangements also facilitates her fantasizing.

When considering the role of fantasizing about labor, it is important to determine the type of fantasy being experienced at each level of development. Some relevant questions include the following: Is the fantasy being used to reach a reasonable level of confidence so that obsessive thinking about the risks of labor diminishes? How does the gravida's fantasy change over time?

For example, in the third trimester most women change their focus of concern from the baby to labor and what it will be like (Maloney, 1985). Usually there was only intermittent concern about the imminence of motherhood. Ms. Allen, in talking about her changed concerns during the third trimester, said:

> New ones [areas of concern] come up as each stage of the pregnancy goes along. It seems like...things that bothered you before aren't problems now.... I am not really focusing on the breast feeding so much anymore as I am on the delivery part. And I guess when that's over then I'll probably be worried about the other one.

One of Ms. Yuth's diary entries indicated her increasing focus on labor.

> Lately, I've been thinking more and more about going into labor and the delivery of my baby. I feel I am ready for it and can handle it, but at times I wonder what will happen if I lose control.... I feel I am prepared for labor and anything that goes with it. I am really looking forward to the birth of our child and anything I have to go through will be worth it when our child finally arrives.

Ms. Uman, who appeared to be exceptionally well prepared for labor, was less able to fantasize about the baby and became preoccupied with thoughts about labor.

> I now project myself into a more realistic setting. I find myself thinking more in terms of time spent in the labor room as well as trying to picture the actual delivery. It is still difficult to imagine myself in the role of a new mother.

In fact, she went on to say:

> [I am]...plagued by a sense of disbelief. It is much harder now to accept the fact that in a few weeks the baby will actually be here.

The focal point of her thoughts about labor varied. Ms. Uman visualized labor in terms of a scene with her husband and herself in a room. She said:

> I think a lot about that setting and us working together and doing the contractions together and trying to manage together.... I worry a lot about transition and that kind of thing, ...about losing control and not maintaining my perspective..... I think quite a lot about what the experience would be like of pushing the baby out and seeing the baby born, and I can imagine it would be very exciting and very thrilling.

During the third trimester, it was a common experience for many participants to fantasize about labor with some anxiety, to think about working with contractions, breathing properly, handling transition and pushing, maintaining control, and to think with excitement, about the baby being born. The anxiety of these women generally was balanced by their excitement.

It was not uncommon for some women to pass over thinking about labor and delivery and think only of the baby. Several women in the project sample avoided thinking about labor, often because intense anxieties were aroused. Ms. Tell was terrified of labor and had not thought about it yet "because I don't want to."

Another woman, Ms. Dann, claimed that she seldom thought about labor and did not think about delivery.

> Whenever I think about it, I think about being in the labor room. I never think about delivery. There's two ways I visualize myself in the hospital. I visualize myself either in the labor room, like on my side or something, going through contractions, ...going through labor. Or I visualize myself afterwards...after the baby is born, like upstairs in the postnatal room.

Ms. Dann often wished that she were not pregnant because she was apprehensive about sustaining both her career and her marriage. She also was concerned about mothering her child, but she accepted the fact that it was too late to do anything about it. She admitted that as far as problems were concerned, "mine [my way] is not to deal with them, but just wait."

Ms. Penn was aware that her inability to visualize herself in labor or with her child was tantamount to her general "unreadiness" to have a baby. This inability concerned her, and in her diary she wrote:

> I keep thinking about my unreadiness for this baby – both mentally and materially. It seems so unreal at times. It's almost as though these months of growing, kicking, etc. will end, but I have a very hard time visualizing us with a child, a family. Maybe this is common with 'first-timers,' but regardless, it is something I must come to grips with myself; Jim can't really help on this one.

Ms. Carre found it hard to picture labor because she did not like to dwell on unpleasant events.

> ...I really cannot get a mental image of myself actually being there in labor, which I think is just as well because I could really see myself getting in a panic about it...... I have all my life thought it would be so nice if you could have the baby and not have to go through that.... Gee! It's too bad you have to go through all that horrible business to have a baby.... I mean, who would want to go through that!

Even though Ms. Bode had read excessively about labor, she found herself too busy to think about it. Actually, she avoided thinking about labor because "it was a long way off, and I didn't have to think about it too soon." She thought about labor mainly in the interview sessions. Despite attending classes, Ms. Bode was unable to assimilate the information. She admitted in her postpartum interview that she had had "no realistic preparation for labor." In talking about the task of maintaining control in transition, she said: "I'm sure it was introduced in the class, but I must not have registered with that particular fact, which is an important one."

A number of women never thought about labor, but only of their babies. Ms. North not only refused to talk to other women about labor but, with no apologies, also refused to think about labor. "I just think about the baby. I don't think about any pain or nothing [sic]. I just think about the baby."

Ms. Ely "never" thought, she said:

> ...of things being related to labor.... My thoughts and feelings... are much more directed toward after the baby is born because labor is such a temporary process; and I'm much more concerned about how we're going to treat the baby afterwards and take care of it and teach it.

Ms. Hayes freely admitted that she avoided thinking about labor. Instead she said: "[I will focus] on the child after delivery." She went on to say: "Other women talk about]…terrible things in labor, ….. I had never given it any thought. I don't know why. Maybe I just blocked it out." Ms. Hayes frequently wished to have her baby without having to go through labor. In fact, she would not have minded having a Cesarean delivery.

Other women did not think about labor, but appeared to think only about delivery. Ms. Vale, for instance, who was obsessed throughout the interviews by the thought that the doctors might injure her with their instruments during delivery, was aware that she was blocking out thoughts of labor.

> I think that the delivery has got me a little bit [afraid]…. Really labor doesn't…. I haven't really thought or even been concerned about the labor part of it. It might be really bad, but that's the part that I haven't really…[thought about].

However, excessive thinking about labor also appeared to interfere with the preparation for labor. Ms. Gale not only overpracticed, but also overprepared for labor in general. She thought about labor continuously.

> When I think about it, I usually am thinking about doing the exercises at the right times or wondering sort of exactly when I'll start using this technique, but feeling fairly confident that I'll know when I need it. Every once in a while I'll think about the monitor, and what that'll be like. I guess the other thing that I wonder is how my husband will do in his coaching role…. In the middle of [the class], I wasn't so sure he was going to be as good as I thought he was at the beginning, and now I have…come around again to thinking that he will be a good coach. But I've had my swings of wondering whether he will do as well as I expect him to, or whether I'll be disappointed, or if he will be disappointed.

Ms. Gale warded off her anxiety about labor not only through obsessive preparation, but also through obsessive thinking and discussing of the pros and cons, vacillating from one position to another. She managed well in labor and delivery, but became unnerved during the postpartum period.

It is important to understand that, in purposeful thinking about labor, a woman begins to prepare herself for separation from the fetus. One indication that she is reaching this stage is when she becomes anxious for the pregnancy to end. Ms. Fair stated that she was impatient about her baby's impending birth.

> I just would rather get it over with. I think that's the point where you know you are going to finally see the baby. And I really want to see the baby; I want a short labor.

Ms. Meta also wrote in her diary about the agony of waiting for the first signs of labor.

> People keep calling and asking when I'm going to have that baby. I could easily get depressed thinking about it, but I try and keep busy so I won't. My husband has been a great help reminding me we are really in no hurry and the baby will come when he or she is ready.

Wanting the pregnancy concluded is not necessarily indicative of the gravida's impatience to see her baby and her successful separation from the fetus. For instance, Ms. Penn assiduously avoided thoughts of labor and was impatient for the pregnancy to be over, but she never appeared anxious to see her child. However, she attempted to look at certain rewards associated with having a baby. She wrote:

> My main feeling right now is just to get the thing going and over with. However, running through my mind have been thoughts about who we'll call and what we'll tell them [about

the newborn]. (Skip over the bad part and look forward to the fun – [I] think psychiatrists refer to that as a defense mechanism!)

As previously noted, Ms. Penn was extremely anxious about mothering and worried that her child might drive her crazy and be a "monster" like other people's children. Her rating on identification of a motherhood role was assessed as low.

Some women who avoided thinking about labor were well prepared, however, for their babies. Often their avoidance of thoughts about labor and their concentration only on the baby were not so much a product of ambivalence about motherhood, as a manifestation of their anxiety that something might happen to their child during labor and delivery. Perhaps their anxiety, which led to both avoidance of thoughts about labor and a preoccupation with labor, was due to the feeling that they did not have adequate information about the process of labor and delivery (Lunenfeld, Rosenthal, Larholt, & Insler, 1984). Rofe, Blittner, and Lewin (1993) referred to this as an approach–avoidance pattern, which indicated maternal conflict related to labor, particularly about the possible consequences of childbirth, such as pain and loss of control. Anxiety appeared as the root of Ms. Meta's ambivalence regarding pregnancy.

> I want the baby, but…nine months is just too long..…. I'm very excited about having the baby, but not about being pregnant or going through labor…. [In some ways] I'm looking forward to going through labor..… I probably wouldn't mind having a spinal or something…. I want to have the feeling of the baby being born…. I think I really want to go through it, but I could stand to be pregnant just a month, and then have the baby.

Ms. Meta had some concern about "safe passage" for her baby. Her dreams suggested some fears of losing her baby during delivery. Thoughts of a perinatal complication which occurred when she was born precipitated her concerns, and her wish to avoid the labor process. Otherwise, it was evident that Ms. Meta eagerly anticipated her baby. Her motherhood role identification rating was high, and as evidenced by her diary, she was simultaneously eager for and dreading the first signs of labor.

A few women expressed the feeling that they would just as soon remain pregnant indefinitely. Despite Ms. Lash's considerable discomfort during pregnancy, she did not feel ready for labor.

> I want labor later. I'm not ready yet. Physically I would not mind having it right now because it would get rid of a lot of physical pain that I've been having, but in terms of other things, I would just as soon that it wait for a while.

By "other things" Ms. Lash meant the responsibilities involved in caring for a baby. Similarly, Ms. Eaden was not "anxious" for her baby to be born for fear that the child would disrupt her marriage. In discussing her anticipation of the baby at delivery, she stated:

> It will be exciting. I look forward to it. I'm not anxious for the baby to come. We're pretty well prepared as far as what we have;… the baby's room is fairly well ready, …but I just cherish these days. I just love them. I wouldn't trade them for anything. I figure these are our last days together and I just can't get over that pretty soon it is going to be three instead of two..… You read so much about babies changing relationships; what if it was a drastic change and it came between us? I hope it doesn't.

Actually, Ms. Eaden was delighted with her baby following delivery and immediately established a strong bond.

Although it appeared that Ms. Bode was readying herself for delivery and separation, she stated that the main reason she wanted her pregnancy to be over soon was so she could ensure her baby's well-being.

> I've enjoyed being pregnant, so it's not that I want to terminate my pregnancy, but I just want to make sure that the baby is all right, then it can go back in and stay awhile. I really want to carry it. I think the health [of the baby] is the big thing that I think of.

Ms. Bode found it hard to think about labor and her baby. She lapsed into what she called "prepartum depression" whenever she thought about being at home alone with the baby. Moreover, she had some difficulty in establishing a motherhood role. Despite these obstacles, she did effect a separation after birth. In her postpartum interview she said:

> It was still one unit, the baby and me, and I don't think it really hit me that there was a baby for a long time – until yesterday [delivery day].... I can now look at her a little bit more as an individual than I could have yesterday even. We named her on Tuesday.

In this statement, Ms. Bode's effort toward separation is apparent, but in her following statement it also is clear that she experienced difficulty with immediate bonding. She claimed to be surprised rather than disappointed.

> It was kind of like I didn't have the instinct because I thought I would be able to treat her more as an individual and less as a part of myself. And I really feel that that is important in raising children, and so maybe that's why it didn't bother me so much that I couldn't part with her.

Ms. Bode, in other words, associated her lack of maternal instinct with her wish to see her child as an individual, apart from herself.

In summary, thinking about labor was a means of trying to understand and prepare for labor, of maintaining control during painful contractions, of envisioning the baby's birth with excitement, and of sharing the experience with one's husband. Such thinking was associated with constructive preparation, even though labor may have been anticipated with a combination of eagerness and dread. Thoughts that were particularly disturbing to mothers, and that may have interfered with constructive anticipatory coping measures included apprehension about becoming a mother, fear of pain in labor, and anxiety about conforming to medical policy. When these concerns occurred, they tended to take precedence in the gravida's thoughts to the exclusion of other aspects of labor. Avoiding thoughts about labor was related to feelings of general unreadiness for motherhood or to a predominant concern for the well-being or "safe passage" of the fetus, a task identified by Rubin (1975). Excessive thoughts concerning safe passage were associated with previous pregnancy loss or deviations from the norm during the gravida's own birth or, as reported by Areskog, Uddenberg, and Kjessler (1981) during the birth of a close relative or friend. Expectant women who experienced obsessive thoughts about "safe passage," either could not absorb and integrate facts about labor or they simply ignored such facts. They usually had a difficult and/or prolonged labor.

In this sample of women, excessive preparation – obsessively thinking and rehearsing for each detail of labor – was related to knowledge of a friend's or family member's previous traumatic experience in labor, as was the case with Ms. Gale, whose mother died shortly after the birth of her second child. Overpreparation was associated with prolonged labor, but this finding was not consistent for all women.

6.3   Congruence Between Fantasy and Reality

The gravida's preparation for labor was evaluated, in part, through comparison of her prenatal description of labor to the reality of the actual experience. The evaluation further depended on how each woman integrated the information she was able to glean, and how imaginative and verbal she was. Of particular interest was her concept of uterine contractions during labor, and how closely her expectations approximated reality.

6.3.1   Labor Contractions

Ms. Santa had an accurate concept of labor. She gave the following criteria for recognizing the onset of labor and how it progresses.

> You'll notice some change like…a change in your bowel habits, or…. your mucus plug will come out, or possibly your water can break and you have small contractions. Generally your contractions are about 15 to 20 minutes apart…. As soon as they are 5 minutes apart for an hour, then you call the hospital and generally they will tell you to come in…. Then your pains will get longer and shorter apart. If your water isn't broken, they'll break your water and put a monitor on you…. About the last hour is transition – that is when your pains are the longest and [with] the shortest amount of time between, ….and they are the hardest….. Transition generally lasts only an hour or two, and then after that you get to push for a while…. And then they take you into the delivery room. Then you get to push and the baby comes out.

Ms. Katen, who had read many accounts of labor, had a better idea than most women of what to expect.

> I have a feeling that it [the contraction] is going to be like a muscle, not a spasm, but an actual muscle movement. I am going to be able to feel something moving from loose to tighter to more relaxed…possibly from back across the front and then subsiding.

Ms. Jabon, a dancer, had a strong sense of her body, and the way she imagined labor was exceptionally accurate.

> [The contractions] build, and then they go back down again and recede, and they grow in intensity. And then also in the course of your labor, not only do the individual contractions grow in intensity, but then the general intensity of the contractions supposedly increase through transition, and then theoretically it is better after…transition. I guess I imagine it will be like menstrual cramps…, only I imagine that they will be quite a bit more intense….. Once you have gone through transition, they are easier to manage, but I would also think that you would be so affected…that youwould be in (a different world or a different sphere.)

Some women had only a vague idea of what contractions or the pattern change of contractions are like. Ms. Ely, for instance, found it hard to imagine what contractions would be like.

> I don't think of them as painful exactly, just like pressure or something like that, ...like the baby is putting pressure on you, ...pushing to get out..... I guess it would be sort of like a bowel movement, only really a lot stronger than that.

Ms. Vale was confused. She felt that contractions would not be much worse than the cramps she was having near term. "[The cramps were like]...a bowling ball was being forced in my stomach. I can't imagine that they would be too much worse than now." She thought that delivery would be either "the most difficult [or]... relieving – which will be really wonderful."

Ms. Dann knew that contractions would be stronger and longer than what she was experiencing with Braxton-Hicks contractions.

> [I think]...the beginning stages are going to be the hardest because towards the end you really can't think about it too much; and if you don't have that much time in between contractions...to think about it, then it's almost like you can deal with it because it's coming so quick.

If agreement exists between a woman's fantasies about labor and the real experience, then she will be better prepared for what is to come. If she is confused, vague, or mistaken about the processes of labor, she will be less prepared for the labor experience. One way of assessing a woman's understanding of labor is to evaluate her concept of contractions. The concept of contractions may be difficult for primigravidas to imagine, because for them the experience of labor is an abstraction, an unknown. Many women used menstrual cramps as an analogy to early labor. Others anticipated a general tightening of the muscles or backaches. Most women knew that contractions become more painful and frequent as transition approaches.

6.3.2 Work and Pain

Another way of evaluating a woman's concept of labor was to assess the extent to which she viewed labor as work and pain. Ms. Santa had a realistic view of labor. She was prepared for work and would persevere. In describing herself, she said:

> [I am]... the kind of person that if I want something really bad, I work at it until I get it. And that's what I feel about my baby. I want it so bad, I'm so excited that I'm going to do it.

Ms. Aaron saw labor as a "working process" in which "the woman does most of the work." When asked to imagine the interviewer as pregnant and to describe labor to her, she said:

> It's important to stay calm through it all. You shouldn't be afraid to show emotion if you feel it. You shouldn't be afraid to talk to your doctor about medication if you need it..... I would tell you not to be afraid, that it [labor] is a very natural process and not to be afraid.

Ms. Katen was prepared for work and an active role during childbirth.

> I want to be able to help during the delivery. I want to be able to push and I don't want
> forceps used unless they are absolutely necessary. So I don't want them to numb me so
> much that I'm of no assistance to them.

Ms. Katen was, however, willing to accept help.

> [To have]... someone to tell you when to push and when to take a breath and when to
> stop.... I'd like it to move quickly and then [get it] over with. I'd like to do a good job.

The desire to be flexible and to play an active role in labor usually was indicative
of good preparation for labor and a positive self-image. However, Ms. Katen, the
woman just quoted, also had fears of losing control, of being coerced, and of losing
self-esteem. Moreover, she was belligerent in asserting her needs. She was under
significant stress and did, in fact, lose control in labor. According to Wuitchik,
Bakal, and Lipshitz (1989), cognitive activity and fears during latent labor are
predictive of the efficiency of both latent and active labor.

Besides anticipation of work, most women anticipated pain. Ms. Cole knew that
labor would be uncomfortable and painful, but felt that she could bear it because of
the excitement of birth.

> I know it's [labor] going to be painful, but I don't know to what extent.... I... really think
> it's wonderful that something like this comes about.... I really feel proud.... I'm... anxious
> right now [about complications] more than anything.

Ms. Eaden said that she was not frightened of the prospect that labor would be
painful.

> I don't think of it [labor] as pain;... it doesn't really bother me. I figure, 'Sure, it's going to
> be there; you can't have a baby without it, so just learn to do the best with it that you can.'

Ms. Yuth also expected some pain during labor.

> [Labor is]... going to hurt some, but I don't think it's going to be as much a painful ordeal
> as some make it out to be. I think I'll be excited and want to see my baby.

Ms. Yuth was confident because she had handled pain well in the past.

Ms. Raaf viewed labor as a natural process that involved pain and work.
She thought:

> [Labor]... is probably going to be hard, but it is perfectly natural. I can get through it okay
> because... that's the way babies have [always] been born. So if everybody else could do it,
> I can do it too.

The perception that the time-limited nature of labor would help with endurance
of pain and discomfort was quite common. Ms. Inis was not afraid of the pain in
labor "because I know that it won't be that long ..... It will be worth it...even if it's
12 hours of pain." Ms. Ely believed she could endure the pain. "[I can]... tolerate
a relatively high amount of discomfort as long as I know there's a limited time
period."

Not all the gravidas were prepared for pain and work. Ms. Hayes wanted to be
as comfortable as possible, wanted no "trauma" in labor, and wanted others to do

the work. She stated that she often wished she did not have to go through labor, and that she did not have a "terrible fear" of a Cesarean. "I sort of look at it and say, "Just knock me out" and it will all be taken care of; it would be easier. I have no desire to go through it if there were a way not to."

Ms. Acton said: "I don't know what it is like for other women. I like to think it's going to be better.... I don't want it to be too hard." She hoped that labor would not last more than "four or five hours."

> [I hope that I will not be]... in any pain at the time, and that things will just sort of happen rather normally and not [present] any problems. And that's what I envision happening.... I don't know if it will.

Ms. Bode also engaged in wishful thinking about labor. She shared her impressions: "[Toward the end of labor the contractions]...are stronger, but I am not sure they are more painful the further you progress into labor." She did not know which part of labor was commonly recognized as the most difficult. As mentioned earlier she did not seem to have heard what was said about transition in labor in her childbirth preparation class.

6.3.3 Risks and the Unknown

Awareness of the risks involved in labor is part of a realistic approach. Ms. Faber was prepared for risks, but this awareness did not overwhelm her. She occasionally thought that something might be wrong with her baby.

> ...you don't always assume that everything is fine,... you have to know that there is a possibility that something might go wrong. I think that if I were to have lost the baby or terminated the pregnancy anytime before the first five months,... I could have handled it a lot better than I could now because I'm really excited about it, much more attached to it.... I don't think that anything is wrong; I think that once in a while you have to think of the possibilities.

Ms. Xana was frightened of labor, but handled her anxiety by telling herself that she had no alternative. In her postpartum interview she recalled: "[At the onset of labor I was]... excited,... but in the back of my mind scared because this was really it. There was no turning back."

Ms. Katen felt that the "unknown elements" of labor were "scary." In fact, she had no idea what contractions would be like, what the pain would be like, or how long labor would last.

> There are a lot of factors that you just don't know about when you first conceive, and won't know about until it's toward the end and all over, and even then medical people can't tell you when you are going to deliver... or what your labor is going to be like;... it varies from woman to woman.... I can talk to and have questions answered by my physicians.... I think a lot of women go into this blind, and they are scared to death; and they are alone.... I have an advantage I think because I know more and I've done that exploration.

Ms. Katen was realistic about the "unknown elements" and coped with anxieties by finding out as much about labor as she could beforehand.

Ms. Santa described her initial thoughts about labor as "... facing the unknown."

> You were going through something that you have never been through before and it was
> going to hurt. It was more or less 'what's it going to be like?'... People tend to exaggerate.
> [You think], 'Is it as bad as what everybody says?' But I never was really scared or anything.
> I was never really afraid.

Although the unknowns of labor did not frighten Ms. Santa, Ms. Eaden was affected by the uncertainty of labor. She said:

> Not knowing tends to be upsetting I think. You want to find out more about it.... I can't
> say... I was really afraid of the idea of it. It's mostly not knowing what would happen.

Ms. Allen realized that "[Labor is]... different for everyone, so I really can't say how it is going to be for me." Accepting the unknowns in labor meant accepting potentially wide variation in the labor experience.

6.3.4 Doubts and Fears About Labor

Being realistic about labor and accepting work, pain, risks, and the unknown inevitably triggers doubts and fears. When a woman avoids or represses these normal emotions, it is expected that she will be poorly prepared for events in labor. What matters is not the doubts and fears, but their intensity and pervasiveness and how she handles them. When fears were intense, it was interesting to observe if women used reality testing to reduce the pressure which resulted from their feelings.

A majority of women reported that they had concerns about themselves and their babies, but that these concerns were fleeting, not obsessive. Ms. Cole, for example, although occasionally worried that she might have a stillborn, did not dwell on this concern; she looked forward to labor and felt that her major strength was her positive attitude.

Many women believed that a fetal anomaly, a Cesarean delivery, or a prolonged labor were the worst circumstances that could befall them, whereas others felt that the worst possible outcome was the possibility of not sharing the experience with their husbands which, by comparison, reflected a more optimistic viewpoint.

Ms. Uman, aware that fear can intensify the pain in labor, said: "I am more fearful now that labor is approaching, and convinced that my fear will cause pain."

6.4 Level of Confidence Regarding Labor

Overall, the feelings expressed by these gravidas indicate that the best psychological preparation for labor is a healthy awareness of the realities of labor – an acknowledgment of work, pain, and risk, balanced by a sense of excitement and expectation of the final reward. When there is obsessive fear or strong ambivalence about the reward, the process of labor may be either dreaded or regarded with superficial optimism untempered by a realistic grasp of the situation. In either case, the woman's level of confidence and her feeling of preparedness are low.

Essentially, the gravida's level of confidence is tied to her self-image and hence to her ability to crystallize a motherhood role. Consequently, high expectations for her performance do not ensure that a woman will handle labor well. High expectations sometimes can result in fears of losing control and self-esteem, and make labor more difficult than it otherwise might have been for the gravida. For example, Ms. Bode read a great deal, but did not transfer her knowledge to an anticipation of what childbirth would be like for herself, or how she would cope with challenging events. She experienced a more lonely, frightened, and longer than average labor.

Ms. Raaf was more realistic about the demands of labor and cautiously optimistic about her ability to handle it. She felt that she would do as well as other women in labor.

> ... and that might be bad, because I'm sure there will be problems that maybe I have anticipated, but pushed to the back of my mind.... I'm probably more optimistic than I should be, but I just sort of feel that we can do it.

Ms. Oaks was confident of her high tolerance of pain. She viewed labor as a natural event and felt that she was keeping it "all in perspective." She said: "I have cultivated, hopefully, a positive, healthy, natural-event type attitude that would help me through labor." Ms. Oaks fully believed that her mental attitude would make labor less difficult.

Ms. Banor considered labor to be a small price to pay for the baby, and "not even really a price to pay because it's kind of like a new experience."

Looking forward to labor with high anticipation is characteristic of mothers who welcome their babies with little ambivalence and who plan for labor. This also indicates that psychological separation from the fetus is occurring. Ms. Inis felt that "planning" and "looking forward to" labor were factors that would make it "easier."

Several woman who had attended childbirth classes viewed labor and delivery experiences as some of the most important moments in their lives, and they wanted to be aware of what was occurring throughout. For them, labor was rewarding. Ms. Inis, for example, said that she would not take medication:

> [I don't]... want to be groggy and not able to do what I'm going to learn and what I'm going to practice.... I just don't want to miss it. Even if it hurts, it's not going to be for that long, and I really want to experience it. I would never want to be put out.

The idea that labor and delivery are natural, exciting, and mysterious was common. One expectant mother, Ms. Uman, referred to the concept of children witnessing their siblings' deliveries.

> I think actually it would be a good deal because it would dissipate a lot of fears that children have formed about birth for one.... I mean it would certainly dispel the old cabbage-patch theory.... If you present the situation to them as being very natural and exciting, they are going to find it very exciting. If you present it to them as being something that is awful, they are going to react in [that] way.

Far from anticipating labor with excitement, a number of women had wishes, fantasies, and dreams of having their babies without labor. This did not mean that they were not prepared for labor, but for reasons associated with anxiety, particularly fears of injury and death, labor was not seen as exciting or rewarding but as something to be met by "gritting your teeth and facing the worst." Ms. Meta often wished that she could have her baby without going through labor. She had worked through the developmental task of establishing a motherhood role for herself, and she perceived conflict only in her relationship to her mother. Because her mother had predicted the worst for her in labor, it was not surprising that Ms. Meta avoided thinking about labor.

Ms. Zeff, who felt frightened and unprepared for labor, wrote in her diary:

> I know that I will never have another child until I get in to the correct state of mind. I was always quite independent, slim, active, the women's lib type. Several people have told me that they never imagined me being pregnant. Next time I plan to enjoy the experience. I will have to be ready next time.

It is evident that preparedness for labor is, in part, a state of mind that can be developed. A case in point was Ms. Penn who dreaded labor, but was able to use classes to develop a more positive attitude. Ms. Penn said:

> I don't dread it [labor] as much as I used to. I think I'm becoming more accepting of it. I think the classes are helping me to understand what's happening... and why you'll have these feelings because it is all necessary.... I don't have a choice;... it's something that is going to happen whether I want it to or not.... At this point you can't out. But I'm not looking forward to it, no.

Eventually she came to see labor simply as an unpleasant task.

> I get more and more awkward every day – but on the other hand I'm kind of afraid of the whole thing. No choice though, so I hope it is soon. I've always been that way about things I really don't want to do but have to – get it over with as soon as possible!

Moreover, Ms. Penn expressed no sense of reward at the end of labor. It was noted previously that she was not ready to separate from the fetus because, in reality, she was not ready for the baby. In Ms. Penn's case, labor could not be viewed as a rewarding and exciting experience because the end result, the baby, was not greatly desired.

6.5   Envisioning the Challenges of Labor for Oneself and the Fetus

For most of the gravidas, thoughts during labor focused predominantly on how they would fare in labor; however, prior to and during the experience there were variations in the extent to which gravidas thought about the fetus and the trial of labor. Asked if she had feared for herself when she was in labor, Ms. Eaden replied:

> [I]... pushed it out of my mind, not intentionally; it just drifted out.... There were times that I worried about the baby, our baby when I was in labor, and I'd think things aren't going quite as well, quite as fast as they should, especially when I was pushing. And I'd tend to become a little frightened then, [thinking] the baby should be born, but the doctor knew what he was doing.... It did run through my mind the baby was having a hard time.... It's difficult for a baby to be born.

Several women expressed concerns about the possible adverse effects of analgesia and anesthesia on the fetus. Ms. Ely said that she would not like to have a caudal.

> [The medication]... can get into the baby's bloodstream and I'd... rather avoid that if I could 'cause I feel the baby is going to have a hard enough time, you know, coming out into this strange new place'.

In general, the women either maintained a flexible stance or were adamant about not receiving medication in labor.

Ms. Hayes, however, insisted prenatally on caudal anesthesia in order to ensure a relatively easy time in labor. "[I am]... going to let the doctor and the nurse worry about the baby, and I am going to hang in there until it's born."

There appeared to be a relationship between the amount of thought and caring about the fetus-newborn and identification of a motherhood role. High anxiety and fears for oneself tend to preclude consideration of the fetus. In addition, the gravida's own self-esteem is related to her concern for the fetus-newborn.

In cases where the mother's foremost thought was the well-being of the fetus-newborn, due to a history of abortion or other complications, her concern about labor both before and after the event was minimal. Ms. Aaron said in the postpartum interview:

> Once the baby was born, I quit thinking about that phase of the whole affair [problems of control and breathing in labor] and started thinking ahead to what this all meant now that our lives were changed and that we had this baby finally.

Her residual doubts about adequacy as a mother also diminished with the birth of a healthy newborn.

Several mothers whose thoughts had not dwelled on the fetus were sometimes compelled to reconsider when the medical-nursing staff noted fetal heart rate deceleration. Recalling this moment, Ms. Gale said that she did not feel "panicky." Instead she said:

> [I]... was glad he [the doctor] had ruptured my membranes because I knew that that would speed things along. I guess I really became aware about the baby... I guess I really started thinking about the baby and that was the most important thing, and I thought to myself, 'Gee, I wonder if the baby is going to be in trouble and I have to do something drastic,' if they have to do surgery. And if they said that I needed a cesarean, I would have said, 'fine.' I guess I became really aware of the baby.

The shift in focus away from herself and her fear of death was facilitative for Ms. Gale.

> The direction of my efforts changed because I wanted to cooperate completely with them – whatever they were doing for the baby's sake.... I just wanted to cooperate with labor as much as I could. And... I think that also... I was concentrating better – that even though the contractions were stronger and it was harder and harder work, all the time I felt that I could do it.

Despite her tremendous fears, this experience actually enabled Ms. Gale to broaden her outlook and to adapt.

6.5.1 Dreams About Labor

It was common for the gravidas to dream about labor in the third trimester, especially if labor was a conscious preoccupation during the daytime.

Several women had what could be called "journey" dreams, in which they traveled down dark roads or dark corridors to unknown places. These dreams were about the journey to be taken in labor, or, more generally, about the journey or step to be taken in order to reach the state of motherhood, or about empathy with their own birth or the birth of their infant.

A few women actually dreamed of labor itself and these dreams could be termed "labor rehearsal" dreams. Ms. Gale recorded a dream about delivery in which she remembered "working hard to push the baby out."

> My husband and my doctor were both there. It seems the dream was repeated several times but I can't remember the details. It seems like maybe the dream was a rehearsal of the work I would have to do.

A significant number of women who dreamed about labor had what could be called "labor anxiety" dreams. The feeling of threat often took the form of a person (usually a man) who broke into the woman's house or who followed her. Ms. Fair dreamed that a burglar tried to get into the back door of her house.

> It scared me really badly and when I went to scream I found that I couldn't and I was also unable to move to wake up John. I felt like I was going to pass out when I woke up and found myself sitting up in bed looking at the door and no one was there.

In discussing her dream, Ms. Fair said:

> [The dream may have meant]…that I'm fearful of being in labor and unable to do anything or ask John for help. The dream left me with a really helpless, down-and-out feeling that lasted a long time.

Ms. Fair's ratings on the scales of fears of injury and death and fears of loss of control and self-esteem indicated high conflict. Her motherhood role identification and preparation for labor ratings were extremely low. In another very detailed dream, Ms. Fair was in the labor ward with other women and her husband was coaching her. A doctor tried unsuccessfully to dismiss her husband and then gave her saddle block anesthesia without her knowledge. Ms. Fair suggested in her associations that her dream meant she felt prepared to deliver by herself, and that the doctors would not have their way (regarding her husband's presence or the use of anesthesia). In fact, Ms. Fair was fearful and mistrustful of "hard," "uncaring" doctors and nurses, and wished to function alone; at the same time she was afraid of being alone.

Ms. Uman had several journey dreams, one of which seemed to express her uneasiness with the unknowns in labor. In this dream she, "an inadequate swimmer," was canoeing downriver. "As we go downstream I am very nervous and fearful as there are no life jackets, and I am afraid of moving water. We have to duck under several old, rusted bridges. As the dream continued, Ms. Uman transferred herself to a lagoon which was safe, but she was alone. [I]… cannot find those who accompanied me. I am fearful they have been swept downstream and, panicking, run searching for them."

She offered an explanation: "The river, with its unpredictable currents, resembled both the irrigation canal near the farm where I grew up, and the Huron River. In both places there have been incidences of drowning due to the current." Because Ms. Uman saw her fears of the unknown in childbirth as the most difficult aspect to handle, the dream may have depicted her fear of the unpredictable facets of labor and her anxiety about being helpless in the face of unknown dangers ahead.

Ms. Zeff was frightened by the approach of labor and became anxious when she found herself alone at home. Her rating on identification with a motherhood role was low, and ratings on her fears of injury and death and loss of self-esteem and control were high. Ms. Zeff also was fearful of harming her baby. Many anxieties were reflected in her dreams. For example, Ms. Zeff had a nightmare in which a vampire was chasing her.

> ... that a vampire was after me.... He was actually one of my neighbors; I was pregnant but living at home with my parents, and he lived next door. He was always looking at me whenever I left the house and I could sense that he wanted to bite my neck and make a zombie out of me. I wouldn't ever stay home alone but one day I had to. The vampire broke in and bit me. After that he disappeared and I wasn't affected by the bite. A few days later my baby was born with no face.

The fear of becoming a "zombie" signified almost overwhelming feelings of helplessness. As a result of being attacked in the dream, she gave birth to a baby with no face – that is, no identity. Ms. Zeff had a sense of some relentless evil being perpetrated against herself and her baby. At one point, she described strong feelings of revulsion toward the fetus.

Another of Ms. Zeff's dreams, presented in an earlier chapter, was of "hiding her baby in a neighbor's garden." This dream revealed her strong ambivalence toward the coming child. One other labor dream clearly expressed her reluctance to go into labor.

> Last night I dreamed that our car broke down en route to the hospital and we lived so far away. Actually I live five minutes away from University Hospital. In the dream, the contractions were coming fast and we couldn't find a cab. I awoke before the dream concluded, and I was very relieved to know that I was at home and still not in labor.

Ms. Yuth dreamed that she went into labor, but in the dream she was worried because her husband could not be reached. In reality, he worked odd shifts and she was concerned that she might have to go to the hospital by herself.

In another "labor anxiety" dream, Ms. Fair saw herself climbing a long, dark stairway littered with obstacles. She was laden with suitcases and she was very tired. When she finally reached the top, she encountered a woman who would not let her pass.

> [I had to]... jump onto the rail at the other side and then onto the platform in front of the door. I was very scared and hesitated for a moment ... I went down on the other side. I was terribly relieved that I had made it.

Ms. Fair interpreted her dream as follows:

> I guess the dream represents how I feel about labor and delivery–I'm scared, but I know I can do it. I have to do it alone and maybe I'm having to carry most of the burden, but I won't complain (if I can)....[It] was like a reward for having made the jump across the pit maybe that's how I see the baby once it's in my arms – as my reward for nine long months and a lot of hard work.

The "jump across the pit" is akin to the developmental step that some women make during labor itself, a step in which they take full responsibility for facing labor and delivery. Ms. Fair's dream also carried the meaning of "mature dependency" in that she realized that, despite the support of those around her, it essentially was her and no one else who would do the work in labor.

Labor dreams were of the wish-fulfilling type when women dreamed of labor as an experience with no stress. Such dreams could be termed "euphoric labor" dreams. Ms. Hayes dreamed that she was in the dentist's office to have a front tooth treated, "and they had to numb a nerve from the top of the skull and remove it from the scalp down. They used Novocain and there was no pain. I was awake and just had to rest two hours after."

Earlier, it was described how Ms. Hayes avoided thinking about labor and wanted a caudal, or to be "knocked out," because she feared that she would fall apart under the stress of labor. She rejected any thought of "problems or anxieties" in labor, and none appeared in her dream.

Ms. Banor had several labor anxiety dreams as well as euphoric labor dreams. In one dream she was in labor, "surrounded by lots of equipment and machinery and lights flashing. This seemed to continue forever. I don't know if anything was wrong with it [the baby] or not. I never saw it." Ms. Banor was afraid to buy baby things for fear that the baby would die in childbirth. She told of one apparently compensatory dream. "I was]... in labor and I saw the baby come out and it was a girl with a bow in her hair. Labor was fun." Ms. Banor wished for an easy labor and a healthy baby girl.

The gamut of euphoric dreams included several dreams in which babies appeared without labor – also a product of wishful thinking. Ms. Oaks had dreams in which she "missed everything," labor and delivery included. One recurrent dream is that of the baby having arrived "in full bloom," "as it were, without my having completed preparations, that is, buying the baby things yet needed." Ms. Oaks felt that her dream was "straightforward" in expressing her lack of preparedness for labor. She described another dream: "The baby's arm came out of my side, like through the rib cage. It was ready to be born and they had to put the arm back and say, 'you're not ready yet.'"

Ms. Tell stated that she had dreams all the time about waking up and finding babies without labor. "I just walked in the house and there they [the babies] were. At one time I dreamed that I had five babies and I just went out of the house for something and I came back, and they were all there just born."

Ms. Carre was aware that her dream of a baby without labor was connected with her tendency to avoid thinking about labor.

> I really cannot get a mental image of myself actually being there in labor.... I had a dream that I had delivered this baby, only I knew... that I was only four months pregnant, and it just didn't seem right,... but there was this nice normal, regular baby and I had to take care of it... there was no business of actually delivering it; it was just pop! there!

One dream, reported by Ms. Penn, could be called a "no-labor, no-baby" dream.

> I had had the baby and was still in the hospital, but the baby did not have any part in the dream at all. It was just me in the hospital, non-pregnant. In fact, I can't recall any of the other people (doctors, nurses) referring to the baby at all. I guess it all goes back to the inability to actually visualize myself having a baby – it is so hard to imagine.

In this dream, Ms. Penn seemed unwilling to go through labor or to have a baby. In fact, she had an extremely low rating on the identification with a motherhood role scale, she seemed to be ambivalent if not hostile about having children, and she was greatly concerned about interrupting her career.

It is understandably difficult for many women to fathom the unknown. The propensity to structure a concept of what labor will be like from abstract notions about pain, uterine contractions, time in labor, and endurance varies among women. Although such notions are not the only ingredients constituting preparation, the interest and ability to pursue them can substantially enhance feelings of preparedness and confidence.

As is the case in fantasizing about labor, dreaming about labor performs a vital function in a woman's preparation for labor by giving her the opportunity to rehearse labor, to express her anxieties about labor, or to reveal her wish to avoid labor. The expectant woman's dreams can inform her about her attitude toward labor, whether optimistic or pessimistic, realistic or euphoric, and they can prepare her for the anxiety that she may experience in labor.

6.6 Summary

Preparation for labor means preparation for the physiological processes of labor (cervical dilation, contractions, pushing, and so on) as well as the psychological processes of separating from the fetus and becoming a mother to the child. Because most women have some anxiety about facing the unknown, one way that they cope with this anxiety is to learn as much as possible about labor beforehand through classes, reading, and talking to other women. When specific fears emerge, many women try to test their fears against reality; this requires a certain degree of honesty and self-confidence to admit to and address these fears. Preparation for labor also can be seen in the way that a woman balances her expectations and general attitude against reality, in her concrete daily behaviors as well as in her fantasies and dreams. Severe doubts or intense and obsessive fears about performance in labor can interfere with a woman's preparation. If she wants her baby but is afraid of labor, she may procrastinate in practicing exercises, and avoid listening in class, reading books, and if possible, thinking about labor. She also may overprepare. If she is ambivalent about being a mother or about the baby interfering with her life, she may wish to postpone labor or prolong pregnancy. Her ambivalence can lead to guilt which, in turn, can intensify her fear of labor and delivery.

Fear may hamper mental preparations the gravida needs to undertake in order to trust her body's ability to perform successfully in labor (Kennedy & Shannon, 2004). Rubin (1975) described the need for the gravida to seek safe passage by gaining knowledge and performing behaviors during pregnancy that allowed herself and her baby to emerge from pregnancy and childbirth intact and healthy. The process requires a giving of oneself that includes a willingness to make personal sacrifices. Preparation for labor signals an important process in a woman's progressive maternal adaptation. In the last trimester of pregnancy Rubin (1975) described a process in which a pregnant woman develops a sense of boundary between herself and the baby that has not occurred up until this point. The process of elucidating separate identities for oneself and for the baby requires an immense investment of oneself (Rubin, 1975). A woman who is self-centered or has low self-esteem may find it especially difficult to make the transition to motherhood. Such a woman may find it difficult to take responsibility not only for her own life, but also for the life of her child. Thus, in several ways, the primagravida's preparation for labor bears analogy to preparation for motherhood.

A woman remembers her childbirth experience for the rest of her life (Trainor, 2002).

References

Aaronson, L., Mural, C., & Pfoutz, S. (1988). Seeking information: Where do pregnant women go? *Health Education Quarterly, 15*, 335–345.

Areskog, B., Uddenberg, N., & Kjessler, B. (1981). Fear of childbirth in late pregnancy. *Gynecologic and Obstetric Investigation, 12*, 262–266.

Crowe, K., & von Baeyer, C. (1989). Predictors of a positive childbirth experience. *Birth, 16*, 59–63.

Delke, I., Minkoff, H., & Grunebaum, A. (1985). Effect of Lamaze childbirth preparation on maternal plasma beta-endorphin immunoreactivity in active labor. *American Journal of Perinatology, 2*, 317–319.

DiMatteo, M. R., Kahn, K. L., & Berry, S. H. (1993). Narratives of birth and postpartum: Analysis of the focus group responses of new mothers. *Birth, 20*, 204–211.

Greenfield, D., & Tepper, S. (1981). Childbirth preparation at urban clinics. *Journal of the American Medical Women's Association, 36*, 370–376.

Hodnett, E. D., & Fredericks, S. (2003). Support during pregnancy for women at increased risk of low birthweight babies. *Cochrane Database of Systematic Reviews*, Issue 3. Art. No.: CD000198. DOI: 10.1002/14651858.CD000198. (Article appears to no longer be available to readers).

Joyce, K., Diffenbacher, G., Greene, J., & Sorokin, Y. (1984). Internal and external barriers to obtaining prenatal care. *Social Work in Health Care, 9*, 89–96.

Kao, B., Gau, M., Wu, S., Kuo, B., & Lee, T. (2004). A comparative study of expectant parents childbirth expectations. *Journal of Nursing Research, 12*, 191–201.

Kennedy, J. P., & Shannon, M. T. (2004). Keeping birth normal: Research findings on midwifery care during childbirth. *Journal of Obstetric, Gynecologic, and Neonatal Nursing, 33*, 554–560.

Kuczynski, J., & Thompson, L. (1985). Be prepared! *Nursing Mirror, 160*, 26–28.

Lederman, R. (1996). *Psychosocial adaptation in pregnancy: Assessment of seven dimensions of maternal development* (2nd ed.). New York: Springer.

Lederman, R., Harrison, J., & Worsham, S. (1995). Differences in maternal development in primigravid and multigravid women. The Society of Behavioral Medicine, San Diego, CA.

Levy, J. M., & McGee, R. K. (1975). Childbirth as a crisis. *Journal of Personality and Social Psychology, 31*, 171–179.

Lin, C. T., & Cho, F. H. (2008). A comparison of maternal psychosocial adaptation among pregnant women with different gravidity. *Hu Li Za Zhi, 55*(6), 28–36.

Lunenfeld, E., Rosenthal, J., Larholt, K., & Insler, V. (1984). Childbirth experience – Psychological, cultural, and medical associations. *Journal of Psychosomatic Obstetrics and Gynaecology, 3*, 165–171.

Mackey, M. C. (1990). Women's preparation for the childbirth experience. *Maternal-Child Nursing Journal, 19,* 143–173.

Maloney, R. (1985). Childbirth, and education classes: Expectant parents' expectations. *Journal of Obstetric, Gynecologic, and Neonatal Nursing, 14,* 245–248.

Melzack, R. (1984). The myth of painless childbirth (the John J. Bonica lecture). *Pain, 19,* 321–337.

Nilsson, A., Uddenberg, N., & Almgren, P. E. (1971). Parental relations and identification in women with special regard to paranatal emotional adjustment. *Acta Psychiatrica Scandinavica, 47,* 57–78.

Norbeck, J. S., DeJoseph, J. F., & Smith, R. T. (1996). A randomized trial of an empirically-derived social support intervention to prevent low birth weight among African-American women. *Social Science and Medicine, 43,* 947–954.

Rautava, P., Erkola, R., & Sillanpää, M. (1991). The outcome and experiences of first pregnancy in relation to the mother's childbirth knowledge: The Finnish family competence study. *Journal of Advanced Nursing, 16,* 1226–1232.

Rofe, Y., Blittner, M., & Lewin, I. (1993). Emotional experiences during the three trimesters of pregnancy. *Journal of Clinical Psychology, 49,* 3–12.

Rubin, R. (1967a). Attainment of the maternal role. Part I: Processes. *Nursing Research, 16,* 237–245.

Rubin, R. (1967b). Attainment of the maternal role. Part II: Models and referents. *Nursing Research, 16,* 342–236.

Rubin, R. (1975). Maternal tasks in pregnancy. *Maternal-Child Nursing Journal, 4,* 143–153.

Schachman, K., Lee, R., & Lederman, R. P. (2004). Baby Boot Camp: Facilitating maternal role adaptation in military wives. *Nursing Research, 53,* 107–113.

Stolte, K. (1987). A comparison of women's expectations of labor with the actual event. *Birth, 14,* 99–103.

Trainor, C. L. (2002). Valuing labor support. *Lifelines, 6,* 387–389.

Wuitchik, M., Bakal, D., & Lipshitz, J. (1989). The clinical significance of pain and cognitive activity in latent labor. *Obstetrics and Gynecology, 73,* 35–42.

Chapter 7
Prenatal Fear of Pain, Helplessness, and Loss of Control in Labor

Fear of pain, helplessness, and loss of control in labor have been the subject of a number of research studies (Beebe, Lee, Carrieri-Kohlman, & Humphreys, 2007; Entwisle & Doering, 1981; Gagnon & Sandall, 2007; Hodnett & Osborne, 1989; Pacey, 2004; Raefael-Leff, 2001; Scott-Palmer & Skevington, 1981; Sherwen, 1983; Willmuth, Weaver, & Borenstein, 1978; Windwer, 1977). As regards fear of loss of control, some of these investigations, however, focused on locus of control – external or internal – or on political, social, and environmental control rather than maternal emotional and physical control. Research on locus of control is contradictory concerning its relevance to prenatal adaptation or outcomes. Entwisle and Doering (1981) used and then entirely dismissed the measure of locus of control because it was unrelated to other childbearing variables. Sherwen (1983) reported that body image attitudes following attendance at childbirth class were not influenced by locus of control, whereas Scott-Palmer and Skevington (1981) reported a relationship between locus of control and length of labor. In the research projects discussed in this book in Chapter 1 (and Chapter 11), the emphasis is on control as it pertains to a woman's body and emotions and, to a lesser extent, on social control with regard to maintaining interpersonal status and respect. This focus reflects the content of the gravidas' expressed apprehensions concerning control in labor and delivery.

Women have many choices today regarding the management of labor, including both analgesia and anesthesia. It should be noted that most women in our research projects did not receive epidural anesthesia in labor, which is currently more common. Thus, the content of this chapter, and the maternal concerns and common themes identified may be more applicable to women anticipating a more natural childbirth experience, with or without the use of analgesia.

The variable, fear of loss of emotional and physical control in labor, was a conspicuous concern among participants in our research projects and in other research samples (Beebe et al., 2007; DiMatteo, Kahn, & Berry, 1993; Pacey, 2004; Slade, MacPherson, Hume, & Maresh, 1993; Trad, 1991; Willmuth, 1975). In the research projects presented in Chapter 1, it was moderately correlated with other variables: fear of loss of self-esteem in labor, relationship to husband, and preparation for labor – and highly correlated with fear of helplessness in labor. Thus, we have combined fears concerning control, pain, and helplessness in to one psychosocial dimension. Fears of pain, helplessness, and loss of control also were correlated to

R. Lederman and Weis, *Psychosocial Adaptation to Pregnancy*,
DOI 10.1007/ 978-1-4419-0288-7_7, © Springer Science+Business Media, LLC 2009

uterine activity and duration of labor In this regard, Chertok's (1969) extensive work on behavior and pain showed that "good control" versus loss of composure favors a "good confinement." Slade et al. reported that satisfaction with labor was associated with the parturient's ability to control panic, as well as other aspects of personal control, such as control of pain and the use of exercises. The range of coping strategies nulliparous women use to manage pain and anxiety in labor is similar to those employed in prior prepregnancy nonlabor pain experiences of their past, and can be identified as potential labor resources prenatally. They included a wide range of coping resources encompassing cognitive and behavioral strategies (Escott, Spiby, Slade, & Fraser, 2004). In contrast, childbirth education classes focus almost exclusively on learning a novel set of behaviors and skills. The pain of labor was seen by the women as threatening in itself, but it also was perceived as a trigger for the loss of control, especially if the pain became intolerable. DiMatteo et al. (1993) reported that loss of control and autonomy, and the unexpected pain of childbirth were common themes of laboring women. It was notable that the ability to maintain control assumed such a great deal of importance in the way the women thought about themselves in labor, a stressful situation in which it could be expected (within given cultural limits), that there would be some external expression of distress. Other common themes pertaining to anxiety regarding labor are concerns about the baby during labor, the length of labor, fears of pain or the return of pain, fear in anticipation of the approaching second stage of labor, fear of alterations in body image, and loss of dignity during childbirth, even in the presence of successful anesthesia (Capogna, Camorcia, & Stirparo, 2006).

Coping methods and the maintenance of control are important factors in maternal anticipatory management of labor. It is noteworthy that Beebe et al. (2007) report that childbirth self-efficacy (maternal self-confidence in being able to perform recommended relaxation or coping techniques in labor) was significantly related to levels of maternal trait anxiety, to the total score on the Lederman Prenatal Self-Evaluation Questionnaire (PSEQ), as well as to three of the PSEQ scales used in the research project: Concern for Well-Being of Self and Baby in Labor; Preparation for Labor; and Fear of Pain, Helplessness, and Loss of Control in Labor. The results showed that the greater the lack of maternal self-efficacy, the more anxiety the gravida experienced in relation to dimensions pertaining to labor fears and concerns. In addition, the three PSEQ scale scores were significantly predictive of a number of different pain management measures in labor.

Most methods of childbirth preparation emphasize the importance of control: breathing properly with contractions, pushing effectively at the right time, and using learned strategies to cope with the pain of labor and avoid medication (Lothian, 2006). In this context, however, control is understood to be flexible rather than rigid behavior, for here the intention of control is to cooperate with the body in order to facilitate labor. All but two women in our original research projects attended childbirth preparation classes; these two women attended two clinic classes taught by the nursing staff.

This analysis is an attempt to discern the meaning of control in labor in terms of the psychological dynamics and the extent of conflict that the gravidas expressed.

A distinction is made between women who maintained control for its beneficial effects, and women who suppressed, sublimated, or projected powerful feelings because their feelings were too frightening to contemplate, or because they felt a sense of resignation toward childbirth as an ordeal. The critical questions posed to the gravidas were the following: How and for what reasons did they wish to maintain control? What were their characteristic methods of coping?

In this section, maternal attitudes toward the following factors are assessed:

1. Loss of control over the body
2. Loss of control over emotions

Then, attitudes that suggest a fear of loss of control are examined. In particular, this discussion includes the following:

1. The mother's ability to trust the medical-nursing staff
2. The mother's attitude toward being awake and aware and toward the use of medication (analgesia and anesthesia) during labor.

7.1 Loss of Control Over the Body

Many women in our sample, aided by their childbirth preparation classes, were prepared for labor – for pain, work, risk, and the unknown – and they were excited about the coming events of labor. On the one hand, the women were prepared to maintain control when they could; on the other hand, they were well aware of some events that lay beyond their conscious control, such as when Braxton–Hicks contractions would appear, when the bag of waters would break, when transition would occur, and when they would deliver. They were prepared to be attentive to their bodies and to adjust their responses accordingly. The prevailing thought among the women was that labor is a natural event which takes its own course. Some women brought a habit of self-discipline to labor, one that was not rigidly conceived and that enabled them to work with their bodies. The fact that labor and delivery is time limited enabled many women to comfort themselves in moments of doubt, so that they did, in fact, find the strength to carry on – to persevere when labor proved more taxing than anticipated.

An example of someone who maintained masterful and unerring physical control during difficult labor was Ms. Jabon, the dancer. She was trained to expect high standards of performance from her body. When in labor and approaching transition, she was aware of preparing herself mentally for the critical point. "I think I was getting psyched up to get the show on the road, and I kept looking at the clock thinking, "Oh, I'll bet that it will only be another hour." The anticipated hour became several hours. When she reached the pushing stage, her concept of teamwork was well expressed.

> I thought that the nurse... was really fantastic and was extremely helpful, and I always thought that I pushed better when she was going through her whole thing of 'Take a breath in and breathe out, and push, push, push!'... I felt like I was being trained for a track match or something;... having that kind of support was really good.

In retrospect, she felt that her experience as a dancer had been helpful in maintaining control.

> I think probably there's the sense of discipline that maybe comes from having been in dance, that the show must go on, and you play your part, and you do your role;... it's like a performance you know. I'm sure that I was partially performing for him [my husband]. Mainly I knew that I had no alternative;... there was the recognition that what else could I do if I didn't keep breathing, or didn't try to keep thinking about that, I would have been just going nuts. Maybe that's the best answer: that if I didn't have... something I was assigned to do, or something to structure the experience, then what else would I have done?

When referring to a structured situation, Ms. Jabon meant using the right style of breathing at the right moment. She knew that if she breathed properly, as taught, she would maintain control; if she stopped breathing, then she might lose control.

Ms. Allen also had a positive attitude toward the coming labor.

> I am hoping that I'll be able to control the contractions, or be able to work with them. Some people say they are not all that bad, and other people say they just couldn't take the pain anymore. I don't know how I'll be reacting at the time. I guess it's something really hard to say since everybody is different.

She was afraid that if she was sedated or became fatigued, she might lose control over contractions. Fatigue was a common concern, especially if the labor should be of long duration, because fatigue sometimes led to a loss of control. A fear of fatigue is an indirect way of expressing doubts about the strength of one's body to endure.

Women were concerned about their ability to relax during contractions, which they had learned was important from their Lamaze childbirth classes (Melzack, 1984). Such a concern can prompt a cycle of projections, in which the more one worries about relaxing the harder it becomes. Ms. Vale described herself as a tense person and said that if she could only relax her body, labor would be easy.

> My first reaction was always just to tense up. I was just always tense whenever I'd have a female examination or anything like that.... If I could just relax with that [labor], I think that it would probably be a breeze.

Ms. Hayes he was afraid that she might be torn apart if she did not relax.

> I talked to Dr._____, and he had said that he feels that some women who go through natural and are not relaxing the pelvic floor properly, are probably tearing things. And that's why if you're not really into the whole thing, you should really have some anesthesia, because Dick and I were thinking you would probably be torn apart if you're that tension likely.

Ms. Hayes was not at all disconcerted about receiving anesthesia because she had little confidence in her ability to relax properly and maintain control during her contractions.

Women who lack confidence to cope with labor at home tend to come to the hospital in the very early stages of labor due to expressed uncertainty, pain, and anxiety Cheyne et al. (2007). Several women feared that they might lose control of the breathing exercises they were taught, as was the case with Ms. Jabon. Using the correct breathing techniques at the appropriate times is emphasized in childbirth classes (Melzack, 1984). Ms. Xana, for example, feared losing control of her breathing.

> I've kind of thought that I might lose control of the breathing. I can't picture myself screaming or anything like that.... It would be okay if I got right back on with the breathing, but to lose it altogether, I'd feel bad.

She imagined herself losing control: "getting all tight and not relaxing and... crying or something like that." Ms. Xana felt that losing control over her breathing would lead to fatigue and that, in turn, to giving in to her emotions.

To push at the correct time and not when the urge first appears – to control the urge to push – is stressed in childbirth classes (Beck & Siegel, 1980). The women had mixed feelings about this task. Some were a little anxious, hoping that they would be able to hold back, but then cooperate at the right moment. Ms. Santa said that nothing would hold her back from pushing because she was so eager to see her baby. Ms. Inis saw pushing as the most exciting part of labor. Ms. Zeff, on the other hand, had some qualms. She had harbored fears of injuring or tearing herself during this stage, but had overcome her fears by seeking further information.

> At the very beginning while I was pregnant, long before now, I did have the feeling of hurting myself.... But since then I've found out that there'll be local anesthesia and... things will be taken care of. I won't just rupture myself to death. And I have had the feeling of, in pushing down, maybe letting out excretion.

However, she felt that if she did lose control in this way, it would not be "the end of the world."

Ms. Bode was extremely worried that she might defecate during pushing which would signify a loss of control over her body, and that when the right time came she might hold back because of fear of embarrassment. Actually, she maintained good control during labor (which was important for her self-esteem), but lost it altogether in transition and demonstrated no inclination to regain it.

Recalling her labor, another woman, Ms. Raaf, said that she felt she was losing control at a certain point.

> [the staff was]... telling me not to push... and they were examining me. I was really close to losing control then. It was horrible because here I had my legs spread wide apart and they're telling me not to push... and I don't have any way to control [pushing]; it was really hard not to control it.

Ms. Raaf always liked to be in control of everything, and she very much feared losing control in labor.

One woman, Ms. Fair, said that she would not hesitate to push if she had the "urge," even if it was too early. In this respect, she was nonadaptive. Interestingly, however, Ms. Fair obtained high ratings, indicating relative mastery of fears of loss of control, loss of self-esteem, and injury and death in labor.

A generalized concern that the childbirth process itself might control the body was expressed occasionally and has been noted by Trad (1991) as well. Ms. Quins felt that there were obvious limits to her responsibility for the course of labor.

I've so little to do with the process really.... I'm used to controlling most of the things in my life, not everything of course, but you feel that you have some kind of control over the quality of what's going on. And if something bad happens, 90 percent of the time it is because you caused it someplace. And this – I have almost no control over it and it just really frightens me. If the child is deformed or ill, what can I do? I can't do a thing. I can take my vitamins every day. I just have to trust completely. It's out of my control. But in a way it goes on without me. I can't do much about it, and it usually turns out anyway which is really a miracle.

Although Ms. Quins surrendered to the mystery of birth, which emanated from precepts in her religion, she nonetheless wanted control over the events of labor.

Similarly, Ms. Ely found it distressing to tolerate lack of control over childbirth. She stated:

One of the main reasons that I wanted to take ... some kind of prepared childbirth training was because I don't like that feeling of being at the mercy of some kind of unknown force. And I think I'll feel much more confident about the whole thing if there is something that I can do about it...having some kind of control over the whole process.

Ms. Ely was anxious that medical decisions during labor and delivery might be made without her knowledge. Control was a theme that ran throughout all her interviews, including fears that she might lose control not only over labor, but also over herself, her baby, and her husband. Mothers' chief fears during pregnancy often involve themes concerning loss of control, pain, complications during labor, and the baby's needs for care (DiMatteo et al., 1993; Gillman, 1968).

In her diary, Ms. Ely recorded the following dream: "[I] had a dream that Tom and I were... on one of those tiny motorcycles like a Honda 50. For some reason, I had to drive it, but we were too heavy for it and I could barely control it, especially going up the little hill." In her associations, Ms. Ely said that if conflict existed between her and her husband over the baby (she had admitted earlier that she was afraid of losing ground with her husband), then the child would suffer: ".. the weight of it would fall on the kid, not on us, and maybe the baby won't be able to hold up under that, if we allow conflict between ourselves over the baby." Ms. Ely also was afraid of having a screaming baby because it would mean that she had lost control over the infant.

In summary, fear of the loss of control over the body meant the loss of control over contractions – not working with contractions, failing to relax between contractions, failing to breathe properly with contractions, or succumbing to exhaustion. The notion existed that if one lost control in these ways, regaining it would be exceedingly difficult. Loss of control also could mean pushing before second-stage labor or holding back at delivery. Loss of control sometimes was viewed as the consequence of either pain or fatigue, which indirectly conveyed doubt about the strength of the body to endure. In a few cases, loss of control was manifested as fear that the biological process itself might control the woman. It can be concluded, therefore, that there is an association between intolerance of the unknown and fear that the events of labor can take possession of one's body. In this regard, Wuitchik, Hesson, and Bakal (1990) found that women who reported greater prenatal fear of pain, helplessness, and loss of control were found to experience higher levels of pain and distress-related thoughts in labor. Beebe et al. (2007) reported similar findings.

7.2 Loss of Control Over the Emotions

Closely associated with loss of control over the body was loss of control over the emotions, such as crying, becoming hysterical, or being hostile to the husband or the medical staff. The unexpected emotional responses occurring in labor is a common theme in mothers' descriptions of labor (DiMatteo, 1993). Some women felt that if they lost control over their bodies during the labor process, they also would lose control over their minds or emotions or vice versa. There was conscious awareness of the symbiosis between body and mind. Ms. Uman, for instance, felt that too much anxiety might increase her pain in labor. Most women who had attended childbirth preparation classes accepted the concept that they could work with their contractions and handle the pain better through conscious control of breathing, so that medications might not be necessary.

A few women were confident that they would not lose control over their emotions in labor, particularly those who knew that they tended to remain calm in crises. Ms. Carre, for example, had no fear of losing her composure, because she knew that she would just "plug along" even under arduous circumstances.

The majority of women who felt confident in their ability to control their emotions, however, did not rule out the possibility that they might lose control in labor. Ms. Quins said, with regard to fatigue and stress, that "...I stand up better than most people. If I'm going on some camping trip or some disaster befell, everybody else falls apart and I usually can handle it." However, she qualified her stance.

> The thing that I don't know about is how much pain I can take. I'm an emotional person, so I think that that would make it difficult. When other people just don't say anything, I say it. I know my feelings. I show my feelings more than most.

Ms. Quins felt that if she did lose control in labor, she "would have every right."

> If you lose control, don't worry because that happens to a lot of people. But I can stand it [labor] because I could go on for a week. I can stand it, I'm sure.

While expressing tolerance, Ms. Quins at the same time viewed her characteristic of openly showing her feelings as a personal flaw.

Ms. Katen felt that she had good control over her emotions. "I'm generally calm in crisis situations where other people are freaking out.... I've been told that I'm a more calming influence or more logical about those kinds of things, like family distress or whatever." For her, losing control meant being irrational. But if she did happen to lose control in labor, Ms. Katen expected people around her to respect her state of mind and allow her to use her own coping devices to regain control.

> When I'm very angry, I don't like people around me being very, very nice…. I'd rather be
> alone or left to calm down a little bit rather than have somebody come around being sweet
> and trying to change me or the way I feel at the time.

Ms. Katen hoped that if she lost control, "it wouldn't last too long, but I think that it's an acceptable thing, and it'll be over with. Because I don't stay angry or irritated that long. It's like it happened, or it happens, and in time it will take care of itself." Ms. Quins and Ms. Katen exemplified the combining of control with flexibility. They were confident in their ability to maintain control, but if they did not succeed they would not flagellate themselves.

Several women believed that it would be quite natural to lose control, especially in transition. Ms. Fair, for instance, accepted a loss of temper as a potential natural outlet for herself. "If I lost my temper, oh, you'd know it. I have a good Irish temper, Italian and Irish together! I would just probably very bluntly and loudly tell everybody to get out and leave me alone." Ms. Fair did not think it so important to maintain control of her emotions in labor, and it was not temperamentally like her to do so.

Many women were not happy at the thought of losing their tempers because then they would lose face. Ms. Raaf stated that she could handle crises, but that she had delayed reactions. "Usually when I fall apart in a crisis is after everything is over. Then I sit and I just shake…. Usually during the crisis I handle it well." She definitely was more concerned about how she would behave in labor than about pain. Ms. Raaf said that she always liked to be in control, and she hated the idea of screaming women.

> I think I am more worried about the way I will act. I don't like to put on a show so to speak;
> I just don't like that. Plus, I always like to be in control over everything, and when I am not
> in control, I really feel uncomfortable with the situation. I don't want to lose control is the
> biggest thing I think.

Another woman, Ms. Lash, did not want anesthesia because she feared loss of consciousness, which was analogous to entrapment and death for her. She related a situation when she had been given gas by her dentist.

> … I went very, very far under with the gas; it was a bad feeling. I felt like I was being
> trapped, and I couldn't get out. I couldn't even talk; I couldn't make any noise because
> I was so far under. And I could just barely hear these voices in the back of my mind – of
> the dentist and his nurse – and I couldn't really make them understand that I was going to
> just zonk out any minute.

Losing control of the situation and of one's behavior also took the form of wanting to give up, of fantasizing about going home in the middle of labor, and of not being able to persevere against what might be mounting odds. These were common fantasies. Ms. Uman, who was anxious about the possibility of losing control, was able to counter her concern with her sense of excitement about the coming baby. Ms. Quins said that she imagined giving up and going home, but realized that she would have no choice but to go on. Ms. Fair said that she would feel badly if the thought of giving up occurred in labor.

> I think I've been preparing myself for a long labor and hard work long enough so that
> [wanting to give up] won't come in, but if it does, that would be it. Then I would get
> frustrated and say, 'Oh, to hell with it all. I want out!'

If she did lose control in this way, Ms. Fair said:

[I would not]... be too pleased with myself, but that would be the fear that I have of losing control.... Then if I lost control after that, then I would feel bad that all the exercising and all the practicing and reminding myself that it [labor] isn't a picnic – then that was all for nothing.... That would make me uneasy.

Several women feared that they would "fall apart" in labor or go crazy. Ms. Vale was afraid not only that she would be unable to relax, but also that if she did not relax she might "go crazy" with the pain as she did with menstrual cramps. She recounted how she lost control when she had had an abortion.

I just perspired, screamed – I just didn't think I could take the pain. I thought that I might die. I couldn't catch my breath.... But I just hope that I can keep it together [in labor] because if it's just that horrible, I guess I'll have to have something, or they'll have to alleviate it somehow, or I'll have to.

Ms. Vale admitted that she also "freaks out" at needles, and then proceeded to recount a nightmare in which men strapped her to a table. I don't know if they were going to operate on me, or if they were going to,... if I was in a crazy house.... I don't know." For Ms. Vale, loss of control was associated with the fear of becoming helpless, of being immobilized so that "things might be done to her" (i.e., that she might be maimed or killed by instruments). She had, in fact, been hospitalized for brain surgery at the age of four. According to Slavazza, Mercer, Marut, and Shnider (1985) being "in control" connotes active participation in labor, while being "out of control" connotes feeling useless or helpless, relinquishing completion of the delivery process to the hospital staff.

Similar to Ms. Vale, Ms. Hayes was afraid of losing touch with reality. In her diary, she wrote: "The description of what to expect in transition frightened me, as it was described as a time where you can "lose touch with reality and self-control." Later in her diary, just before her due date, she wrote: "I am getting anxious to have the baby. I'm somewhat 'falling apart' and not too willing to do anything. Ms. Hayes felt that she probably would panic or become hysterical in transition and not be able to "get hold of myself.' Thus, she wanted caudal anesthesia and felt that without it she could not maintain control. She also was concerned that she might go into a depression and not pull out of it.

I have had periods of depression in my life, and I'm afraid that if something really irritates me and I get depressed, I will get a little uncommunicative. It was a very horrible way of getting at people by not talking to them, or being mean – which I learned from my parents. I have made an extremely big effort to overcome that, but I don't want to get into that because I can get to the point where I cannot pull myself out of it and control it.

Ms. Hayes also feared that bodily damage might occur in labor if she was unable to relax.

The sense of being overwhelmed – of being bombarded in labor with too many happenings – was anticipated and dreaded by Ms. Tell. She felt: "Everything is going on at one time... the baby coming, trying to breathe, nurses and doctors, and examinations."

Ms. Vale was afraid that she would find it difficult to relax in labor: [There will be]… a lot of commotion.… I think that the less commotion around me, the more calm I can stay.… I have to always know what is going on… my concentration isn't real good. In this case, losing control meant losing control over reality as it became increasingly fragmented and chaotic (Richardson, 1984).

In summary, fear of the loss of control over emotions meant a wide range of things: simply showing feelings (seen as a weakness), childish behavior (seen as a regression), irrational behavior, inappropriate behavior (screaming, crying), hysterical behavior (panicking, "falling apart," "going bananas"), bizarre behavior (acting crazy), loss of consciousness, and depression (loss of activity). A number of women felt that if they lost control in these ways, they would be embarrassed and ashamed, a finding reported by others (DiMatteo et al., 1993). Deutscher (1970) reported that women looked upon labor and delivery as a "test to be passed," and a predictor of mothering ability. If they lost control, the women thought (1) it might prove that they were worthless, and decisions regarding themselves and their babies might be taken out of their hands; (2) they might be rendered helpless or trapped; (3) they might lose control over events or over a reality that could become increasingly fragmented.

Other women felt that a loss of control in labor was "natural" and even healthy because of unique circumstances, and that they would feel no sense of devaluation if they lost control. Nevertheless, they were determined to try their utmost to maintain control, to persevere, and to do "a good job."

7.3   Ability to Trust the Medical/Nursing Staff

Another measure of a woman's fear of loss of control was the extent to which she could trust the medical/nursing staff, her husband, and other people. It first was determined whether this trust was (1) a naive trust based on wishful thinking, (2) a mature trust based on reality, or (3) a lack of trust based on skepticism or paranoia. In addition, the interviewer distinguished between skepticism based on past negative experiences with hospitals and/or the medical/nursing staff, and skepticism based on misinformation or fantasy.

It was expected that women with naive trust would exhibit excessive dependency needs and little autonomous behavior. In mature trust, there is a balance between independent behavior and acceptance of reasonable dependency needs. In the absence of trust, there often is a belligerent exaggeration of independence and a refusal to accept any dependency behavior – usually accompanied by a need to be in control at any time and place, or there may be suspicion of the medical/nursing staff and of hospitals.

A frightening experience during hospitalization, especially when the person was a young child, can have lasting effects on attitudes toward hospitals and doctors. It can be terrifying from a child's point of view when doctors, presumably with powers of life and death, "take over" and "do horrible things" with instruments. In some women, particularly those who had had such early experiences, the fear of having contact with hospitals assumed phobic proportions.

However, most women felt at ease with the medical/nursing staff. Ms. Eaden believed that the staff demonstrated concern for her emotional as well as her physical needs.

[The nurses]... are great. They've all been very helpful; they answer questions,... they always ask; they don't wait for you to say if you have something on your mind and you don't really have the nerve to say it; they'll ask.

Ms. Meta was pleasantly surprised with the care she received from the hospital staff.

There's more attention than I figured would be given out. There's more concern that the doctors have than I had expected that they would have had. Dr._____ has been just great in answering questions.... I feel that I am in real good hands, and so I'm not worried about the doctors at all.

The medical equipment at the hospital gave Ms. Aaron confidence. "What was reassuring was to see all the equipment they had in the [labor] room... all the things that they had just in case something was needed." This was to be Ms. Aaron's first extended stay in a hospital. "I've never been operated on at all, and I only spent one night in the hospital itself, so the whole idea of a hospital is sort of an exciting new type of experience for me."

Trust in the judgment of the medical staff to make appropriate decisions does not imply passivity. Ms. Santa was happy with the medical care she received at the clinic because she felt that her wishes were respected.

I just feel really at ease. All the personnel, the nurses... with the clinic are really friendly, and they always ask you if you have any questions. The doctors are always eager to answer any questions that you have. They have a class beforehand. The public health nurse shows films and you can ask questions, and they have a nutritionist that you can talk to. If you go to a private doctor a lot of times, you don't get these little extras and I really appreciate them.

Although Ms. Santa was quite prepared to work hard at bringing her baby into the world, she also recognized her limitations and appreciated help; that is, she was at ease with her dependency needs. When asked what might make it more difficult for her to go through labor, she answered:

Sometimes it's easy for me to change my mind and want to give up if it gets really difficult. I guess it depends on my frame of mind, how I go at it. But if I have encouragement... I'm the kind of person, if someone is patting me on the back, it helps.

Ms. Santa felt that encouragement and support would help her maintain control.

Ms. Cole wished to maintain her independence as much as possible, but at the same time she talked about what she called "natural dependence" on "my husband, my folks, my family." "It's just a natural dependence that children have for their parents. I know my brothers depend on me to take them swimming and to take them fishing because my folks don't get out that much with both of them working...." Ms. Cole had to struggle to accept her "natural dependence" on people. She could not (with good reason) trust her husband and was wary of being placed in a dependent role for fear of being let down. She believed that one must ultimately rely only on oneself.

The ability to trust and to accept reasonable dependency needs implies cooperation with the medical staff as well as with the husband, who presumably is working with his wife as a team in compliance with what he has learned in classes. Many women felt that this supportiveness from their husbands in the labor room made a significant difference in the way that they conducted themselves in labor. Most American women indicate that the presence of their partner increased the meaning of their labor and delivery experience. Even if partners do not participate actively, women report their presence as important and special to the birth process (Ballen & Fulcher, 2006; Lavender, Walkinshaw, & Walton, 1999). What seemed most helpful was to have someone or several people, preferably those "close" to the woman, who always were present, and not coming and going during the course of labor. The presence of a supportive person or companion in labor has been associated with lower reported pain scores and lower state anxiety scores during labor (Hofmeyer, Nikodem, Wolman, Chalmers, & Kramer, 1991). In addition, women with continuous intrapartum support are less likely to have intrapartum analgesia and operative deliveries, or to report dissatisfaction with their childbirth experiences (Hodnett, Gates, Hofmeyr, & Sakala, 2003).

When reminiscing about her labor, Ms. Katen saw her husband as helpful, but only when "getting commands from two or three different voices of what to be doing."

> [The student nurse]... was there telling me to squeeze her hand, and she was saying Breathe, breathe, breathe! with him [my husband]. He was yelling at me, but I was yelling at everybody too.... It was just that she was there the whole time. She never left once she came in the room, whereas the other people were in, they'd look at the machine, and then they'd go out, or they'd come in, they'd look at something, and they wouldn't tell you what they were looking at unless you asked them.

Although frightened of loss of control, injury, and death in labor, Ms. Katen was well prepared. She found her husband generally was interested in discussing labor, but that he had difficulty acknowledging her physical limitations in pregnancy and meeting her special physical needs during labor. Therefore, it was not surprising that she found the nurse's coaching and care more helpful to her during labor.

A number of women expressed varying degrees of distrust associated with hospitals. At one time, Ms. Raaf had endured a traumatic experience with an abortion, during which she said that the medical staff seemed interested only in her money and made her feel as if she was merely a number. She described her suction abortion.

> ... and I told them that it was really hurting. And the doctor... just as much called me a liar. You don't even know what you're talking about.... the people that were there to help – there just wasn't any understanding or compassion or nothing whatsoever. I thought my back was going to break in half.... I've never had a feeling of pain like that before. I suppose that scared me, and the more scared I got, the more tense I got, and the worse everything was. It was horrible!

Ms. Raaf also had a "hospital dream" that took place in an intensive care ward.

> I dreamt I was taking care of a man on a respirator, who was unconscious. I don't know whether he was in RICU [Respiratory Intensive Care Unit] where I used to work, or E.R. [Emergency Room]. He suddenly awoke and started pulling his endotracheal tube. I tried to stop him, but wasn't physically strong enough and started yelling for someone to come and help me. No one would come and the man starting pulling on the rest of his tubes: foley, I.V.'s [Intravenous tubes], etc. I was still yelling when I awoke.

Although she gave no associations, Ms. Raaf clearly had an anxiety dream in which she was abandoned, no one came, and no one listened; this dream expressed the fear of being helpless in a crisis situation. Dependency-independency conflicts often are present in the dreams of pregnant women, and dreams about the unborn child generally occur in a context of anxiety, particularly during the last trimester (Van de Castle & Kinder, 1968). In light of her professional background as a nurse in an emergency room, it was interesting to note that Ms. Raaf associated the hospital paraphernalia with death and injury, in contrast to Ms. Aaron, for whom the medical equipment inspired confidence. Ms. Raaf stated that she typically handled crises well, but tended to fall apart afterward. Despite her nursing education, she had great personal anxiety about medical procedures. She also was afraid of losing control in labor, of making a spectacle of herself, and perhaps of alienating the doctors who were to make decisions concerning her. Nevertheless, Ms. Raaf managed to have some positive feelings about the clinic that she attended. She stated that she had confidence in the clinic. "[I know]… the reputation of this place and I know they have all the latest equipment." She also believed that not all doctors and nurses are uncaring. "There are good nurses and there are bad nurses, in the same way there are good doctors and bad doctors. I don't know any of the nurses here, so I don't know what it is like. In other words, Ms. Raaf was prepared to keep an open mind.

Ms. Fair did not trust doctors, finding them unfeeling, incompetent, noncommunicative with their patients, uncooperative, and negligent. About her own doctor, she said: "I hope he's not there by the time I deliver. I think he's a real lulu! He's the one who told me I was four months [pregnant] when I was three months…. I just think he doesn't know what he is talking about.

Ms. Fair appeared to have had bad experiences with doctors in the past, and even during her present pregnancy there had been some confusion regarding whether she was pregnant. She was quite prepared, however, to assert her rights. While pregnant, Ms. Fair went into the hospital for an appendectomy. Her husband said that she was "…really obnoxious on the recovery table." "He [my husband] said the doctor came in to tell me I wasn't pregnant, and I tried to climb out of the bed and hit him cause I knew I was. Ms. Fair admitted, albeit unwillingly, that the clinic was good.

> I think they try. Even the doctors, the questions that I do have and I ask, they are very considerate about it. Whether they think it's stupid or not, they'd never let me know… and they give me pretty straight answers most of the time, and I think that they have your welfare very much in mind all the time.

Other women also felt threatened that doctors might take control. Ms. Ely was concerned by what she viewed as male dominance.

> Sometimes they [doctors] are patronizing. I want to feel like I have some kind of control. I don't want the doctor to feel like he is running everything. I don't think I'll run into that here though. I haven't ever so far, not at the clinic.

Consequently, she was happy at the clinic.

> [the resident and interns]… are more open to you. Their egos aren't that involved. They haven't been in practice for 20 years. You don't feel like you are challenging their authority if you say you don't like some- thing, or you want to know more about something.

As previously noted, Ms. Ely was uneasy about being dependent in any way and fearful that she might become the victim of unknown forces. Her fears of loss of control were wide ranging. She tried, however, to develop confidence in the doctors.

Ms. Lash was fearful that doctors would rob her of her autonomy.

> I keep thinking that they would yell at me and give me an anesthetic or something and say, If you're not going to cooperate, we're going to put you out.... I guess I'm very leery of doctors; I'm very leery of what they're going to do to me while I'm not looking,... like putting me under when I don't want to go under, or like giving me pills to dry me up when I want to nurse, things like that....

As far as her care was concerned, Ms. Lash admitted that she preferred the personalized attention of her family doctor in the clinic.

> ... the only thing that has sort of been worrying me is that perhaps they [the doctors] are not really terribly aware of exactly what's happening with me since I don't have the same person every time. They are not so terribly oriented with knowing my situation personally.

A few years earlier, Ms. Lash had been in a hospital in a strange city and had felt very much abandoned and alone.

Many gravidas felt that hospitals tend to be over-mechanized and over-routinized, places where patients receive no personal attention. Ms. Uman, for instance, recalled a dream in which she found herself, following the birth of her baby, in a huge barn "which appears to be some sort of prison." In some women, the bodily sensations of pregnancy can produce "persecution dreams" in which they dream of being surrounded, caught, or in danger (Gillman, 1968). In that dream, someone explained the procedures involved when babies are brought to their mothers.

> A man behind the wire explains we will only be allowed to have the babies twice, each time for one hour. The scene changes, and I am still pregnant and outdoors. My mother has sent me over [to] the family doctor's house to see if he will accompany me to my next doctor's appointment, since he has retired and can no longer treat me.

Ms. Uman explained her dream.

> The barn probably represents in some form the hospital, where my activities will be somewhat restricted due to regulations and my physical condition after birth. Having the family doctor accompany me on my appointment probably symbolizes my mother's fear of American medical technology which she claims is far advanced where machines and dispensing pills is concerned, but lacking in basic common sense. Our family doctor, who just retired, is a compassionate man whose concern for his patients is genuinely personal.

A number of women who distrusted doctors altogether were not able to keep an open mind. Ms. Vale bluntly stated: "I just do not trust doctors and I don't trust nurses, and that's where it's at. If I had a little bit of faith in them, it would be another story. But it's really hard for me to find somebody whom I have any faith in whatsoever." Male doctors were regarded as authoritarian, "hard," "forceful," and as performing their duties in a mechanical way compared with female doctors, who were viewed as "gentle" and "caring." Ms. Vale once had an experience with a doctor who had made a serious mistake with medications. She had an extreme fear of instruments – needles in particular – and of being immobilized by straps or anesthetics.

Ms. Vale had been a "breech baby" and had had a series of brain operations at an early age because of a cyst that she understood had resulted from her own delivery. In recounting the details of these early operations, she said: "I hated that doctor. I was afraid of him. And he was very nice, just very clinical.... I don't ever remember any pain being inflicted on me; I just had to have my booster shots and things like that." Later, she had undergone a tonsillectomy and a facial operation to remove cysts. Each time that she was wheeled into the operating room she "freaked out."

> ... when they started putting those rubber things on, you know those cardiogram things [EKG electrodes]....I'm frightened of the instruments. I don't know where it's from... I guess I used to pass out when I used to get shots. But now shots don't bother me.

Ms. Vale became upset when she recounted these details, finding it difficult to separate one episode from another. Clearly, her early brain operations were responsible for her uncontrollable suspicion of doctors and hospitals, and she was not able, on a deeper level, to distinguish between her forthcoming hospitalization and the earlier ones.

At the other extreme was naive trust, wherein some women expressed unquestioning faith in doctors and felt that they themselves had no power of decision making at all. These women tended to be dependent and passive women. Ms. Zeff was terrified at the thought of being alone in labor, as well as later on at home, for fear that something would happen. The thought of having medical staff around her was comforting.

> I just don't think I'd be able to handle things, especially during the last part of labor. If I were alone, I'd just lay back and say Lord, take us both!... I picture doing something wrong. I picture something going wrong. I picture a hemorrhage, or the cord being wrapped around the baby's neck, or not knowing what to do if it came, or being sick to my stomach or something like that.... And my mother had delivered alone at home, you know. Maybe I should have talked to her about it, but I just never.... I'm never around her. I don't see her that much.

Ms. Zeff was afraid of being alone because she might lose control, "do something wrong," and harm herself and the baby. She felt that if left to her own devices, she was bound to do something wrong. Her fear of her own aggressive drives left unchecked apparently is what led to her dependency. Ms. Zeff's mother did not seem to serve as an adequate role model for labor, and had not been a supportive or available person during the pregnancy; Ms. Zeff felt that her mother did not care.

When asked if anything would prevent her from pushing during labor, Ms. Penn answered:

> No, because the doctor is not going to tell you to do it until it is okay to do it, when he has made sure, you know, the episiotomy or whatever, that you are not going to hurt yourself.... And hopefully when it gets down to that situation [pushing] I would be a little bit more aware that they are not going to tell me to do something that's not good, at least not on purpose.

Ms. Penn was not happy about having to take responsibility for her actions in labor. It was her husband who had taken the initiative in practicing breathing exercises and in most other matters in their life together.

In conclusion, the women trusted the medical/nursing staff when doctors and nurses answered or anticipated questions, gave individual attention, and respected their needs. Also, the staff was trusted when they were understanding and compassionate, made wise decisions, were reliable and responsible, and were available. The women hoped or expected the medical/nursing staff to treat them as adults, not as children, and to allow for maneuverability, flexibility, and some degree of autonomy. If a woman was suspicious because of a close relative's or her own negative experiences with hospitals, she often tried to keep an open mind because she knew that her situation was different from all past experiences. Women who could trust generally did not fear either loss of control or self-esteem, or injury and death during labor.

7.4   Attitudes Toward Being "Awake and Aware" and the Use of Medication

Control in labor without pharmacological aids is taught as a primary goal in many childbirth classes. According to Annandale (1987), the essential elements of patient control during labor and delivery include having all available information required to make informed decisions, and having the potential ability to make decisions contrary to staff preferences without incurring their disapprobation.

Fear of being given medication and anesthetics and lack of trust in the medical/nursing staff seemed to be parallel concerns, originating perhaps partly in prenatal classes. However, this combined fear of medication and anesthesia and distrust of the medical/nursing staff did not necessarily result in a woman fearing the loss of control. It was possible that she could lack confidence in her own ability to maintain control and still trust others. What appeared to be important was whether a woman feared that she would lose control and therefore felt responsible for problems that could arise, or whether she perceived natural causes or unknown medical factors as responsible for problems should her behavior deviate from expectations. Van den Bussche, Crombez, Eccleston, and Sullivan (2007) found that women who choose to use epidural analgesia during labor express a greater desire to "enjoy their childbirth," and "have a pain-free and relaxed childbirth." Importantly, the women electing to have epidural analgesia described a greater fear of being overwhelmed by pain during childbirth. The women choosing not to use epidural analgesia reported having more confidence in their ability to tolerate labor pain.

A wide variety of attitudes toward medication and anesthesia were observed, ranging from adamant refusal to explicit acceptance of any medication. The women gave various personal reasons for their cautious attitudes about drugs. The most common reason for a woman's ambivalence about drugs was that they might harm the baby (Lowe, 1989). Because a woman's attitude toward being awake and aware, aside from her concern about the baby, is a function of her basic perception of labor, her acceptance of dependency needs, her trust in the medical/nursing staff, and her self-image, it is important to learn not only whether she decided to have medication or anesthesia, but also the reasons for her decision.

A common reason for not wanting medication or anesthesia was that the woman was interested in and curious about childbirth, and did not want to miss anything; she wanted to be aware of all the events – to experience a great moment (Lowe, 1989). If anesthesia was given or a cesarean delivery became necessary, the women tended to feel keen disappointment. The following quotations are indicative of the responses given to the question: "How awake and aware do you want to be in labor?"

Ms. Wooly certainly wanted to be awake and aware. "I think it's [childbirth] one of the big moments in your life. I would kind of like to be around and know what's going on. I don't want to have people tell me how it was. I want to know for myself."

Ms. Aaron wanted to be alert. "It's going to be one of the most exciting experiences of my life and I can't imagine wanting to miss it."

Ms. Raaf wanted: "to be able to feel the baby and know when it first comes and be able to hear it cry."

Ms. Xana hoped to see the baby being born. "[I want to]… be able to breathe and do everything that I'm supposed to."

Ms. Fair said that she would feel cheated if she were not awake during labor.

I've waited so long for it, I just can't see missing out on the birth of the baby…. I put enough time and effort into… creating the thing and carrying it around with me. I… would really be upset if I didn't see it, and then all of a sudden 'here's your kid.' Oh really!

Ms. Banor wanted to be totally aware because she wanted to "know everything that's going on."

… First of all I feel it gives the baby a better chance cause… most medications are safe, but still it's better if you can do it without any for the baby. And then I think I'll be more responsive to my husband's directions if I'm totally aware. And the things that I've read… say that you have more of a feeling of excitement afterwards if you have been aware and experienced it, than if you have been drugged or anything.

Among her many reasons for not receiving anesthetics, Ms. Banor placed a high value on teamwork with her husband. All these gravidas looked forward to labor and delivery with much anticipation.

Many women stated that they did not want medication or anesthesia because they might lose control of their breathing pattern. For example, Ms. Xana said:

I've heard that doctors give women sedatives in the night so that they can get a really good sleep, but I don't want any because if I should go into labor in the night, I don't want to be drowsy and not be able to breathe right or something like that.

Ms. Xana wanted to be brave, and she also feared the effect of medications on the baby. Similarly, Ms. Allen was concerned about maintaining good control.

I feel that if I am sedated in any manner I am going to have a much harder time controlling the contractions and keeping on top of things…. I hope I don't get so exhausted that I am going to want to sleep because that too prevents you from keeping on top of things.

Ms. Quins did not want medications.

… It's only for one day; you can stand anything. If I can stand going to the dentist, I can probably stand this. It's only just time, and it's over with. I might lose control during the time, but I wouldn't give up – I mean you can't give up. I have no choice.

Ms. Quins was more concerned with her ability to endure labor than her capacity for control in labor.

Ms. Lash said that she would refuse medication for discomfort.

> I would rather just do it by myself than have any sort of drug in my body.... If they said that you are really going to have problems if you don't do this, or the baby is going to have problems, then.... But if they said you would probably be more comfortable, I wouldn't... basically because I don't feel that one should take any kind of unnecessary drugs. Like I stay away from aspirin or anything like that as much as I possibly can.... I've never been one to really need a lot of medication and my mom never was. It's sort of the feeling to tough it out rather than take the easy way out.

In other words, Ms. Lash said that she would refuse medications, not necessarily because of the baby, but because of her own high expectations of herself. She appeared to be patterning herself after her mother, who did not "take the easy way out."

Ms. Cole would agree to accept medication if the pain became unbearable, but stated that she would feel badly. "I think I'd call myself a chicken deep down inside, because you couldn't take... the pain." Ms. Cole also said that she would feel badly if she lost control in labor or if she lost her temper.

Ms. Inis wanted no medication for pain because she did not want to sleep between contractions.

> ... like they [in ... class] were talking about sometimes being offered a sleeping pill at the very onset of labor. I just think that would be really weird to do that. I'm just really quite sure that I'd never take anything. I can't imagine it being that bad that I would have to give in because I really wouldn't want to.

Here, again, taking medications meant "giving in." Ms. Inis wanted to be awake and aware to experience the entire birth, especially delivery. She looked forward to labor and did not want medication of any type. In addition, she was afraid of anesthesia, particularly the needles, that"... something would go wrong because of it, like paralization [sic] or something. I just didn't like it. I don't know what it is."

Several women refused anesthetics, not because they wanted to experience the entire birth process, but because they feared losing control. They did not look forward to the experience of labor; instead they feared injury or, in some cases, death. Ms. Bode wanted to be "mentally alert," not in order to see the baby born, but so that she could watch out for herself. "It's not so much that I [have] ... this overwhelming feeling to see my baby born. It's just to watch out what is happening to myself I think." Ms. Bode was anxious about losing control and specifically expressed a fear of bodily injury during labor and delivery. She had "always hated doctors."

Ms. Vale wanted to be aware during labor.

> ... because I'm afraid of anesthetics. If I wasn't so afraid of being put out – and like spinals and things like that – they really frighten me. I think that they would affect the baby. I felt that way before [childbirth classes] or anything like that. I think that that would be a horrible thing.

As previously noted, Ms. Vale, due to surgery in early childhood, was terrified of being injured, was frightened of doctors, instruments, and needles, and feared that she might be assaulted in some way if she were anesthetized.

Ms. Lash was afraid of being "knocked out," thereby losing control over her body.

> I'd rather have control of what's going on than not. I know just from talking to women who have fallen asleep between contractions. You wake up and you're right in the middle of a contraction. There's nothing you can do about it and you are at the mercy of the contraction at that point. And I would rather be in control of the whole thing rather than just sort of helplessly riding along.

It may be recalled that Ms. Lash was "mortally afraid of the dentist" because she had been given gas and had felt trapped. The worst thing that could happen to her in labor would be to "… forget everything I learned, for Gerald to forget everything we learned, and so just simply lose the whole thing, have to have an anesthetic, and that would be it." Loss of control was equivalent to loss of consciousness induced by anesthetics. Despite this overwhelming fear of anesthetics, Ms. Lash seemed relatively confident in the outcome of delivery, mainly because of her "ability to perform under stress" and her faith in her husband.

Paradoxically, some women who voiced many fears, particularly the fear of loss of control, were able to cope well with labor. Ms. Zeff was terrified of being alone and of losing self-esteem; she also was frightened of pushing and of being injured or dying in labor, as well as losing control. In addition, when talking of her doubts about mothering, she stated that she was afraid of harming her baby through negligence.

> I'll be the same way with my child. I'll leave her for a minute laying on the bed, and run to do something knowing full well she could fall off. You know like I said, I don't mean to do it to be cruel, but sometimes you just say Nothing can happen in that split second and sometimes it does, and I just hope and pray that it doesn't.

Despite Ms. Zeff thoughts that something terrible would happen either in labor or to the child if she turned her back for a "split second," she actually functioned well in labor. Excessive attention to detail, perhaps out of fear of impending disaster, can mask a fear of losing control. In fact, such women can function well in labor because they often make an intense effort to be prepared and maintain control of the dreaded event. According to Janis (1958), preoperative patients demonstrated that the "work of worry" – experiencing some anxiety and seeking information – helped them face stress and develop coping patterns before surgery, which subsequently enabled them to be more cooperative and adaptive. In this context, primigravid women who attended a psychoeducational program designed to alleviate labor fears and anxiety had significantly decreased fears: for themselves in labor, of coping during labor and delivery, concerning their babies, and decreased signs and symptoms of anxiety (Sharma, Sangar, & Bajwa, 1998).

Another group of women assumed a more moderate position and attempted to go through labor without medication and anesthetics, but were willing to accept them if necessary. This group tended to be more flexible and less judgmental of themselves for failure to achieve their goals.

Ms. Fair stated that she would not be upset if it became necessary to accept medication during labor.

> I don't expect to use it [medication]. In fact, I can't even foresee it happening, but if I thought I needed it, I wouldn't hesitate to ask for it, and I wouldn't feel bad about it.

Ms. Fair was reasonable about medication in spite of her suspicions of the medical/ nursing staff.

Ms. Yuth would accept medication, but was afraid of the effect on her baby.

> I'm kind of afraid that if I get medication for it [the pain], then it's going to influence the baby because it's just a little tiny thing. I'm a bigger person, and they'll give me an adult dose. Then it might go into the blood stream of the child and hurt it or something.

Reassured that medication generally does not harm the baby, Ms. Yuth said that she "wouldn't feel so bad" if she had to take it. This reaction was common. In her diary, Ms. Carre wrote: "I'd like to think I can get through labor without anesthetics; however, I can see where I'll probably be forced to ask for some." That moment might come, she felt, when "you're looking around frantically for something to get your mind off the pain." Ms. Carre expected that the fetal monitor might give her something to "focus on" and help take her mind off the pain.

At the other extreme were a few women who said they would accept anything offered. Ms. North was accepting of medication for discomfort because "I figured they know what they're doing." Ms. Penn had no reservations about accepting medication.

> If the doctor felt that it was necessary, yes, I'm not going to question what the doctor would say. I figure he knows more what's going on than I do.... I would hope he would suggest it.... I have no hatred of the idea to say the least, so we'll see what happens.

These two women demonstrated what we termed "naive trust;" that is, they did not plan to exercise any decision making on their own.

Ms. Dann was not entirely convinced that labor would be a "memorable experience," and would not have minded being "spaced out" except that it would interfere with the experience of the delivery.

> Like if I had a choice of being completely – not completely out of it – but drowsy, and not feeling that it would affect my baby, and kind of spaced out, it wouldn't bother me terrifically as far as remembering.... One thing that I'd really want to feel is the delivery. I want to be completely aware, and I want to push the baby out. I don't want somebody to snatch it out of me. I definitely don't want to have my body dead.

Ms. Hayes was resolute in wanting to be "knocked out," insisted on a caudal, and would not have minded a cesarean delivery. She showed no concern about the effect of anesthesia on the baby. She wanted an easy birth with no trauma. As noted, Ms. Hayes was afraid of panic, depression, and pain, and feared that without pharmaceutical aids she would lose control. Ms. Hayes and Ms. Tell, who both were convinced that they would lose control in labor, did. They appeared to bring to the childbirth experience the opinion that self-discipline was difficult and that it was not important.

7.5　Summary

Childbirth education encourages a woman to develop techniques of control during labor and delivery in order to help her cope with pain and render her less likely to need medications (Beck & Siegel, 1980; Hodnett, & Osborn, 1989; Lamaze, 1970). Consequently, women who attend classes seem to become conditioned to the need for control. Concerns about the risks of labor and fears of injury and death tend to occupy a less central position in their mental preparation for labor.

Fear of loss of control was engendered by doubts about bodily endurance and emotional stability. An analogy sometimes was made by the gravidas between these doubts and their doubts regarding their potential as mothers. Fears of loss of control were assuaged by general confidence in oneself (Beebe et al. (2007), trust in others, and anticipation of reward – the baby. However, greater prenatal fears regarding well-being of self and baby, and fears of pain, helplessness, and loss of control were associated with greater pain in labor and more distressing thoughts (Beebe et al.; Van den Bussche, Crombez, Eccleston, & Sullivan, 2006; Wuitchik et al., 1990). Such women may seek early admission to the labor unit (Cheyne et al., 2007) and may have a greater likelihood of postnatal depressive symptoms (Fairbrother and Woody, 2007).

Usually a woman who is confident that she will maintain control – within reasonable limits – is confident in other areas of her life as well and is more likely to perceive greater control in labor (Hodnett & Osborn, 1989). She has a healthy sense of self, having been tested in other stressful situations, and knows that she can handle crises. At the same time, she has set reasonable expectations for her performance in labor and will not be self-punishing if she does not achieve her goals, because she realizes that too many factors are unknown in childbirth.

Apart from the effect on the baby, those women who said that they would refuse medication and anesthesia wanted to be "awake and aware" for the entire childbirth experience, feared they might lose control of their bodies in the activity of labor, or felt that they otherwise would be taking the path of least resistance. They were inclined to have a high level of confidence in their ability to manage labor. A maternal prenatal expectation of having control in labor was related to the use of less medication, and women who did not use medication in labor had a shorter labor (Hodnett & Osborn, 1989). Entwisle and Doering (1981) found that increased awareness at birth, due to preparation and limited medication, significantly enhanced a positive perception of birth.

Another group of women said that they would refuse medication because losing alertness or consciousness in labor could trigger fears of paranoia, of being rendered helpless, or of being at the mercy of the hospital staff, or because loss of consciousness was equated with death. A few women feared that if they lost consciousness, they might be victimized by their bodies. These women tended to have a rather low level of confidence in their ability to manage labor.

At the other extreme was a third group of women who were willing to accept drugs without hesitation or who insisted on medication, feeling that it was the only way to maintain control in labor; or they accepted medication simply out of faith in the authority of the medical/nursing staff. This last group generally suffered from a low level of confidence in their own ability to progress through labor. In a state of unawareness they would not face the ordeal of labor, but neither would they enjoy the excitement of delivery. This tradeoff did not appear to be a source of concern for these women. In this regard, Engle and associates (Engle, Scrimshaw, Zambrana, & Dunkel-Shetter, 1990) reported that higher prenatal anxiety was associated with less desire for control and an active role in labor and delivery.

In between the two extremes were women who, although they did not welcome medication or anesthetics, were not upset at the prospect of using them. They would try to go through labor without pharmacological aids, but would not be disappointed if pharmacological assistance became necessary. Such women enjoyed a high level of confidence and could more easily appreciate their human limitations.

Reviews of research literature on the effects of antenatal education for childbirth indicate that they remain inconclusive or unknown regarding effects on knowledge acquisition, anxiety, control, pain, childbirth support, breastfeeding, or infant care abilities (Gagnon & Sandall, 2007). Other studies suggest that childbirth education management methods may be more effective in early labor than late labor (Van den Bussche, 2006). The variety and range of coping strategies employed by women in labor appear to be more encompassing than the methods taught in childbirth education classes, and are often based on women's past experiences in coping with pain and anxiety (Escott, 2004). In addition, the use of more coping strategies is associated with a report of less pain in labor (Beebe et al., 2007). These findings suggest individual approaches, as well as group approaches, to the management of prenatal and intrapartal fears of pain, helplessness, and loss of control in labor. Complementary and alternative therapies for pain management in labor, including hypnosis and acupuncture (Smith, Collins, Cyna, & Crowther, 2006), and music therapy (Podder, 2007), have been effective in reducing pain perception and medication usage (analgesia and anesthesia) Cyna, McAuliffe, and Andrew (2004), and deserve further consideration. Prenatal psychoeducation on coping strategies in labor also was effective in reducing anxiety in labor (Sharma et al., 1998).

Another area worthy of continued research is the father's concerns and fears of labor regarding his own experience and that of his partner. Although research is emerging in this area, there still remains a dearth of literature that includes inquiry into paternal conceptions, experiences, factors influencing and modifying role formulation and satisfaction, and supportive measures, all of which are factors influencing the dynamics of maternal preparation for and responses in labor (Capogna et al., 2007; Eriksson, Salandar, & Hamburg, 2007; Greening, 2006).

References

Annandale, E. (1987). Dimensions of patient control in a free-standing birth center. *Social Science and Medicine, 25*, 1235–1248.

Ballen, L. E., & Fulcher, A. J. (2006). Nurses and Doulas: Complementary roles to provide optimal maternity care. *Journal of Obstetric, Gynecologic, & Neonatal Nursing, 35*, 304–311.

Beck, N., & Siegel, L. (1980). Preparation for childbirth and contemporary research on pain, anxiety, and stress reduction: A review and critique. *Psychosomatic Medicine, 42*, 429–447.

Beebe, K. R., Lee, K. A., Carrieri-Kohlman, V., & Humphreys, J. (2007). The Effects of childbirth self-efficacy and anxiety during pregnancy on prehospitalization labor. *Journal of Obstetric, Gynecologic, and Neonatal Nursing, 35*, 410–418.

Capogna, G., Camorcia, M., & Stirparo, S. (2006). Expectant fathers' experience during labor with or without epidural anesthesia. *European Journal of Anaesthesiology, 23*, 611–617

Capogna, G, Camorcia, M., & Stirparo, S. (2007) Expectant fathers' experience during labor with or without epidural anesthesia. *American Journal of Obstetric Anesthesia, 16*, 110–115.

Chertok, L. (1969) *Motherhood and personality: Psychosomatic aspects of childbirth*. Philadelphia. PA: Lippincott.

Cheyne, H., Terry, R., NIven, C., Dowding, D., Hundley, V., & McNamee, P. (2007). 'Should I come in now?': A study of women's early labour experience. *British Journal of Midwifery, 15*, 604–609.

Cyna, A. M., McAuliffe, G. L., & Andrew, M. I. (2004). Hypnosis for pain relief in labour and childbirth: A systematic review. *British Journal of Anaesthesia, 93*, 505–511.

Deutscher, M. (1970) Brief family therapy in the course of first pregnancy: A clinical note. *Contemporary Psychoanalysis, 7*, 21– 35.

DiMatteo, M. R., Kahn, K. L., & Berry, S. H. (1993). Narratives of birth and postpartum: Analysis of the focus group responses of new mothers. *Birth 20*, 204–211

Engle, P. L., Scrimshaw, S. C. M., Zambrana, R. E., & Dunkel-Shetter, C. (1990). Prenatal and postnatal anxiety in Mexican women giving birth in Los Angeles. *Health Psychology, 9*, 285–299.

Entwisle, D. R., & Doering, S. G. (1981). *The first birth: A family turning point*. Baltimore: The Johns Hopkins University Press.

Eriksson, C., Salandar, P., & Hamburg, K. (2007). Men's experiences of intense fear related to childbirth investigated in a Swedish qualitative study. *The Journal of Men's Health and Gender, 4*, 409–418.

Escott, D., Spiby, H., Slade, P., & Fraser, R. B. (2004). The range of coping strategies women use to manage pain and amciety prior to and during first experience of labor. *Midwifery 20*, 144–156.

Fairbrother, N., & Woody, S. R. (2007). Fear of childbirth and obstetrical events as predictors of postnatal symptoms of depression and post-traumatic stress disorder. *Journal of Psychosomatic Obstetrics and Gynaecology, 28*, 239–242.

Gagnon, A., & Sandall, J. (2007). Individual or group antenatal education for childbirth or parenthood, or both. Cochrane Database of Systematic Reviews, 3 CD002869.

Gillman, R. D. (1968). The dreams of pregnant women and maternal adaptation. *American Journal of Orthopsychiatry, 38*, 688–692.

Greening, L. (2006). And – how was it for you dad? *Community Practitioner, 79*, 184–187.

Hodnett, E. D., Gates, S., Hofmeyr, G. J., & Sakala, C. (2003). Continuous support for women during childbirth. *Cochrane Database of Systematic Reviews, 3*, CD003766.

Hodnett, E. D., & Osborn, R. W. (1989). Effects of continuous intrapartum professional support on childbirth outcomes. *Research in Nursing & Health, 12*, 289–297.

Hofmeyer, G. J., Nikodem, V. C., Wolman, W., Chalmers, B. E., & Kramer, T. (1991). Companionship to modify the clinical birth environment: Effects on progress and perceptions of labour, and breastfeeding. *British Journal of Obstetrics and Gynaecology, 98*, 756–764.

Janis, I. L. (1958). *Psychological stress*. New York: Wiley.

Lamaze, F. (1970). *Painless childbirth, psychoprophylactic method*. Chicago: Regnery.

Lavender, T., Walkinshaw, S. A., & Walton, I. (1999). A prospective study of women's views of factors contributing to a positive birth experience. *Midwifery, 15*, 40–46.

Lothian, J. (2006). Birth plans: The good, the bad and the future. *Journal of Obstetric, Gynecologic, & Neonatal Nursing, 35*, 295–303.

Lowe, N. (1989). Explaining the pain of active labor: The importance of maternal confidence. *Research in Nursing & Health, 12*, 237–245.

Melzack, R. (1984). The myth of painless childbirth (the John J. Bonica lecture). *Pain 19*, 321–337.

Pacey, S. (2004). Couples and the first baby: Responding to new parents' sexual and relationship problems. *Sexual and Relationship Therapy, 19*, 223–246.

Podder, L. (2007). Effects of music therapy on anxiety levels and pain perception. *Nursing Journal of India, 98*, 161.

Raefael-Leff, J. (2001). *Pregnancy. The inside story*. London: Karnac.

Richardson, P. (1984). The body boundary experience of women in labor: A framework for care. *Maternal-Child Nursing Journal, 13*, 91–101.

Scott-Palmer, J., & Skevington, S. M. (1981). Pain during childbirth and menstruation: A study of locus of control. *Journal of Psychosomatic Research, 25*, 151–155.

Sharma, S., Sangar, K., & Bajwa, G. (1998). A psycho-educational programme for the primigravidae: Effect of psycho-educational programme (Related to labor and delivery) on primigravidae's level of anxiety during their third trimester of pregnancy. *The Nursing Journal of India, 89*, 53–55

Sherwen, L. N. (1983). An investigation into the effects of psychoprophylactic methods training and locus of control on fantasy production and body cathexis in the primiparous woman. In L. N. Sherwen and C. Toussie-Weingarten (Eds.), *Analysis and application of nursing research: Parent-neonatal studies.* Monterey, CA: Wadsworth Health Sciences Division.

Slade, P., MacPherson, S. A., Hume, A., & Maresh, M. (1993). Expectations, experiences and satisfaction with labour. *British Journal of Clinical Psychology, 32*, 469–483.

Slavazza, K., Mercer, R., Marut, J., & Shnider, S. (1985). Anesthesia, analgesia for vaginal childbirth: Differences in maternal perceptions. *Journal of Obstetrics, Gynecologic, and Neonatal Nursing, 14*, 321–329.

Smith, CA, Collins CT, Cyna AM, Crowther CA. Complementary and alternative therapies for pain management in labour. Cochrane Database of Systematic Reviews, 2006;Oct 18, (4):CD003521.

Trad, P. (1991). Adaptation to developmental transformations during various phases of motherhood. *Journal of the American Academy of Psychoanalysis, 19*, 403–421.

Van den Bussche E., Crombez, G., Eccleston, C., & Sullivan, M. J. L. (2006). Why women prefer epidural analgesia during childbirth: The role of beliefs about epidural anesthesia and pain catastrophizing. *European Journal of Pain, 11*, 275–282.

Van den Bussche E, Crombez G., Eccleston, C., & Sullivan, M.J.L. (2007). Why women prefer epidural analgesia during childbirth: the role of beliefs about epidural analgesia during childbirth: the role of beliefs about epidural analgesia and pain catastrophizing. *European Journal of Pain, 11*, 275–282.

Van de Castle, R., & Kinder, P. (1968). Dream content during pregnancy. *Psycho-physiology, 4*, 375.

Willmuth, L. (1975). Prepared childbirth and the concept of control. *Journal of Obstetric, Gynecologic and Neonatal Nursing, 4*, 38–41.

Willmuth, L., Weaver, L., & Borenstein, J. (1978). Satisfaction with prepared childbirth and locus of control. *Journal of Obstetric, Gynecologic and Neonatal Nursing, 7*, 33–37.

Windwer, C. (1977). Relationship among prospective parents' locus of control, social desirability, and choice of psychoprophylaxis. *Nursing Research, 26*, 96–99.

Wuitchik, M., Hesson, K., & Bakal, D. A. (1990). Perinatal predictors of pain and distress during labor. *Birth, 17*, 186–191.

Chapter 8
Prenatal Fear of Loss of Self-Esteem in Labor

The gravida's concept of self is central to a consideration of preparation for child-birth. In attempting to elucidate each woman's self-image, the interviewer arrived at an understanding of the woman's unique character with its particular personality traits and tensions. This understanding helped explain her personal experience of childbirth.

In varying degrees, many women fear that they will lose self-esteem in labor. The degree of fear depends on the stability of their sense of self. It is expected that a young mother who is reasonably confident about her new role will know who she is and will have a healthy sense of her own worth. However, the reverse is not necessarily true; that is, a woman with high self-esteem may not wish to have a baby or may not have an opportunity to have a child for one reason or another. A woman's sense of self-worth is not necessarily determined by her need or ability to "nurture." However, if she does need to "nurture" and has no child, she may seek satisfaction by working in the service professions, by serving the community on a volunteer basis, or by expressing her creativity through various activities and personal interests.

8.1 Overview

Results of the project (Lederman, Lederman, Work, & McCann, 1978, 1979) indicated that an extreme fear of losing self-esteem, as well as the willingness to lose it, affected a woman's performance in labor. A particular woman may not make an effort in labor because she "knows" that she will fail, or she may misinterpret helping gestures and counter every effort to help her. When a woman feels threatened, it is important to assess the following factors:

1. Source of the threat.
2. Intensity of reaction to the threat.
3. Response to the threat.

First, it is necessary to know the source of threat to self-esteem. Does it emanate from within or is it external to the women? Or, is the threat perhaps imagined?

R. Lederman and K. Weis, *Psychosocial Adaptation to Pregnancy*,
DOI 10.1007/978-1-4419-0288-7_8, © Springer Science+Business Media, LLC 2009

With an internal threat, the aggressive act is associated with self-blame or guilt. When the source of the threat is external, aggressiveness is experienced as being directed at oneself. As for an imagined threat, the aggressive act again originates from within, but is projected in such a way that the aggressor appears to be external. Second, it is important to learn how the gravida reacts to an aggressive act. Does she attempt confrontations and seek additional information and assistance, or does she respond with denial, self-denigration, guilt, or some other negative response?

Finally, it is important to determine whether the intensity of a wound to self-esteem is commensurate with the intensity of the stressor. Is the effect on self-esteem short lived or does the woman tend to brood over feelings, whether imagined or real? A woman who accepts self-devaluation as just punishment for imagined wrongs – for example, for earlier wishes to abort the fetus – might grasp the opportunity to derogate her own self-esteem. In addition, someone who is alert for a possible offense, often from an unknown source, would tend to be frightened of losing the semblance of self-esteem.

There is ample evidence for a relationship between self-esteem and depression. Research shows that symptoms of depression are far more likely to be seen in mothers with low self-esteem than in those with high self-esteem (Hall, Kotch, Browne, & Rayens, 1996). In a study by Fontaine and Jones (1997), low prenatal self-esteem was associated with moderate depression at two weeks postpartum.

The Fear of Loss of Self-Esteem in labor is closely analogous to the Lederman Prenatal Self-Evaluation scale on Fear of Pain, Helplessness, and Loss of Control in Labor. Low prenatal self-esteem is related to marked or moderate maternal insecure attachment, which is also related to prenatal and postpartum depression (Bifulco, Moran, Ball, & Lillie, 2002; Ritter, Hobfoll, Lavin, Cameron, & Hulsizer, 2000; Berthiaume, Saucier, & Borgeat, 1998). Low self-esteem and concerns about having a higher risk pregnancy and pregnancy outcomes may occur more frequently in women experiencing pregnancy after a period of infertility (Covington & Burns, 2000) and in women with complications during pregnancy (World Health Organization, 2003).

8.2   Measures of Self-Image

One way of learning about the status of a woman's self-image was to ask how she felt about herself. At times a woman's self-image could be readily determined. Usually, however, it was determined indirectly by discovering how accepting she was of herself and how empathic she was toward others. Self-acceptance referred to whether she liked, respected, and was tolerant of herself, and to whether she acknowledged her strengths and accepted her weaknesses. It usually followed that the self-accepting woman tended to exhibit acceptance toward other people. In short, she was empathic. If a woman liked herself to an extreme, she tended to like others only if they fueled her protected image; she may have been absorbed in thoughts of herself to the exclusion of others, and devoid of altruistic or empathic attitudes. Conversely, the woman who disliked herself tended to indulge in self-blame and guilt, and was willing to endure humiliation. She tended not to be empathic because she was consumed by thoughts of her injured self. Both the narcissistic and the denigrating women were inclined not to "hear" what others said and, therefore, could not empathize. Each group of women feared loss of self-esteem, but for different reasons.

In this chapter, the self-image of the gravidas is first discussed in general terms. Then, the chapter focuses on the loss or gain of self-esteem as reflected in the following behaviors:

1. Tolerance of self.
2. Value of self and assertiveness.
3. Body image and appearance.

Other behaviors that were indicative of self-esteem included:

1. Empathy, discussed here in relationship to the gravida's mother and her husband.
2. Trust, discussed in terms of the fear of loss of control.
3. Perseverance, discussed in relation to preparation for labor. Perseverance also was seen as an indicator of self-esteem, in the sense that the women who proceeded toward goals in the face of obstacles were presumed to possess a fair degree of self-confidence.

All these behaviors appeared to overlap one another and were related to other personality variables. Consequently, self-esteem as a behavioral variable did not lend itself to independent assessment to the same degree as did the other prenatal personality variables previously discussed. Furthermore, even if a woman appreciated herself as she was or had only fleeting fears of losing self-esteem, her positive sense of self did not preclude certain areas of vulnerability in which she was likely to fear the loss of self-esteem. In addition, women who suffered from self-denigration sometimes unexpectedly exhibited strength in certain areas. Such parallel behaviors were evident in the women's remarks that are used as illustrations.

8.3 Evaluation of Self-Worth

When considering self-esteem and its relationship to what is understood as a healthy sense of self-worth, it is useful to begin by determining how the woman evaluates herself. It is important to know, for example, whether she bases her identity mainly on her own assessment, or whether she is more dependent on others for her identity.

If a woman accepts responsibility for the way in which she defines herself, then her self-image is likely to be strong and stable (Giblin, Poland, & Sachs, 1987). In our study, two women typified such autonomy. Ms. Cole said: "I have my own ideas and I really don't like to follow anybody else that much,… especially if I don't agree with them."

Ms. Allen recognized that her own feelings would ultimately determine the way that she would handle labor, although support from others would be welcomed. Ms. Allen said: "[If I am offered assistance by anyone during labor,]… it would help, but I think the most important thing is telling myself – hearing it from inside – that I can do it because that's helped me through a lot of things." Regarding the welcome support from others, it is recognized that the availability of support from close family members during pregnancy helps assuage low self-esteem and depression (Patel, 2003; World Health Organization, 2003).

On the other hand, when a woman depends on others for her identity her self-image tends to be subject to the approval or disapproval of others, and she is more likely to succumb to self-devaluation. The "vulnerability hypothesis" proposes that individuals with low self-esteem have fewer positive self-cognitions than individuals with high self-esteem and are therefore more vulnerable to statements of disapproval (Hobfoll, Nadler, & Leiberman, 1986). The research literature on attachment supports this finding (Monk, Leight, & Fang, 2008; Rholes, Simpson, Campbell, & Grich, 2001; Wilson, Rholes, Simpson, & Tran, 2008). Many women in the study were worried about what others would think of them if they did not behave "correctly." They feared that others would think poorly of them and this caused their self-esteem to plummet. When compared with individuals having high self-esteem, those with low self-esteem tend to feel more threatened by elements of inferiority and dependency associated with seeking and receiving help (Giblin et al., 1987; Hobfoll et al.). In response to the question, "What about you as a person will make it easier or more difficult for you to cope with labor and delivery?" Ms. Gale defined her strengths in terms of her husband's strengths and her marital relationship. She did not identify any positive self-attributes, even when the question was posed to her in various ways to give her that opportunity.

Some women masked their vulnerability with an appearance of independence when they actually were dependent on others' assessments. Ms. Katen, for example, became irritated when she thought that people were trying to "change her" during periods of anger. In her diary, she stated that she would resist being "pushed into doing something without full knowledge of what I'm getting into." Ms. Katen's irritation seemed to stem from a fear of attacks on her integrity. She appeared noticeably defensive in the interviews. Later it was discovered that she actually was rather dependent on others' opinions for a sense of identity, and she worried that she had not "measured up." In labor, she thought that the doctors and nurses rating of her self-esteem was "zero for yelling and screaming."

Ms. Aaron was conscious that she tended to be unsure of herself and that she lacked confidence. She said:

> I tend to worry about myself,…that I don't measure up. I tend to compare myself with other people around me. I always have…I just worry that I don't measure up to other people…I worry [that] …I will be the one that fails,…fails my child.

Ms. Aaron's self-image vacillated. She worried about imparting feelings of insecurity to her child, and about failing herself, her infant, and others.

It is important to determine whether a woman's image of herself is primarily positive or negative. A positive image means that a woman appreciates both her strengths and her weaknesses. A negative image means that the woman chiefly tends to devalue herself, or to inflate herself, which can, mask devaluation. Women in the study who had identity problems fell into the first category and tended toward devaluation. For example, Ms. Gale found it difficult to identify either her strengths or her weaknesses; Ms. Aaron was confused about who she was; Ms. Tell viewed herself negatively, as "insecure, introverted, shy, lacking confidence." All these women were rated high on the fear of loss of self-esteem in labor.

In summary, a woman with a negative self-image generally is pessimistic about the outcome of events and tends to fear and dread labor, especially the possibility of injury and death. On the other hand, a woman who does not have an abnormal fear of losing self-esteem is likely to have an optimistic attitude toward events – in this case, childbirth. As discussed in Chapter 6, these women usually look forward to labor with excited anticipation and do not expect complications, yet are realistic enough to understand that complications could occur.

8.4 Behaviors that Reflect Self-Esteem

8.4.1 Tolerance of Self

The degree to which the gravida is realistic – how reasonable her perceptions of cause and effect are – can determine the way in which she sees herself. A mother might have high expectations of herself indicating high self-esteem, but she also should be aware of risks and of the unexpected. If she does not live up to her expectations, can she handle failure without devaluing herself?

In the study, a gravida's attitude toward herself was partly assessed by asking how she thought she would feel if anything went unexpectedly wrong in labor. Ms. Meta's reply revealed tolerance of herself. "Maybe I would have to have a cesarean or something. I'm not afraid of it; I know I will feel disappointed, but I wouldn't blame myself."

Although Ms. Quins had a conflict between continuing her career and caring for the baby, she had little guilt.

> I feel kind of upset about it, but circumstances have forced me into it so I am going to try to do the best I can...I'm not used to being at home at all. I feel very torn. I want to stay home and bake bread and take care of my baby because I've never done that in my whole life. And I can't [don't know how to] do it. Sometimes I get really resentful. But it might work out fine.

Several other women tended to blame themselves for anything that went wrong in their lives. Ms. Aaron admitted that she tended "to worry about" herself, that she disliked making mistakes because it "embarrasses" her, and that she was afraid she would "make a spectacle" of herself. If something happened in labor, she wondered:

…what are we going to do with all these [baby] things…How will I feel? And I know that I would blame myself. I tend to do that anyway. I did it a lot with my miscarriage last summer…I would feel it was something that was in my control and that I blew it, even if it wasn't really the case. So the feelings don't happen a lot, but when they do sometimes they are very depressing.

In her postpartum interview, Ms. Aaron mentioned that because she had "lost" a few contractions in labor, she "felt kind of like a failure…really shook up." This response reflected a tendency toward depression and a rather fragile sense of self. Even though Ms. Aaron believed that she was resilient and would be able to block out anxieties in order to persevere in labor. She later said: "[I am]… not a very patient person. I don't like to wait, and I am afraid that I'll get impatient and tense and tired. These are the things that worry me most of all." As discussed earlier, her worries were so severe that they interfered with her sleep. Although she demonstrated considerable insight, Ms. Aaron was not able to control or modify her underlying feelings of self-doubt, intolerance of failure, and dependency.

Similarly, Ms. Lash said: "[I am]…inadequate in a lot of areas…There are times when I go off the deep end and sit down and say, "Oh, what is going to become of me? Oh, woe is me!" She had many areas of doubt.

About my physical ability to do things, like am I really a good actress? Am I really a good director? Or have I been kidding myself all these years?… Do I give everything I can give? Or am I being lazy? Am I just telling myself I don't feel like doing it and using that as an excuse not to?

Ms. Lash indulged in excessive preoccupation with self, particularly while home alone during her third trimester.

I get very lonely because my husband is away all day, and all my neighbors work, and so I'm sort of sitting there talking to myself and listening to the radio. Consequently…those kinds of feelings come up when I'm alone and brooding.

While alone she found it difficult to control the punitive part of herself. Her fears about present and future loneliness triggered depression.

Ms. Cole went even further in her self-blame. If she were to have a stillborn, she stated: "Maybe I'd say: 'Well, you shouldn't have worked so long, or you shouldn't have done that…' I'd blame myself…I'd feel very disappointed…like a convicted murderer or something.

Guilt, which is an extreme form of self-blame, was a common experience among the participants. Ms. Uman, in describing occasions when she wished that she was not having a baby, said that she felt guilty immediately after such thoughts. She reported:

[I blame]…certain things on my husband that weren't his fault…and within one or two minutes I know…the truth and I tend to feel very guilty. So even though I might still be a little mad, I explain to him that I realize that I'm at fault and he isn't.

Ms. Uman's anger and subsequent guilt feelings were short lived, probably because she knew about her tendency to project. Women with low self-esteem were less resilient in recovering from self-doubts and experienced more prolonged depression.

It was more difficult for Ms. Xana to overcome her guilt feelings because she occasionally wished that she was not having a baby at this time. "I really have a guilty feeling about not working. I think it's because my husband is in dental school and [we] don't have a lot of money …. I just feel that I really should have helped out." Ms. Xana seemed quite vulnerable and was frequently concerned with how others viewed her.

Ms. Tell felt that her child would be like she was: "… a spoiled, rotten, overprotected kid who can't handle himself outside the house." When speculating on why she thought that she was spoiled and overprotected, Ms. Tell said:

[My father]…gave me [too much] – not materially – [but in that] I depended on him too much. He was all I ever needed. He was right there. I didn't have to go out of the house or anything…I dug while I was a kid, but now I realize that I shouldn't have done that;… It was all my fault. I knew that I was his favorite. I guess he just loved me too much, and I took advantage of it. I didn't bother having any kind of relationship with anybody else, just him.

When asked what she thought her reaction to pain in labor would be, Ms. Tell replied:

[I am]…not worried about it…When I was in high school and college, I had this…persecution complex…where I used to get mad at myself and pound my hands…I always think of pain like a punishment, so I don't mind it. I think I deserve it [for]…doing something wrong.

She thought that she would do worse in labor than other women because she would "never be in control." Ms. Tell appeared to suffer from extreme self-loathing and felt a need to punish herself. She was genuinely concerned that her child would repeat her experience. Her dreams, too, were typical of a severely depressed person. As discussed earlier, Ms. Tell often appeared in her dreams as "a fat ugly kid."

A number of women had trouble accepting failure, perhaps as a result of living in an achievement-oriented society. Ms. Jabon, a dancer, called herself a "worry-wart" and said that she "took things hard." She feared "…any sort of failure….I'm probably… achievement oriented. In my family there is a lot of emphasis on academic achievement." Fear of failure was associated with disappointment in herself and concern about what people thought of her. Recalling labor in the postpartum interview, she said:

I really think that I had a sense that I was supposed to play the role and to do my bit, to do my part, and that to act out or to complain or to scream or whatever would have been disappointing myself… I think that probably I…am too concerned about what other people think…I really didn't want the…people there thinking, 'Boy, she sure falls apart at the seams under pressure.'

Ms. Uman worried about failing, but thought that this frame of mind was counterproductive.

I wouldn't want to have my children afraid of failing. We have to learn to accept failure too as a part of life. I never was able to. I had to be best; I had to achieve everything. There's still that fear hanging over me now I guess.

Both Ms. Jabon and Ms. Uman demonstrated considerable insight, which seemed to help them handle this punitive part of themselves.

8.4.2 *Value of Self*

The women who liked themselves had a healthy sense of self-survival and were inclined to set limits on those who devalued them, but not in a belligerent, aggressive way. Ms. Katen, who was typical of this group, was concerned that her wishes be respected by the medical staff.

> I think that taking the Lamaze course or something else buffers that [hospital authority] a little bit and tells you that you do have more rights than the hospital is going to tell you… you do in terms of seeing your baby after it is born,…putting it on a demand feed schedule, and that kind of thing.

Ms. Carre thought that most people recognized her independence of mind. When asked, "Have your parents helped you make any decisions about caring for the baby?" she answered:

> No. With my parents it's definitely a hands-off business, especially my mother [regarding breast vs. bottle feeding]. I don't get much of an opinion on that. People know that I am a fairly opinionated sort of person and people know they can't sway me easily, and they mostly don't try.

The expectation that others will respect one's feelings and needs depends on the ability to trust others, and the ability to assert that one has certain human rights. In the literature, it generally is viewed as a healthy way of handling aggressive drives. Valuing the self depends on knowing oneself and being able to identify and respect one's feelings. Openness with oneself and others provides a tool for dispelling irrational doubts and fears that can beset anyone. Honest communication permits the testing of reality. The ability to assert oneself tactfully and make decisions allows one to acquire needed background information and arrive at solutions for change.

The women who worried excessively about others' opinions were dependent on those opinions for their sense of identity, and tended to devalue their own needs, feelings, and ideas. Ms. Yuth felt that she might lose control in labor and "throw a temper tantrum." If this were to happen, she said that she would feel like "a fool," and she feared that she might embarrass her husband. The concern that she might create stress for others seemed more crucial to her than her own welfare.

> The only thing I want to mention is…about being brave in labor. I've been kind of a frivolous person; I've always been accused of being too silly and making a fool of myself…It's always been important to me not to make a fool of myself…I guess that's why I brought in the word 'brave,' because that signifies…to me a very strong, stoic kind of person…I don't want to be a screamer or cause any undue stress for anyone around me.

Ms. Xana expressed guilt about having rested a great deal during her pregnancy and about not having worked. "It bothers me a lot because I feel a lot of women work when they're pregnant, and I'm just taking it easy. I guess I feel I shouldn't." She dreamt about a pair of earrings that she wanted to buy, but in the dream she refused to indulge herself because then she would "feel guilty buying a pair of earrings for myself."

Passivity, as noted, was a trait exhibited by a number of gravidas. They avoided taking responsibility and looked to others to initiate action on their own behalf.

Ms. Penn said that she always waited for her husband to suggest practicing their exercises. She thought of herself as "slip-shod." She also was prepared to leave all decision making about her pregnancy to the doctor, and demonstrated what might be termed "naive trust" in people. Ms. Zeff had little confidence that she could manage on her own. Her passivity and dependency appeared to be intensified by isolation. Thus, she thought that the worst thing that could happen to her in labor was "to be alone."

> As long as someone's there, no matter what's happening, at least somebody's there to go get so and so...I think the worst thing that could ever happen to me is to have a baby alone...I'd panic and both of us would just die, I know. Even if it's somebody who doesn't know anything about babies, I'd feel a lot better.

This concern is commonly recognized in the research literature (Clark & Affonso, 1979; Reeder, Mastroianni, Martin, & Fitzpatrick, 1980), but it was not commonly mentioned by these project participants, perhaps because all of them attended some type of labor preparation class and expected their husbands to be a companion in labor.

Ms. Zeff related vague fears that she would harm herself or that something bad would happen to her. "I usually won't go out anywhere I'm going to be alone. I will not go to the supermarket alone at 11 o'clock at night. I do not want to be alone .... I'm watching everything, and I won't ignore anything.

Ms. Zeff's and Ms. Yuth's concerns may have been intense, yet they were inclined to voice vague or abstract fears more commonly than they voiced concrete fears. Perhaps feelings of vulnerability and superstition – or fear of acknowledging the reality of danger – partly explain this type of expression.

A few women, like Ms. Katen, were afraid of becoming dependent in any way and pushed help away when it was offered. This may have been a defense against fears of abandonment to which Ms. Katen openly admitted.

A number of participants in the study demonstrated good insight and were able to experience and show their feelings. They also were able to act on their insight. Many others, however, seemed unaware of their feelings, were afraid of them, or kept them hidden. In response to many questions during interviews, Ms. North simply answered "I don't know." She avoided, denied, or perhaps repressed her feelings. Ms. Raaf said that she did not like to "put on an emotional show," preferring to see herself as "stoic." Ms. Hayes clearly feared her feelings. She tried to confront this problem due to the fear of "going crazy," but although she generally was talkative, she avoided more sensitive areas of inquiry regarding possible complications. Ms. Meta found it difficult to express anger and said that she would feel badly if she did. Ms. Bode could not remember ever losing her temper. Ms. Zeff thought that if she did not assert herself, she might be abandoned or that some other type of retribution would follow.

Many of these women admitted to a tendency to "bottle up" their feelings. Unfortunately, if a woman is too timid or finds it difficult to directly express feelings, she can be thwarted in clearly communicating her needs to others. A number of women who suppressed their feelings were hurt, because they thought that their feelings were either trampled on or ignored. They seemed to expect others to intuit their unverbalized thoughts. In addition, they were fearful of their own anger and aggression, and perhaps expected retribution for expressing these feelings. Conversely, a woman like Ms. Katen who tended to be belligerent, demanded respect, and loudly insisted on her rights, may have been suspicious and fearful that others would control her if she did not always remain watchful.

8.4.3   Body Image and Appearance

The interview schedule did not include questions on body image, but because body image was spontaneously mentioned by many participants, it is discussed briefly. Body image is clearly an aspect of self-esteem and an indication of attitudes about the pregnant self (Iffrig, 1972; McConnell & Daston, 1961; Norris, 1970).

A woman who respects her body and "listens" to it has high expectations of body performance and is likely to think well of herself. Norris (1970) similarly refers to gaining mastery through skillful monitoring and increasing awareness of the pregnant body.

In contrast, some gravidas felt ugly and disgusting: "like the side of a barn," like a "circus animal," or "like an elephant." This type of self-image could be an acculturated response in the United States where slimness is admired. Some gravidas thus experienced lowered self-esteem because of their changed shape. Moore (1978) also reported a poorer maternal self-image in advanced pregnancy. Some women, such as Ms. Lash, disliked their appearance whether pregnant or not. "I still get upset about my looks sometimes. You know, I look in the mirror, and think, Gah! What an awful looking person."

One woman worried that childbirth would cause her to begin to age like her mother, while another worried that her husband would no longer find her attractive because of her "big tummy." These women had difficulty not just in accepting their pregnant state, but in accepting themselves altogether. Few women in the last trimester could sustain themselves with a sense of awe about the approaching birth. Endurance, when observed, more often took the form of relief that the pregnancy would soon terminate and that the much-awaited child would be born.

The way in which a woman takes care of her body probably is indicative of her self-respect. Many gravidas looked forward to attractive maternity clothes to dress up their altered shapes. Others were resentful that their old clothes no longer fit, and were upset about whether they would ever be slim again and about stretch marks; a few let their appearance go altogether.

Ms. Faber, who equated physical activity with attractiveness and health, said:

> The more I try to stay physically active, the better I'll feel. When I go jogging and play tennis and softball...I think I'll have more energy and I think...the delivery will be better... I think the more active you are, the less tired you get...I don't like to sit around.

Several other women also referred to body image in terms of activity or work accomplished.

8.5 Summary

Women who showed high self-esteem during pregnancy tended to find integrity in terms of recognizing their needs and limitations. They tactfully asserted independence in searching for solutions to concerns and questions, and persevered in defining and attaining goals for themselves. They were relatively self-confident, adjusting to the unexpected and unknown, accepting risk as a reality, and tolerating future uncertainty. Their self-confidence and inquiring nature enabled them to recover from threat and insult quickly, demonstrating resilience instead of depression.

Gravidas with low self-esteem lacked an adventurous outlook, and avoided confrontation or the concrete expression of their fears. They were inclined to be more passive, often hoping that others could anticipate and answer their unverbalized concerns, and they experienced depression when this did not occur. Articulation of concerns was absent usually because of dread of revealing fears. These women tended to deprecate themselves more, were intolerant of their weaknesses, and were unable to identify their strengths. They had more self-doubts and were prone to guilt. Women with low self-esteem experienced prolonged rather than short-lived periods of depression, which were triggered by loneliness, and they lacked introspection and the capacity to devise solutions for change (Hobfoll et al., 1986). They were more likely to find themselves feeling helpless and alone, and to conceal their anger and aggressive impulses when these feelings arose. These women were fearful of their dependency and, overall, their self-image was confused (Hobfoll et al.).

Characteristics of high and low self-esteem often coexisted instead of occurring as discrete phenomena. The proportions of high and low self-esteem varied in different women, and were closely related to the other personality variables measured during pregnancy. Pregnancy is filled with feelings of self-doubt that Rubin (1984) described as destabilizing dissonance. With prenatal maternal adaptation and attachment there is a desire to protect the unborn baby and meet his or her needs even at the expense of the mother's own needs (Condon & Corkindale, 1997). Thus, a woman's self-esteem is an encompassing dimension that correlates with other prenatal personality variables, and reflects and influences the achievement of other important developmental tasks throughout pregnancy.

References

Berthiaume, M., Saucier, D. H., & Borgeat, F. (1998). Correlates of pre-partum depressive symptomatology: A multivariate analysis. *Journal of Reproductive & Infant Psychology, 16,* 45–56.

Bifulco, A., Moran, P., Ball, C., & Lillie, A. (2002). Adult attachment style. II. Its relationship to psychosocial depressive-vulnerability. *Social Psychiatry and Psychiatric Epidemiology, 37,* 60–67.

Clark, A. L., & Affonso, D. D. (1979). *Childbearing: A nursing perspective* (2nd ed.). Philadelphia: Davis.

Condon, J. T., & Corkindate, C. (1997). The correlates of antenatal attachment in pregnant women. *The British Journal of Medical Psychology, 70*, 359–372.

Covington, S. N. & Burns, L. H. (2000). Pregnancy after infertility. In L. H. Burns & S. N. Covington (Eds.), *Infertility counseling*(pp.430–432). New York, Informa Health Care.

Giblin, P., Poland, M., & Sachs, B. (1987). Effects of social supports on attitudes and health behaviors of pregnant adolescents. *Journal of Adolescent Health Care, 8*, 273–279.

Fontaine, K. R., and Jones, L. C. (1997). Self-esteem, optimism, and postpartum depression. *Journal of Clinical Psychology, 53*, 59–63.

Hall, L. A., Kotch, J. B., Browne, D., Rayens, M. K. (1996). Self-esteem as a mediator of the effects of stressors and social resources on depressive symptoms in postpartum mothers. *Nursing Research, 45*, 231–238.

Hobfoll, S., Nadler, A., & Leiberman, J. (1986). Satisfaction with social support during crisis: Intimacy and self-esteem as critical determinants. *Journal of Personality and Social Psychology, 51*, 296–304.

Iffrig, M. C., Sr. (1972). Body image in pregnancy. *Nursing Clinics of North America, 7*, 631–679.

Lederman, R., Lederman, E., Work, B. A., Jr., & McCann, D. S. (1979). Relationship of psychological factors in pregnancy to progress in labor. *Nursing Research, 28*, 94–97.

Lederman, R., Lederman, E., Work, B. A., Jr., & McCann, D. S. (1978). The relationship of maternal anxiety, plasma catecholamines, and plasma cortisol to progress in labor. *American Journal of Obstetrics and Gynecology, 132*, 495–500.

Lederman, R. P., Weis, K., Brandon, J., Hills, B., Mian, T. (2002) Relationship of Maternal Prenatal Adaptation And Family Functioning To Pregnancy Outcomes. Poster presentation at the Annual Meeting of the Society of Behavioral Medicine. April 3-6, Washington, DC.

McConnell, O., & Daston, P. (1961). Body image changes in pregnancy. *Journal of Projective Techniques, 25*, 451–456.

Monk, C., Leight, K. L., & Fang, Y. (2008). The relationship between women's attachment style and perinatal mood disturbance: implications for treatment and screening. *Archives of Women's Mental Health, 9*, 117–129.

Moore, D. S. (1978). The body image in pregnancy. *Journal of Nurse-Midwifery, 22*, 17–26.

Norris, C. M. (1970). The professional nurse and body image. In C. M. Norris & C. Carlson, (Eds.), *Behavioral concepts and nursing intervention*. Philadelphia, PA: Lippincott.

Patel, V. (2003). *Where there is no doctor*. London: Gaskell.

Reeder, S. R., Mastroianni, L., Jr., Martin, L. L., & Fitzpatrick, E. (1980). *Maternity nursing* (14th ed.). Philadelphia, PA: Lippincott.

Rholes, W. S., Simpson, J. A., Campbell, L., & Grich, J. (2001). Adult attachment and the transition to parenthood. *Journal of Personality and Social Psychology, 81*, 421–435.

Ritter, C., Hobfoll, S. E., Lavin, J., Cameron, R. P., & Hulsizer, M. R. (2000). Stress, psychosocial resources, and depressive symptomatology during pregnancy in low-income, inner-city women. *Health Psychology, 19*, 576–585.

Rubin, R. (1884) Maternal Identity and the Maternal Experience" New York, Springer.

Wilson, C. L., Rholes, W. S., Simpson, J. A., & Tran, S. (2008). Labor, delivery, and early parenthood: An attachment theory perspective. *Personality and Social Psychology Bulletin, 33*, 505–518.

World Health Organization. (2003). *Managing complications in pregnancy and childbirth*. Geneva, World Health Organization.

Chapter 9
Prenatal and Postnatal Psychosocial Adaptation in Military Women[1, 2]

9.1   Part 1. Prenatal Adaptation

While the military family has existed throughout time and dealt with continual military operations and deployments, little is known about the military family and even less about the pregnant military wife. Notably, maternal adaptation is a progressive process that does not occur in isolation from one's environment. The ability to adapt and identify with the concept of being a mother, particularly for the first-time mother (versus the second or third), requires self-socialization and a testing of self-definitions (Deutsch, Ruble, Fleming, Brooks-Gunn, & Stangor, 1988). For military wives attempting to accommodate new maternal self-definitions, there may be increased conflict because of the isolating factors associated with the military.

Military families share the same life course issues faced by all members of our society. However, there are challenges that set military families apart (Martin, 2000). Frequent deployments and separations potentiate stress within the family (Martin, Mancini, Bowen, Mancini, & Orthner, 2004). Moreover, for military families faced with relocations, there may be less opportunity or desire to form friendships or participate in community activities, which tends to increase feelings of isolation and reduced social well-being (Kelley, Finkel, & Ashby, 2003). The importance of informal social support in promoting the physical, psychological, and social well-being of individuals has been established for both military and civilian communities (Bowen, Martin, Mancini, & Nelson, 2000). The following findings underscore the significance of the community network, adaptability of one's family, and deployment separation to the gravida's maternal adaptation process. The results are presented in two parts: Part 1 pertaining to prenatal data results and Part 2 pertaining to postpartum results.

---

[1] The content and conclusions expressed here are those of the authors and do not necessarily reflect the views of TriService Nursing Research Program, the Department of Defense, or the U.S. Government.

[2] The military-related results discussed in Chapters 1 and 9 were the findings from a project sponsored by the TriService Nursing Research Program, MDA-905-00-1-0039.

9.2 Part 1. Research Questions: The Relationship of Community Support and Family Adaptability to Prenatal Maternal Adaptation

Weis (2006) followed 421 primigravid and multigravid women married to military servicemen across all trimesters of pregnancy and through delivery in order to answer the following research questions:

1. Does the gravida's perception of her community's support have an effect on the level of conflict and anxiety experienced and on maternal change over time for prenatal psychosocial adaptation?
2. Does the gravida's perception of her family's adaptability (flexibility) have an effect on the level of conflict and anxiety experienced and on maternal change over time for prenatal maternal psychosocial adaptation?

9.2.1 Method

Of 503 women consented for participation in the study, 421 women completed all portions of the prenatal phase of the study, from first trimester through delivery. The women were 18–35 years old and were recruited from four military treatment facilities. The participants were met in each trimester of pregnancy and asked to complete a booklet of questionnaires containing Lederman's *Prenatal Self-Evaluation Questionnaire* (PSEQ), the *Social Support Index* (SSI) (McCubbin, Patterson, & Glynn, 1982), and *FACES II* (Olson, 2000; Olson, Sprenkle, & Russell, 1979).

The PSEQ was developed to measure a woman's prenatal maternal psychosocial adaptation to pregnancy over the course of the three trimesters of pregnancy. The instrument contains 79 statements which comprise seven scales measuring different dimensions of maternal prenatal adaptation. All items have four Likert response options. The respondent is able to reflect on how she feels regarding the statement by circling, *"Very Much So," "Moderately So," "Somewhat So,"* or *"Not At All."* Higher scores on a scale indicate greater anxiety or conflict related to the formulation of the motherhood role. The scores do not necessarily indicate a positive or negative adaptation to pregnancy, but rather the level of anxiety the woman is experiencing relative to the particular dimension. Descriptive statistics for the Prenatal Self-Evaluation Questionnaire scales are presented in Table 9.1. Cronbach's alpha coefficients for the scales range from $\alpha = 0.75$–0.92 (Lederman, 1996). The instrument has shown good reliability ($\alpha = 0.83$–0.94) in an intervention study with military wives (Schachman, Lee, & Lederman, 2004).

The Family Adaptability and Cohesion Evaluation Scales (FACES II version) is a 30-item self-report instrument designed to measure adaptability and cohesion within the family system (Olson, 2000; Olson et al., 1979). The items are answered on a Likert-type scale with response options indicating (1) *"Almost Never"* to (5) *"Almost Always."*

Table 9.1 Descriptive Statistics for the Prenatal Self-Evaluation Questionnaire

PSEQ scale	1st trimester M (SD)	2nd trimester M (SD)	3rd trimester M (SD)
Acceptance[a]	20.47 (6.51)	19.46 (6.06)	19.58 (5.77)
Identifcation[b]	18.72 (4.24)	18.97 (4.12)	18.77 (4.19)
Well-being[c]	15.87 (4.71)	15.60 (4.46)	15.25 (4.59)
Preparation[d]	18.11 (5.58)	18.20 (5.65)	17.19 (5.40)
Helplessness[e]	16.77 (4.37)	16.70 (4.41)	16.48 (4.39)
Relationship/Mother[f]	18.72 (4.24)	14.15 (5.99)	13.82 (5.69)
Relationship/Husband[g]	14.07 (4.68)	14.40 (5.19)	14.52 (5.54)

[a] Acceptance of Pregnancy scale
[b] Identification with a Motherhood Role scale
[c] Well-being of Self and Baby in Labor scale
[d] Preparation for Labor scale
[e] Fear of Pain, Helplessness, and Loss of Control in Labor scale
[f] Relationship with Mother scale
[g] Relationship with Husband scale

The Family Adaptability scale contains 14 items that measure the theoretical concepts of assertiveness, leadership, or control, negotiation, roles, and rules within the family. The reliability coefficient for the adaptability scale for a sample of 2,543 adults across the life cycle was $\alpha = 0.80$. Test-retest at four weeks was $r = 0.80$. The scale is proposed to measure a curvilinear concept of balance or that of a linear relationship along a continuum. Numerous studies identified a linear relationship with respect to family health (Alexander & Lupfer, 1987; Curtiss, Klemz, & Vanderploeg, 2000; Finello, Litton, deLemos, & Chan, 1998), and a linear scoring approach is recommended (Olson, Bell, & Portner, 1992) and will be used for data analyses. In terms of the Adaptability scale, mean scores from 46 to 54 indicate a "flexible" family; mean scores from 40 to 45 indicate a "structured" family, and scores from 15 to 39 indicate a rigid family structure. Theoretically, the family is considered to have stable roles and a democratic style of leadership and negotiation with scores ranging from 40 through 54 (Olson, 1995).

The Social Support Index (SSI) (McCubbin et al., 1982) is a 17-item instrument designed to measure the degree to which families are integrated into the community, view the community as a source of support, and feel that the community can provide emotional, esteem, and network support. The instrument uses a 5-point Likert scale ranging from "*Strongly agree*" (5) to "*Strongly disagree*" (1). A higher score indicates more perceived anticipated social support. The SSI was found to have a validity coefficient of .40 with the criterion measure of family well-being (McCubbin et al.). Construct validity was assessed in a study with over 1,000 families and the perceived support was positively correlated with a family's sense of fit within the community ($r = .40$). The fit was significantly related to successful family adaptation. The internal reliability of the SSI was reported as $\alpha = 0.82$ and test-retest reliability as $r = 0.83$ (McCubbin et al.).

Deployment status was defined as the departure, travel, and arrival to some destination where temporary living quarters and work environments are established for the purpose of supporting a defined military mission for a specified minimum time and duration of thirty days. The women were asked in first trimester whether their spouses were currently deployed. In the last trimester they were asked if at any time during the pregnancy their husband had been deployed. The first trimester dichotomous variable for deployment was scored: (1) Yes, the spouse was deployed during the first trimester, and (2) No, the spouse was not deployed during the first trimester. The scores were used in two separate conditional growth curves, in which the effect of deployment on individual change over time was assessed for *Acceptance of Pregnancy* and then *Identification with a Motherhood Role*.

9.2.2   Data Analysis

Descriptive statistics were obtained from the prenatal and postpartum dataset. Differences for the two groups on the outcomes variables were assessed using one-way ANOVA. There were no significant differences between the two groups on any of the outcomes variables, so the two datasets were combined for questions pertaining to the prenatal variables. (The postnatal questions follow this section).

To answer the proposed questions, two-level conditional individual linear growth models were created: (1) a model with the covariate of Community Support (SSI) in each trimester and (2) a model with the covariate of Family Adaptability in each trimester. The individual linear growth models were used in order to account for the individual differences in intercepts not possible with a repeated measures approach. The Level 1 of the models represented linear individual growth, and Level-2 expressed variation in parameters from the growth model as random effects (Singer, 1998). The models contained fixed effects for the intercept and for the effect of TIME (trimesters of pregnancy). The random effects statement within each model allowed for variation in intercept, TIME slope, and the within-person residual. An unstructured covariance matrix for within-person error was determined to be the best fit.

9.2.3   Results

9.2.3.1   Community Support and Prenatal Self-Evaluation Questionnaire (PSEQ) Scale Scores

Tables 9.2–9.5 show results for Community Support (SSI) regressed on each PSEQ dimension over time. For the first trimester, the results in each of the Tables 9.2–9.5 reflect a significant relationship between a network of community support and a decrease in conflict for each dimension of individual prenatal maternal adaptation except for *Relationship with Husband*. For the second trimester, the results in each of the Tables 9.2–9.5 reflect a statistically significant negative effect for Community Support (decreased conflict) for all the dimensions except *Well-Being of Self and Baby in Labor* (Table 9.3), which had borderline significance ($\beta = -0.07, p \leq 0.06$).

Table 9.2 Coefficients for Acceptance of Pregnancy and Identification with a Motherhood Role trajectories with Community Support (SSI)

Parameter	Estimate	SE	df	t	p
Acceptance[a]					
Intercept	41.11	1.72	836	23.87	<0.001
Linear trend	−1.02	1.54	1031	−0.66	
SSI(1)	−0.14	0.04	837	−3.15	<0.01
SSI(2)	−0.16	0.05	836	−3.44	<0.001
SSI(3)	−0.10	0.05	836	−1.91	<0.10
Time*SSI(1)	0.08	0.04	1029	2.08	<0.05
Time*SSI(2)	0.01	0.04	1030	0.13	
Time*SSI(3)	−0.08	0.04	1031	−1.74	<0.10
Identification[b]					
Intercept	33.62	1.12	836	30.13	<0.001
Linear	0.11	1.03	972	0.11	
SSI(1)	−0.14	0.03	836	−5.10	<0.001
SSI(2)	−0.10	0.03	836	−3.39	<0.001
SSI(3)	−0.03	0.03	836	−1.02	
Time*SSI(1)	0.07	0.03	978	2.63	<0.01
Time*SSI(2)	−0.01	0.03	979	−0.21	
Time*SSI(3)	−0.06	0.03	979	−2.2	<0.05

Note. Numbers in parentheses indicate the trimester of pregnancy

[a]Trajectory for Acceptance of Pregnancy across each trimester of pregnancy

[b]Trajectory of Identification with a Motherhood Role across each trimester of pregnancy

Table 9.3 Coefficients for Preparation for Labor and Well-Being of Self and Baby in Labor trajectories with Community Support (SSI)

Parameter	Estimate	SE	df	t	p
Preparation[a]					
Intercept	33.59	1.57	833	21.46	<0.001
Linear	0.68	1.43	1,001	0.48	
SSI(1)	−0.23	0.04	834	−5.84	<0.001
SSI(2)	−0.15	0.04	834	−3.52	<0.001
SSI(3)	0.09	0.04	833	2.07	<0.05
Time*SSI(1)	0.07	0.04	998	2.04	<0.05
Time*SSI(2)	0.01	0.04	998	0.13	
Time*SSI(3)	−0.10	0.04	1,000	−2.47	<0.01
Well-being[b]					
Intercept	26.77	1.32	836	20.51	<0.001
Linear	1.01	1.21	981	0.84	
SSI(1)	−0.11	0.03	836	−3.25	<0.001
SSI(2)	−0.07	0.04	836	−1.91	<0.10
SSI(3)	−0.03	0.04	836	−0.80	
Time*SSI(1)	0.05	0.03	980	1.61	
Time*SSI(2)	−0.01	0.03	981	−0.2	
Time*SSI(3)	−0.01	0.03	981	−1.97	<0.05

Note. Numbers in parentheses indicate the trimester of pregnancy

[a]Trajectory for Preparation for Labor across each trimester of pregnancy

[b]Trajectory of Well-Being of Self and Baby across each trimester of pregnancy

Table 9.4 Coefficients for Fear of Pain, Helplessness and Loss of Control, and Relationship with Mother Trajectories with Community Support (SSI)

Parameter	Estimate	SE	df	t	p
Helplessness[a]					
Intercept	30.7	1.18	835	26.05	<0.001
Linear	0.51	1.11	955	0.46	
SSI(1)	−0.13	0.03	836	−4.18	<0.001
SSI(2)	−0.14	0.03	835	−4.28	<0.001
SSI(3)	−0.01	0.03	835	−0.03	
Time*SSI(1)	0.05	0.03	953	1.82	<0.10
Time*SSI(2)	0.01	0.03	953	0.36	
Time*SSI(3)	−0.07	0.03	954	−2.35	<0.05
Relationship/Mother[b]					
Intercept	34.64	1.65	809	20.99	<0.001
Linear	−0.03	1.53	950	−0.28	
SSI(1)	−0.20	0.04	810	−4.62	<0.001
SSI(2)	−0.17	0.04	809	−3.83	<0.001
SSI(3)	−0.02	0.05	810	−0.38	
Time*SSI(1)	0.01	0.04	951	1.88	<0.10
Time*SSI(2)	0.01	0.04	942	0.08	
Time*SSI(3)	−0.01	0.04	959	−1.67	<0.10

Note. Numbers in parentheses indicate the trimester of pregnancy
[a]Trajectory for Fear of Pain, Helplessness, and Loss of Control across each trimester
[b]Trajectory of Relationship with Mother across each trimester of pregnancy

Table 9.5 Coefficients for Relationship with Husband Trajectory with Community Support (SSI)

Parameter	Estimate	SE	df	t	p
Relationship/Husband[a]					
Intercept	27.43	1.37	822	20.00	<0.001
Linear	0.10	1.37	868	0.07	
SSI(1)	−0.07	0.03	823	−1.76	<0.10
SSI(2)	−0.09	0.04	822	−2.39	<0.05
SSI(3)	−0.10	0.04	822	−2.63	<0.01
Time*SSI(1)	0.08	0.03	864	2.34	<0.05
Time*SSI(2)	−0.01	0.04	864	−0.06	
Time*SSI(3)	−0.08	0.04	863	−1.96	<0.05

Note. Numbers in parentheses indicate the trimester of pregnancy
[a]Trajectory for Relationship with Husband across each trimester of pregnancy

In the third trimester, Community Support had a statistically significant effect on the conflict associated with two dimensions, *Preparation for Labor* (Table 9.3) and *Relationship with Husband* (Table 9.5). Importantly, rather than Community Support in the *third trimester* decreasing the conflict associated with *Preparation for Labor*, it increased the conflict (Table 9.3, $\beta = 0.09$, $p \leq 0.05$). Community Support in the *third trimester* did, however, decrease the conflict the gravida was experiencing relative to her *Relationship with Husband* (Table 9.5, $\beta = -0.10$, $p \leq 0.01$).

Tables 9.2–9.5 further show the interaction of Community Support (in the 1st trimester) with TIME; the interaction results were significant for *Acceptance of Pregnancy, Identification with a Motherhood Role, Preparation for Labor,* and *Relationship with Husband*. These results indicate that perceived community support in the first trimester did alter the trajectory over time for these particular dimensions. The interaction of Community Support (in the 3rd trimester) with TIME was significant for *Identification with a Motherhood Role, Preparation for Labor, Well-Being of Self and Baby, Fear of Pain, Helplessness, and Loss of Control in Labor,* and *Relationship with Husband*. It is important to emphasize that the positive effect for the interaction terms reflects the direction of the trajectory, not the level of conflict. The interaction terms indicate that Community Support does alter the change over time in the dimensions, whereas the findings for Community Support by trimester define the effect of Community Support on the conflict the gravida is reporting for each PSEQ dimension by trimester.

9.2.3.2 Family Adaptability and Prenatal Self-Evaluation Questionnaire (PSEQ) Scale Scores

Tables 9.6–9.9 show the results for *Family Adaptability* regressed on each PSEQ dimension over time. The results indicate a significant relationship between the 1st trimester perceived flexibility within the family and a decrease in conflict

Table 9.6 Coefficients for Acceptance of Pregnancy and Identification with a Motherhood Role Trajectory with Family Adaptability (ADAPT)

Parameter	Estimate	SE	df	t	p
Acceptance[a]					
Intercept	30.82	1.25	817	24.65	<0.001
Linear trend	−0.08	1.17	940	−0.07	
ADAPT(1)	−0.20	0.03	817	−5.99	<0.001
ADAPT(2)	−0.10	0.04	817	−0.24	
ADAPT(3)	−0.02	0.03	818	−0.53	
Time*ADAPT(1)	0.04	0.04	940	1.29	
Time*ADAPT(2)	0.00	0.04	940	0.02	
Time*ADAPT(3)	−0.04	0.03	940	−1.34	
Identification[b]					
Intercept	23.26	1.77	815	13.12	<0.001
Linear	2.13	1.61	985	1.32	
ADAPT(1)	−0.10	0.05	815	−2.26	<0.05
ADAPT(2)	−0.07	0.05	815	1.38	
ADAPT(3)	−0.06	0.04	815	−1.39	
Time*ADAPT(1)	0.02	0.04	984	0.43	
Time*ADAPT(2)	−0.01	0.05	983	−0.20	
Time*ADAPT(3)	−0.06	0.04	983	−1.43	

Note. Numbers in parentheses indicate the trimester of pregnancy
[a] Trajectory for Acceptance of Pregnancy across each trimester of pregnancy
[b] Trajectory of Identification with a Motherhood Role across each trimester of pregnancy

Table 9.7 Coefficients for Preparation for Labor and Well-Being of Self and Baby in Labor Trajectories with Family Adaptability (ADAPT)

Parameter	Estimate	SE	df	t	p
Preparation[a]					
Intercept	38.80	1.82	817	21.26	<0.001
Linear	−1.17	1.65	996	−0.71	
ADAPT(1)	−0.26	0.05	817	−5.36	<0.001
ADAPT(2)	−0.00	0.05	817	−0.05	
ADAPT(3)	0.08	0.04	818	−1.89	<0.10
Time*ADAPT(1)	0.07	0.04	996	1.77	<0.10
Time*ADAPT(2)	0.02	0.05	995	0.35	
Time*ADAPT(3)	−0.08	0.04	995	−1.97	<0.05
Well-being[b]					
Intercept	23.89	1.42	817	16.83	<0.001
Linear	−0.10	1.33	936	−0.01	
ADAPT(1)	−0.16	0.04	817	−4.22	<0.001
ADAPT(2)	0.02	0.04	817	0.57	
ADAPT(3)	−0.01	0.03	818	−0.42	
Time*ADAPT(1)	0.04	0.03	936	1.11	
Time*ADAPT(2)	−0.01	0.04	936	−0.23	
Time*ADAPT(3)	−0.04	0.03	935	−1.08	

Note. Numbers in parentheses indicate the trimester of pregnancy
[a]Trajectory for Preparation for Labor across each trimester of pregnancy
[b]Trajectory of Well-Being of Self and Baby in Labor across each trimester of pregnancy

Table 9.8 Coefficients for Fear of Pain, Helplessness, and Loss of Control, and Relationship with Mother Trajectories with Family Adaptability (ADAPT)

Parameter	Estimate	SE	df	t	p
Helplessness[a]					
Intercept	26.42	1.32	816	20.01	<0.001
Linear	0.71	1.25	925	0.57	
ADAPT(1)	−0.15	0.03	816	−4.19	<0.001
ADAPT(2)	0.04	0.04	816	1.01	
ADAPT(3)	−0.07	0.03	817	−2.23	<0.05
Time*ADAPT(1)	0.03	0.03	925	1.03	
Time*ADAPT(2)	−0.03	0.04	924	−0.67	
Time*ADAPT(3)	−0.02	0.03	924	−0.79	
Relation/Mother[b]					
Intercept	27.36	1.86	789	14.70	<0.001
Linear	0.36	1.75	911	0.20	
ADAPT(1)	−0.27	0.05	790	−5.42	<0.001
ADAPT(2)	0.04	0.06	790	0.76	
ADAPT(3)	−0.01	0.05	790	−0.30	
Time*ADAPT(1)	0.06	0.05	925	1.32	
Time*ADAPT(2)	−0.09	0.05	913	−1.66	<0.10
Time*ADAPT(3)	0.02	0.04	916	0.37	

Note. Numbers in parentheses indicate the trimester of pregnancy
[a]Trajectory for Fear of Pain, Helplessness, and Loss of Control across each trimester
[b]Trajectory of Relationship with Mother across each trimester of pregnancy

Table 9.9 Coefficients for Relationship with Husband Trajectory with Family Adaptability (ADAPT)

Parameter	Estimate	SE	df	t	p
Relationship/Husband[a]					
Intercept	33.53	1.25	815	26.77	<0.001
Linear	0.36	1.16	969	0.31	
ADAPT(1)	−0.18	0.03	816	−5.45	<0.001
ADAPT(2)	−0.12	0.04	818	−3.16	<0.001
ADAPT(3)	−0.06	0.03	817	−1.96	<0.05
Time*ADAPT(1)	0.12	0.03	973	3.78	<0.001
Time*ADAPT(2)	0.06	0.04	981	1.81	<0.10
Time*ADAPT(3)	−0.18	0.03	976	−6.35	<0.001

Note. Numbers in parentheses indicate the trimester of pregnancy

[a]Trajectory for Relationship with Husband across each trimester of pregnancy

associated with all seven dimensions of prenatal maternal adaptation. In the 2nd trimester, the gravida's perceived flexibility within the family does not significantly affect the conflict the gravida experienced relative to any of the dimensions of maternal adaptation, except for Relationship with Husband.

In the *third trimester,* however, perceived flexibility within the family does significantly decrease the conflict the gravida experienced for *Fear of Pain, Helplessness, and Loss of Control in Labor* (Table 9.8), and *Relationship with Husband* (Table 9.9). In addition, in the 3rd trimester the relationship of the gravida's perceived family flexibility approached significance for decreasing conflict associated with *Preparation for Labor* (Table 9.7, $\beta = 0.08$, $p \leq 0.06$).

The interaction of Family Adaptability (in the 3rd trimester) with TIME was only significant for *Preparation for Labor* and *Relationship with Husband.* These results indicate that perceived Family Adaptability in the third trimester did alter the trajectory over time for these particular dimensions. Family Adaptability in all trimesters with TIME had a statistically significant effect on the trajectory of *Relationship with Husband.* Given the relationship between these two variables, this finding is not surprising.

9.2.4 Discussion of Part 1. Prenatal Results

The findings provide evidence for the significance of a network of community support and flexibility within the family for women to resolve prenatal adaptational conflict. Moreover, the findings provide important results regarding the significance of the type of support by trimester. This is an important step toward developing sound intervention theory (Sidani & Braden, 1998).

Researchers have long examined the effect of support on mitigating the physical and emotional strain experienced by the gravida during pregnancy (Dunkel-Schetter, Sagrestano, Feldman, & Killingsworth, 1996; Kalil, Gruber, Conley, & Sytniac, 1993; Liese, Snowden, & Ford, 1989; Norbeck, 1981; Norbeck & Anderson, 1989; Orr, 2004; Pryor et al., 2003). However, the type of support, by whom the support is provided, as well as the timing of the support are often poorly differentiated (Feldman, Dunkel-Schetter, Sandman, & Wadhwa, 2000). The importance of support, especially support from the husband, has been found to correlate with greater prenatal and postpartum adjustment (Lederman, Weis, Brandon, & Mian, 2001; Weiss, 1974; Weiss & Chen, 2002). The concept of adaptability within the family to the woman's changing role has not been well differentiated. For military populations faced with lifestyle changes requiring continual alterations in roles and rules, the impact on maternal adaptation is important to decipher. The aim of this project was to distinguish the support provided by the family in terms of adaptability, from the emotional esteem-building support provided by a community network.

For all dimensions, the emotional-esteem building support from a community network (in the first and second trimesters) had a statistically significant effect on decreasing the conflict the gravida experienced. The findings emphasize the importance of early emotional support for a gravida's healthy maternal development. The descriptive statistics for the SSI, presented in Table 9.10, reflect the perception of a strong community support network for this sample. Neither McCubbin et al. (1982) nor Splonskowski and Twiss (1995) reported as high a score for military samples as those obtained for this sample. Notably, Splonkowski and Twiss sampled military wives at three months postpartum rather than prenatally, and reported a mean score of 38.04, on the SSI compared to the results reported in this study of 52.74–53.90.

As early as the first trimester, the gravida searches for information predominantly about pregnancy (Deutsch et al., 1988). However, she is also beginning the process of disengaging from her identity as a woman without a child to a woman with a child (Lederman, 1996; Rubin, 1984). Information is sought from "women friends" who can share and listen. In the first trimester, the gravida may limit her pregnancy announcement to the father of her baby, her mother, and closest friends. It is this small network of friends and family that are most likely to provide intimate care, protection, and supportive nurturance desired by the gravida (Rubin). Importantly, the findings reflect the importance of the gravida having some type of perceived network of support as early as the first trimester to help address fears she is already experiencing related to her identification of being a mother, fears of childbirth, and her mother's acceptance of her pregnancy. The findings leave little doubt as to the importance for provision of some type of supportive network in the second

Table 9.10 Descriptive Statistics for Measures of Community Support

	Trimesters		
	One	Two	Three
Mean	53.39	52.74	53.90
Mode	57.00	51.00	50.00
Range	24–68	28–68	23–68
SD	7.41	7.88	7.54
α	0.85	0.88	0.88
n	388	388	387

trimester of pregnancy. The gravida's developmental process in becoming a mother continues throughout pregnancy. However, in the second trimester, after feeling the baby move, the gravida begins in earnest to formulate her parenting role and the expected interactions with her infant (Lederman, 1990). This adaptational process requires realignment of kinship and friendship bonds, i.e., tightening of some and loosening of others (Sleutel, 2003). The importance of this cannot be underestimated for the military wife. Because they are more likely to be dislocated from family and life-long friends, they may obtain greater value from community network resources than women living closer to family. Moreover, as the gravida adapts to her maternal identity, she needs esteem-building support. Interactions with others have enduring, cumulative effects on self-esteem (Swann & Brown, 1990), if the person feels cared for and valued (Procidano & Heller, 1983). People absorb information when it complements their existing views or needs (Jacobson, 1986). Clearly, the emotional-esteem building support the gravida needs and seeks in the first and second trimester does significantly decrease her conflict associated with prenatal maternal adaptation. Importantly, the perceived support in the third trimester had a less significant impact on the gravida's overall conflict or anxiety.

The perceived flexibility of the family by the gravida in the *first trimester* significantly decreased her conflict for all aspects of her prenatal maternal adaptation. The findings highlight the significance of the gravida's early prenatal concerns for her family's preparedness (anticipated flexibility) and for her maternal adaptation and the arrival of a newborn. Not surprisingly, the conflict the gravida experiences related to the *Relationship with Husband* dimension is interlinked with her perception of the family's flexibility. The concept of "adaptability or flexibility" within the family is important to maternal development. The shift that occurs prenatally, from a woman without child to a woman with child, requires flexibility within the family to accommodate interdependency rather than dependency in each other. The interplay of the gravida's concerns (evidenced in the third trimester findings) regarding the flexibility within her family, the relationship with her husband, and fears over feelings of helplessness, and possible loss of control are all intrinsically linked to the interpersonal skills desired and needed in her husband. The ability to accommodate the needs of another person and to maintain a balance between providing guidance and caring while also allowing autonomy are qualities identified as being necessary for competency as a good husband and father (Margolin, Gordis, & John, 2001; McHale & Rotman, 2007).

It is significant to note that while the mean scores for the Adaptability scale of FACES II (Table 9.11) indicate that the woman's perception of the family's adaptability during the three trimesters of pregnancy change very little, the early prenatal perceptions of family adaptability have significant effects on prenatal maternal adaptation. Friedman, Utada, and Morrissey(1987) found that for 96 families, the perception of "ideal" adaptability within the family was a score of approximately 52 from the adults in the family. The national norm is 49.9 (Vega et al., 1986). In this sample, the mean across the trimesters ranged from 54.19 in the last trimester to 54.62 in the first trimester. The values indicate the perception of stable roles with a democratic style of leadership within the family (Olson, 1995).

Table 9.11 Descriptive Statistics for Measures of Family Adaptability

	Trimesters		
	One	Two	Three
Mean	54.62	54.36	54.19
Mode	56.00	51.00	55.00
Range	19–67	24–68	25–66
SD	6.84	7.08	7.83
α	0.84[a]/0.91[b]	0.84[a]/0.91[b]	0.85[a]/0.94[b]
n	387	387	387

[a]Cronbach's alpha for FACES II Family version
[b]Cronbach's alpha for FACES II Couples version

These values are indicative of a positive family trait (Friedman et al.), showing very high flexibility in family adaptation in this military sample. Importantly, a lack of perceived flexibility, when it occurred, significantly increased the woman's conflict related to each of the seven dimensions of prenatal maternal adaptation. The results indicate that the gravida's concerns about her pregnancy were inclusive of adjustments she felt must be made within the family. However, rather than desiring greater structure within the family unit to combat feelings of uncertainty and disruption caused by the shifting of roles (Smith & Ingoldsby, 2009), the gravida actually desired greater perceived flexibility within the family. Albeit, the need for increased flexibility may be a by-product of a military population, but it is an important key to the development of intervention theory.

With all seven dimensions of maternal adaptation there was a significant decrease in prenatal maternal adaptational conflict with a perceived increase in family adaptability in the first trimester of pregnancy. The perceived flexibility did not significantly decrease conflict associated with any of the seven dimensions of maternal adaptation in the second trimester. Interestingly, it is in the second trimester that the emotional-esteem support provided by a community network had the most consistent significant impact. Of note, is the importance of the family's support (flexibility) in the third trimester when the gravida is trying to come to terms with increasing anxiety over childbirth, with the fetus ultimately becoming a separate being, and the anticipated parenthood demands following childbirth (Lederman, 1990; Rubin, 1984). A composite family functioning score (adaptability and cohesion) was found to be the best indicator of complicated labor and delivery, and low birthweight infants (Reeb, Graham, Zyzanski, & Kitson, 1987). Women perceiving their families as dysfunctional were at higher risk for both outcomes. In another study of family functioning related to birth and postpartum complications, the psychosocial risk evaluation of family functioning considered in conjunction with individual biomedical risk factors was the most consistent predictor of postpartum complications (bleeding, infection, pain, fever, difficulty with infant feeding, health problems of the infant, and depression) when evaluated with the psychosocial variables of recent life experiences, life changes, and general social support. Importantly, reports of more life changes in the year preceding pregnancy were associated with perceived "good" family functioning.

This finding signifies the importance of continual adaptation within a family unit to confront and cope with the ongoing stressors. It is important to note the sample population for both the prenatal and postnatal findings, to follow, comprised women in their mid 20s ($M = 26.5$, SD = 4.23), educated, married women with solid family incomes, and available prenatal care. Gurung, Dunkel-Schetter, Colllins, Rini, and Hobel (2005) found that older, more educated, higher earning, and married women had significantly more positive attitudes toward pregnancy which attenuated perceived anxiety at all stages of pregnancy. While this study sample of military wives had lower mean scores for the PSEQ than reported previously by Lederman (1996), the flexibility of the family and the emotional, esteem-building support from a community network decreased prenatal pregnancy-related anxiety. Additionally, controlling for age, parity, and ethnicity did not affect the results. Salmela-Aro, Aunola, Saisto, Halmesmaki and Nurmi (2006) found that primiparous and multiparous families experienced similar depressive symptoms and marital dissatisfaction with pregnancy and childbirth. The prenatal pregnancy-related conflicts that a gravida experiences during her maternal adaptation, which include concerns over changes in work and spousal acceptance of the pregnancy are very genuine regardless of one's age, parity, or ethnicity (Lederman, 1996; Nelson, 2003).

9.3   Part 2. Postnatal Adaptation

With the birth of a child there is an immense shift in orientation (Rubin, 1984) from a mother with child to a mother of a child (Lederman, 1996, Rubin). An immediate reconstruction of the self-system occurs to one of a mother-child system, to that of a family system (Rubin). Investigators (Haedt & Keel, 2007; Huang, Wang, & Chen, 2004) have found that prenatal maternal adaptation and fetal attachment predict infant outcomes. Walker and Montgomery (1994) found that maternal identity at 1–3 days and 4–6 weeks postpartum was a significant predictor of a child's socioemotional characteristics at 9 years. Prenatal self-acceptance has been found to positively correlate with acceptance of the maternal role responsiveness to the infant (Shereshefsky & Yarrow, 1973). Halman, Oakley, and Lederman (1995) found significant correlations between third trimester *Identification with a Motherhood Role* and 6-week postpartum measures of *Confidence with Motherhood Tasks* and *Satisfaction with the Motherhood Role*.

The developmental transformation experienced by the gravida during the antenatal and postnatal periods significantly influences the evolution of an attachment relationship with the infant (Trad, 1991). A lack of pregnancy acceptance and poor maternal prenatal adaptation represent an emotional detachment that can have profound effects on maternal-infant attachment (Bloom, 1998; Condon & Corkindale, 1997). Rubin (1984) theorized that the reconstruction of the self that must occur in order to incorporate the child into a mother-child system may not occur until 8–9 months after childbirth. There is a direct relationship between the strength of supportive bonds and the quality of a woman's identification with being a mother

(Rubin). Additionally, the family system's boundaries, roles, and duties must be reorganized in preparation for the new family member (Duvall, 1977; Ingoldsby, Smith, & Miller, 2004; Whitchurch & Constantine, 1993).

Following birth there is continued realignment and delineation of routines and boundaries (Mercer, 2004). Family cohesion and emotional support from one's partner contribute to a woman's postpartum mental health (Weiss & Chen, 2002). There is a need for esteem-building, nurturing support (preferably from family members) throughout pregnancy, in order for the maternal adaptive process to occur (Rubin, 1984). Research related to support from family, specifically the husband, has focused on the woman's perception of support from the husband, but not necessarily the woman's perception of the family accommodations of the changing roles throughout pregnancy. This would seem to be an important step to the formulation of effective interventions aimed at improving maternal role satisfaction.

9.4 Part 2. Research Questions: The Relationship of Community Support, Family Adaptability, and Spousal Deployment to Postnatal Maternal Adaptation

Weis (2006) followed 113 (from $n = 421$ above) gravidas from first trimester through six months postpartum with the purpose of answering three research questions:

1. Are patterns of change over time for certain psychosocial dimensions of prenatal maternal adaptation predictive of postpartum satisfaction and confidence in the maternal role?
2. Does maternal prenatal perception of family adaptability or community support predict postpartum satisfaction and confidence in the maternal role?
3. Does a history of deployment (by the husband), prenatally, affect postpartum satisfaction and confidence in the maternal role?

9.4.1 Methods

One hundred and thirteen (113) women from the original sample of 421 consented to participation in a continuation of the initial study. They consented postdelivery while still in the hospital to participation in an additional data collection point at 6-months postpartum. The women were met at the infant's 6-month pediatric appointment where they were given a booklet of questionnaires comprising the Postpartum Self-Evaluation Questionnaire (PPSEQ) (Lederman, 1981), FACES II (Olson, 2000), and the Social Support Index (SSI) (McCubbin et al., 1982). The women were asked if they had been separated from their spouse or the father of the baby due to deployment since the birth of the baby. Data obtained prenatally regarding deployment separation were used to create a dichotomous variable indicating whether the mother had experienced separation from her husband due to deployment during her pregnancy.

The PPSEQ (Lederman) contains seven subscales, totaling 82 items that measure the woman's perceived postpartum adaptation to motherhood. The seven subscales each represent a dimension of postpartum adaptation developed through qualitative work by Lederman and associates. Similar to the PSEQ, the respondent is able to reflect on how she feels regarding a statement by circling, "*Very Much So,*" "*Moderately So,*" "*Somewhat So,*" or "*Not at All.*" Two of the seven scales (*Confidence in Motherhood Role and Satisfaction with Infant and Infant Care*) were used in analysis because they specifically measured concepts related to the woman's confidence and satisfaction with her adaptation to motherhood and her attachment to the infant. The *Confidence in Motherhood Role* scale (13 items) measures the mother's doubts about her ability to parent, to interpret her infant's behavior, and to meet his or her needs. The Satisfaction with Infant/Infant Care scale (13 items) assesses the mother's pleasure with nurturant activities and her preference for a motherhood role vs. other roles. This scale was developed because data reflected a mother, particularly a multipara, might have confidence in her infant care skills, but not be satisfied with the infant or providing infant care (Lederman, Weingarten, & Lederman 1981). The Cronbach's alpha for *Confidence with Motherhood* Role was 0.73 and for *Satisfaction with Motherhood Tasks and Infant Care* was 0.79 in the reported study. The reliabilities ranged from $\alpha = 0.77$ to 0.93 for a 3-day postpartum measurement, and from $\alpha = 0.66$–0.95 at a 3-week postpartum assessment (Lederman et al.). Reece (1995) showed concurrent and predictive validity for the instrument at 1, 3, and 12 months following delivery. The FACES II and the SSI were administered identical to the processes described prenatally. The reliabilities for each were adequate and similar to those obtained prenatally.

The ability of prenatal psychosocial dimensions to predict postpartum adaptation focused on two prenatal dimensions of the PSEQ: *Acceptance of Pregnancy* and *Identification with a Motherhood Role*. While the PSEQ was administered in its entirety and all scales encompass portions of maternal prenatal adaptation, the desire was to assess longitudinally the ability of early formative thoughts regarding one's pregnancy to predict maternal postpartum maternal adjustment. The *Acceptance of Pregnancy* scale encompasses feelings related to planning and wanting the pregnancy, feelings of well-being and happiness regarding the pregnancy vs. depression and discomforts experienced during the pregnancy and feelings related to body changes. The *Identification with a Motherhood Role* scale is conceptualized as inclusive of the gravida's motivation for motherhood: the ability to envision oneself as a mother, and the anticipation of life changes associated with being a mother.

For this analysis, the multilevel variables (the slopes change over time) of *Acceptance of Pregnancy* and *Identification with a Motherhood Role* created for the prenatal analysis were entered into two separate regression models: one for *Confidence with a Motherhood Role* as the dependent variable and the second for *Satisfaction with Infant and Infant Care* as the dependent variable. The variables of family adaptability and emotional esteem-building community support were entered into each regression model as a variable that reflected the prenatal change over time (prenatal slopes) for each variable.

9.4.2   Results

All the women were wives of military service members (94%) or active duty women. The sample was predominantly Air Force (78%) with some Army (19%) and Navy (3%) military wives. The sample was predominantly White-non-Hispanic (60%), with the remainder of the sample being Hispanic (26%), Black, non-Hispanic (11%), and Asian (3%).

Tables 9.12–9.14 present intercorrelations of the prenatal scales in all trimesters of pregnancy with the postpartum scales. Correlations for Acceptance of Pregnancy with Identification with a Motherhood Role were high across all trimesters ($r = 0.61$, $p \leq 0.01$; $r = 0.63$, $p \leq 0.01$; $r = 0.63$, $p \leq 0.01$, for 1st, 2nd, and 3rd trimesters, respectively). Moderately high negative correlations for both *Acceptance*

Table 9.12 Intercorrelations for First Trimester Pregnancy and Postpartum Scales

Scales	ACCPREG	IDMORO	ADAPT	SSI	CMRT	SIC
Acceptance of pregnancy (ACCPREG)	–	0.61**	−0.37**	−0.37**	0.33**	0.26**
Identification with a motherhood role (IDMORO)	–	–	−0.35**	−0.44**	0.23**	0.25**
Family adaptability (ADAPT)	–	–	–	0.35**	−0.26**	−0.23*
Social support index (SSI)	–	–	–	–	−0.27**	−0.25**
Confidence with motherhood role/tasks (CMRT)	–	–	–	–	–	0.64**
Satisfaction with Infant/Infant Care (SIC)	–	–	–	–	–	–

*$p < 0.05$; **$p < 0.01$

Table 9.13 Intercorrelations for Second Trimester Pregnancy and Postpartum Scales

Scales	ACCPREG	IDMORO	ADAPT	SSI	CMRT	SIC
Acceptance of pregnancy (ACCPREG)	–	0.63**	−0.35**	−0.45**	0.28**	0.21*
Identification with a motherhood role (IDMORO)	–	–	−0.32**	−0.48**	0.45**	0.41**
Family adaptability (ADAPT)	–	–	–	0.32**	−0.07	−0.15
Social support index (SSI)	–	–	–	–	−0.32**	−0.24**
Confidence with motherhood role/tasks (CMRT)	–	–	–	–	–	0.64**
Satisfaction with infant/infant care (SIC)	–	–	–	–	–	–

*$p < 0.05$, **$p < 0.01$

Table 9.14 Intercorrelations for Third Trimester and Postpartum Scales

Scales	ACCPREG	IDMORO	ADAPT	SSI	CMRT	SIC
Acceptance of pregnancy (ACCPREG)	–	0.63**	–0.39**	–0.43**	0.24**	0.22**
Identification with a motherhood role (IDMORO)	–	–	–0.32**	–0.45**	0.45**	0.37**
Family adaptability (ADAPT)	–	–	–	0.36**	–0.18	–0.17
Social support index (SSI)	–	–	–	–	–0.31**	–0.18
Confidence with motherhood role/tasks (CMRT)	–	–	–	–	–	0.64**
Satisfaction with Infant/Infant Care (SIC)	–	–	–	–	–	–

$*p < 0.05$, $**p < 0.01$

of *Pregnancy* and *Identification with a Motherhood Role* with community support (SSI) indicate a strong relationship between increasing community support and decreased conflict with acceptance of pregnancy and identification with a motherhood. The correlations reflect the strongest negative relationship in the second trimester of pregnancy. The correlations for family adaptability to *Acceptance of Pregnancy* and *Identification with a Motherhood Role* are similar to those for community support. The findings indicate that with perceived decreases in flexibility within the family there is a statistically significant increase in conflict with prenatal psychosocial adaptation. Of note, there is a significant negative relationship with prenatal family adaptability in 1st trimester and the two postpartum measures of maternal adaptation. This reflects the developmental changes the woman is experiencing early in pregnancy. In no other trimester is there a statistically significant relationship between these variables. The relationship of community support to the postpartum adaptation variables is statistically significant in all trimesters. Also of note, there is a statistically significant relationship between the prenatal psychosocial adaptive dimensions in all trimesters and the postpartum maternal psychosocial adaptation variables. These results indicate that *Acceptance of Pregnancy* and *Identification with a Motherhood Role* are uniquely different dimensions.

Tables 9.15 and 9.16 show results for the regression models of the prenatal slopes of Acceptance of Pregnancy and Identification with a Motherhood Role on postpartum Confidence in Motherhood Roles and Tasks and Satisfaction with the Infant and Infant Care. The results indicate that the prenatal slope of *Acceptance of Pregnancy* did not significantly affect the woman's *Confidence in Motherhood Roles and Tasks* or her *Satisfaction with the Infant and Infant Care* at 6-months postpartum. However, the prenatal slope of *Identification with a Motherhood Role* did have a statistically significant effect on the woman's *Confidence with Motherhood Role and Tasks* (Table 9.15, $\beta = 1.49, p \leq 0.001$) and with *Satisfaction with Infant and Infant Care* (Table 9.16, $\beta = 1.16, p \leq 0.001$). The findings for change over time prenatally in *Identification with a Motherhood Role* regressed on *Confidence with Motherhood Role and Tasks* presented in Table 9.15 indicate that the intercept for *Confidence with Motherhood Role and Tasks* at 6-months

Table 9.15 Prenatal slopes of Acceptance of Pregnancy, Identification with a Motherhood Role, Family Adaptability, and Community Support regressed on postpartum Confidence with Motherhood Role scale

Variables	Model 1		Model 2	
	Coeff.	SE	Coeff.	SE
Acceptance of Preganancy slope[a]	0.23	0.28	0.28	0.28
Identification Motherhood Role slope[b]	1.49***	0.34	1.21***	0.38
Family Adaptability slope[c]	0.10	0.12	0.14	0.12
Community Support slope[d]	0.20	0.13	−0.28*	0.14
Acceptance* Family Adaptability[e]			−0.00	0.08
Acceptance* Community Support[f]			0.00	0.12
Identification* Family Adaptability[g]			0.28[†]	0.15
Identification* Community Support[h]			−0.27[†]	0.15
Intercept	17.36***	0.29	17.27***	0.33
Critical value	11.25		6.79	
Degrees of freedom	4		8	

$*p < 0.05$, $**p < 0.01$, $***p < 0.001$, $†p < 0.10$
[a]Slope for Acceptance of Pregnancy scale over the course of pregnancy
[b]Slope of Identification with a Motherhood Role scale over the course of pregnancy
[c]Slope for Family Adaptability scale over the course of pregnancy
[d]Slope for Community Support scale over the course of pregnancy
[e]Interaction of the slopes of Acceptance of Pregnancy and Family Adaptability
[f]Interaction of the slopes of Acceptance of Pregnancy and Community Support
[g]Interaction of the slopes of Identification with a Motherhood Role and Family Adaptability
[h]Interaction of the slopes of Identification with a Motherhood Role and Community Support

Table 9.16 Prenatal slopes of Acceptance of Pregnancy, Identification with a Motherhood Role, Family Adaptability, and Community Support regressed on Postpartum Satisfaction with Infant and Infant Care Scale

Variables	Model 1			Model 2		
	Coeff.		SE	Coeff.		SE
Acceptance of Pregnancy slope[a]	−0.15		0.23	−0.09		0.28
Identification Motherhood Role slope[b]	1.16	***	0.28	0.94	**	0.32
Family Adaptability slope[c]	−0.15		0.10	−0.20	†	0.11
Community Support slope[d]	−0.06		0.11	−0.08		0.12
Acceptance Preg* Family Adaptability[e]				0.03		0.06
Acceptance Preg* Community Support[f]				0.16		0.10
Identification Mohd* Family Adaptability[g]				−0.08	†	0.12
Identification Mohd* Community Support[h]				−0.20	†	0.13
Intercept	15.30	***	0.24	15.20	***	0.29
Critical value	8.35			4.53		
Degrees of freedom	4			8		

$*p < 0.005$, $**p < 0.01$, $***p < 0.001$, $†p < 0.10$
[a]Slope for Acceptance of Pregnancy scale over the course of pregnancy
[b]Slope of Identification with a Motherhood Role scale over the course of pregnancy
[c]Slope for Family Adaptability scale over the course of pregnancy
[d]Slope for Community Support scale over the course of pregnancy
[e]Interaction of the slopes of Acceptance of Pregnancy and Family Adaptability
[f]Interaction of the slopes of Acceptance of Pregnancy and Community Support
[g]Interaction of the slopes of Identification with a Motherhood Role and Family Adaptability
[h]Interaction of the slopes of Identification with a Motherhood Role and Community Support

postpartum began at 17.36 and for every unit increase in conflict associated with *Identification with a Motherhood Role* prenatally, there was an increase of 1.49 in postpartum conflict for *Confidence with the Motherhood Role and Tasks*. In Table 9.16 for *Satisfaction with Infant and Infant Care* at 6-months postpartum, the intercept was 15.30, and for every unit increase in the conflict associated with prenatal *Identification with a Motherhood Role*, there was a 1.16 unit increase in the woman's conflict experienced for postpartum *Satisfaction with Infant and Infant Care Tasks*.

The slopes of Family Adaptability and Community Support had borderline predictive value for different aspects of postpartum maternal psychosocial adaptation. The slope of prenatal Family Adaptability had a borderline significant negative effect to a woman's *Satisfaction with Infant and Infant Care* ($\beta = -0.20$, $p \leq 0.07$) and the slope of Community Support had a statistically significant main effect on *Confidence with the Motherhood Role and Tasks* ($\beta = -0.28$, $p \leq 0.05$). Both results indicate that increases in support either through flexibility within the family, or through greater perceived support from the community network, decreased the conflict associated with *Satisfaction with Infant and Infant Care* and for *Confidence with the Motherhood Role and Tasks*.

Results of First Trimester Prenatal Spousal Deployment on Maternal Postpartum Adaptation

Table 9.17 presents the results of individual regression models tested for the effects of first trimester Spousal Deployment with *Acceptance of Pregnancy* and *Identification with a Motherhood Role* regressed on *Confidence with the Motherhood* and *Tasks* as well as *Satisfaction with Infant and Infant Care* (in a separate model). First trimester Deployment and *Identification with a Motherhood Role* predicted *Satisfaction with Infant and Infant Care* (Table 9.17, Model 2). First trimester Deployment and Acceptance of Pregnancy were borderline predictive of one's Satisfaction with Infant and Infant Care ($\beta = 0.97$, $p \leq 0.07$) (Table 9.17, Model 1).

Table 9.17 Coefficients from Regression of Prenatal Acceptance of Pregnancy and Identification with a Motherhood role with Deployment in the first Trimester on Postpartum Satisfaction with Infant and Infant Care

Variables	Model 1. Prenatal Acceptance B (SE)	Model 2. Prenatal Motherhood Identification B (SE)
Intercept	15.09 (0.16)***	15.22 (0.15)***
Prenatal maternal adapt. scales	0.50[a] (0.12)***	1.25[b] (0.13)***
Deployment[c]	0.97 (0.53)[†]	0.95 (0.49)*
R^2	0.07	0.22

*$p < 0.05$, **$p < 0.01$, ***$p < 0.001$, [†]$p < 0.10$
[a]Slope for Acceptance of Pregnancy scale over the course of pregnancy
[b]Slope of Identification with a Motherhood Role scale over the course of pregnancy
[c]First trimester deployment

9.4.3 Discussion of Part 2. Postpartum Results

The individual trajectories of Acceptance of Pregnancy were not found to be predictive of postpartum Confidence with Motherhood Role and Tasks or Satisfaction with Infant and Infant Care. The results for Type I sums of squares did indicate a significant amount of variance explained by Acceptance of Pregnancy. However, Acceptance of Pregnancy does not explain results above those captured by Identification with a Motherhood Role for these variables. Given the high correlation for Acceptance of Pregnancy and Identification with a Motherhood Role, this result could be expected.

The correlation tables provide verification that concepts within Acceptance of Pregnancy are related to aspects of postpartum maternal psychosocial adaptation. Higher correlations for first trimester Acceptance of Pregnancy to the postpartum maternal psychosocial adaptation variables provide evidence of the importance of early prenatal maternal adaptation to postpartum maternal role formulation for the expectant mother. Early in pregnancy the gravida is concerned with changes taking place in her body and the discomforts associated with pregnancy (Rubin, 1984; Lederman, 1996). As the pregnancy progresses, the movement of the fetus is felt, attachment increases (Laxton-Kane & Slade, 2002), and concerns with role identification heighten. Given the high correlation between Acceptance of Pregnancy and Identification with a Motherhood Role, it is evident that concerns over Acceptance of Pregnancy are impacting motherhood role identification. Additionally, accepting the changes that come with pregnancy and identifying with one's role as early as the first trimester appear to be linked with postpartum satisfaction. In this context, the significance of the change across pregnancy in Identification with a Motherhood Role to the prediction of both Confidence with Motherhood Role and Tasks and Satisfaction with Infant and Infant Care is fully recognized. Haedt and Keel (2007) found that body dissatisfaction during pregnancy moderated a positive relationship between maternal attachment and weeks of pregnancy. Identification with being a mother requires an introspection and an understanding of oneself, as well as the separateness of the developing fetus that can only occur with a growing attachment to one's unborn infant (Grienenberger, Bernback, Levy, and Locker, 2005; Haedt and Keel). This developmental process clearly impacts 6-month postpartum Confidence with Maternal Role and Tasks and Satisfaction with Infant and Infant Care. The findings provide validation for the importance of and the appropriate timing for prenatal intervention. The changes occurring in early- and mid-second trimester are often overlooked because of the perception of increased feelings of well-being by the gravida (Arizmendi & Affonso, 1987; Huizink et al., 2002). The findings with this sample of military women reflect the importance of early prenatal adaptive changes to postpartum maternal adaptation. The longitudinal findings for the support variables of family adaptability and community support provide additional unique results regarding the relationship of prenatal support to the gravida's prenatal and postpartum adaptation.

The prenatal slope for community support was a statistically significant predictor of Confidence with Maternal Role and Tasks. In other words, increased values for prenatal perceived network support decreased the conflict experienced in maternal role confidence at 6 months postpartum. The formulation of oneself as a mother continues throughout pregnancy and into the postpartum period. The results provide some evidence that the relationship between prenatal maternal psychosocial adaptation and later postpartum adaptation can be altered by emotional esteem-building support provided by a community network. It is quite possible that military wives, inexperienced as mothers in a military environment and dislocated from family and life-long friends, may obtain greater value from community network resources than women living in closer proximity to family members. While perceptions of available support may not be particularly accurate (Dunkel-Schetter & Bennett, 1990), various studies have indicated that perceived available support buffers the effects of stress, and received support does not (Gottlieb, 1996; Heller, Swindle, & Dusenbury 1986). In this study, prenatal community support had a direct effect on decreasing postpartum conflict and anxiety related to confidence in maternal role and tasks.

The results reported herein include patterns of relationships as well as results achieving statistical significance. The main effect for the slope of prenatal Family Adaptability had a borderline significant effect to a woman's *Satisfaction with Infant and Infant Care*. Increased flexibility from the family prenatally decreased the conflict the woman experienced postpartum for *Satisfaction with Infant and Infant Care*. The support from a community network did not impact this important component of maternal adaptation. Clearly, the family plays an important role in the woman's acceptance of pregnancy, motherhood role identification, and satisfaction with being a mother. Lower trait and state anxiety scores have been found for women with supportive husbands (Kalil et al., 1993; Norbeck & Anderson, 1989). Kalil et al. measured aspects of emotional support, while Norbeck and Anderson measured emotional and tangible support offered from the husband and gravida's mother. Postpartum role adaptation has been found to be significantly associated with a supportive relationship from the gravida's husband (Lederman, 1990; Florsheim & Smith, 2005). Crnic Greenberg, Robinson, and Basham (1984) describe "intimate" support as being the most important predictor of positive maternal attitudes at 1, 8, and 18 months postpartum. Family functioning has been related to maternal-fetal attachment (Fuller, Moore, & Lester 1993). The focus of family support in this study was adaptability rather than cohesion. Adaptability is a supportive element, closely tied to emotional support, but offering additional clarification of the type of support provided. Flexibility within the family in terms of roles and rules clearly impacts the woman's maternal adaptive process. Parity, in this sample, did not alter the study findings.

The findings for prenatal paternal deployment to postpartum maternal psychosocial adaptation are profound. Namely, the significance of the enduring effects of first trimester military deployment on the woman's prenatal and postpartum maternal adaptation must be underscored. The conflict associated with accepting pregnancy compounded with first trimester deployment had positive borderline significance to the mother's *Satisfaction with Infant and Infant Care*. Moreover, the prenatal conflict the gravida experienced related to identifying with her motherhood role in conjunction with first trimester deployment had a statistically significant positive effect on *Satisfaction with Infant and Infant Care*. Deployment causes feelings of isolation and abandonment for the military family (Duckworth, 2003; Wood, 2004). For the pregnant wife, the feelings of abandonment may be compounded because of the need to formulate her maternal identity through communication with her spouse. The pregnant wife may also feel the stress of taking on additional responsibilities at a time when she desires to concentrate fully on her changing role. Military wives voice their despair over feeling totally isolated during their husbands' deployments (Wood). It is important to note that the conflict the woman experienced related to deployment only impacted the woman's cognitive feelings regarding her satisfaction with her maternal identity and attachment with the infant, but not her confidence with her maternal role and tasks. The absence of the husband impacted aspects of maternal identity formation directly related to the attachment the mother had to her infant rather than her competency in the role. This subtle finding has significance for emergency attachment theory. The significance of first trimester deployment to later satisfaction with the infant and the care of the infant provides quantifiable support for the theories of attachment that describe maternal adaptation as a progressive process building on each stage of pregnancy. The process is significantly affected by the absence of the husband.

References

Alexander, P. C., & Lupfer, S. L. (1987). Family characteristics and long-term consequences associated with sexual abuse. *Archives of Sexual Behavior, 16*, 235–245.

Arizmendi, T. G., & Affonso, D. D. (1987). Stressful events related to pregnancy and postpartum. *Journal of Psychosomatic Research, 31*, 743–756.

Bloom, K. C. (1998). Perceived relationship with the father of the baby and maternal attachment in adolescents. *Journal of Obstetric, Gynecologic, and Neonatal Nursing, 27*, 420–430.

Bowen, G. L., Martin, J. A., Mancini, J. A., & Nelson, J. P. (2000). Community capacity: Antecedents and consequences. *Journal of Community Practice, 8*(2), 1–21.

Condon, J. T., & Corkindale, C. (1997). The correlates of antenatal attachment in pregnant women. *The British Journal of Medical Psychology, 70*, 359–372.

Crnic, K.A., Greenberg, M.T., Robinson, N.M., & Ragozin, A.S. (1984). Maternal stress and social support: Effects on the mother-infant relationship from birth to eighteen months. American *Journal of Orthopsychiatry, 54*, 224–235.

Curtiss, G., Klemz, S., & Vanderploeg, R. D. (2000). Acute impact of traumatic brain injury on family structure and coping responses. *The Journal of Head Trauma Rehabilitation, 15*, 1113–1122.

Deutsch, F. M., Ruble, D. N., Fleming, A., Brooks-Gunn, J., & Stangor, C. (1988). Information-seeking and maternal self-definition during the transition to motherhood. *Journal of Personality and Social Psychology, 55*(3), 420–431.

Duckworth, J. (2003). The military culture. *Family Therapy, 2*, 13–17.

Dunkel-Schetter, C., & Bennett, T. L. (1990). Differentiating the cognitive and behavioral aspects of social support. In B. R. Sarason, I. G. Sarason, & G. R. Pierce (Eds.), *Social support: An interactional view* (pp. 267–296). New York: Wiley.

Dunkel-Schetter, C., Sagrestano, L. M., Feldman, P., & Killingsworth, C. (1996). Social support and pregnancy. In G. R. Pierce, B. R. Sarason, & I. G. Sarason (Eds.), *Handbook of social support and the family* (pp. 375–412). New York: Plenum Press.

Duvall, E. (1977). *Family development*. Philadelphia, PA: Lippincott.

Feldman, P. J., Dunkel-Schetter, C., Sandman, C. A., & Wadhwa, P. D. (2000). Maternal social support predicts birth weight and fetal growth in human pregnancy. *Psychosomatic Medicine, 62*(5), 715–725.

Finello, K. M., Litton, K. M., deLemos, R., & Chan, L. S. (1998). Very low birth weight infants and their families during the first year of life: Comparisons of psychosocial outcomes based on after-care services. *Journal of Perinatology, 18*, 266–271.

Florsheim, P., & Smith, A. (2005). Expectant adolescent couples' relations and subsequent parenting behavior. *Infant Mental Health Journal, 26*, 533–548.

Friedman, A. S., Utada, A., & Morrissey, M. R. (1987). Families of adolescent drug abusers are "rigid": are these families either "disengaged" or "enmeshed," or both? *Family Process, 26*(1), 131–148.

Fuller, S. G., Moore, L. R., & Lester, J. W. (1993). Influence of family functioning on maternal-fetal attachment. *Journal of Perinatology, 13*, 453–460.

Gottlieb, B. H. (1996). Theories and practices of mobilizing support in stressful circumstances. In C. L. Cooper (Ed.), *Handbook of stress, medicine, and health* (pp. 339–357). Boca Raton, FL: CRC.

Grace, J. T. (1993). Mother's self-reports of parenthood across the first 6 months postpartum. *Research in Nursing & Health, 16*, 431–439.

Grienenberger, J., Kelly, K., & Slade, A. (2005). Maternal Reflective Functioning, mother-infant affective communication and infant attachment: Exploring the link between mental states and observed caregiving. Attachment & Human Development, 7, 299–311.

Gurung, R. A. R., Dunkel-Schetter, C., Collins, N., Rini, C., & Hobel, C. J. (2005). Psychosocial predictors of prenatal anxiety. *Journal of Social and Clinical Psychology, 24*, 497–519.

Haedt, A., & Keel, P. (2007). Maternal attachment, depression, and body dissatisfaction in pregnant women. *Journal of Reproductive and Infant Psychology, 25*, 285–295.

Halman, L. J., Oakley, D., & Lederman, R. (1995). Adaptation to pregnancy and motherhood among subfecund and fecund primiparous women. *Maternal Child Nursing Journal, 23*, 90–100.

Heller, K., Swindle, R. W., Jr., & Dusenbury, L. (1986). Component social support processes: Comments and integration. *Journal of Consulting and Clinical Psychology, 54*, 466–470.

Huang, H., Wang, S., & Chen, C. (2004). Body image, maternal-fetal attachment, and the choice of infant feeding method: A study in Taiwan. *Birth, 31*, 183–188.

Huizink, A. C., de Medina, P. G., Mulder, E. J., Visser, G. H., & Buitelaar, J. K. (2002). Coping in normal pregnancy. *Annals of Behavioral Medicine, 24*, 132–140.

Ingoldsby, B. B., Smith, S. R., & Miller, J. E. (2004). *Exploring family theories*. Los Angeles, CA: Roxbury Publishing Company.

Jacobson, D. E. (1986). Types and timing of social support. *Journal of Health and Social Behavior, 27*(3), 250–264.

Kalil, K. M., Gruber, J. E., Conley, J., & Sytniac, M. (1993). Social and family pressures on anxiety and stress during pregnancy. *Pre- and Perinatal Psychology Journal, 8*(2), 113–118.

Kelley, M. L., Finkel, L. B., & Ashby, J. (2003). Geographic mobility, family, and maternal variables as related to the psychosocial adjustment of military children. *Mil Med, 168*(12), 1019–1024.

Laxton-Kane, M., & Slade, P. (2002). The role of maternal prenatal attachment in a woman's experience of pregnancy and implications for the process of care. *Journal of Reproductive and Infant Psychology, 20*, 253–266.

Lederman, R. P., Weingarten, C. G., & Lederman, E. (1981). Postpartum Self-Evaluation Questionnaire: Measures of maternal adaptation. In R. P. Lederman, B. S. Raff, & P. Carroll (Eds.), *Perinatal parental behavior: Nursing research implications for newborn health* (Birth defects: Original article series, 2nd ed., Volume 17, Number 6, pp. 201–231) New York: Alan R. Liss, Inc.

Lederman, R. P. (1990). Anxiety and stress in pregnancy: significance and nursing assessment. *NAACOG'S Clinical Issues in Perinatal Women's Health Nursing, 1*(3), 279–288.

Lederman, R. P. (1996). *Psychosocial adaptation in pregnancy: Assessment of seven dimensions of maternal development* (2nd ed.). New York: Springer.

Lederman, R. P., Weis, K. L., Brandon, J., & Mian, T. S. (2001, November 12). *Prediction of pregnancy outcomes from measures of adaptation to pregnancy and family functioning.* Paper presented at the Sigma Theta Tau International's 36th Biennial Convention, Indianapolis, IN.

Liese, L. H., Snowden, L. R., & Ford, L. K. (1989). Partner status, social support, and psychological adjustment during pregnancy. *Family Relations, 38*, 311–316.

Lederman, R. P., Weingarten, C. G., & Lederman, E. (1981). *Postpartum self-evaluation questionnaire: Measures of maternal adaptation.* Paper presented at the Perinatal parental behavior: Nursing research and implications for newborn health conference *17*(6), 201–231.

Margolin, G., Gordis, E. B., & John, R. S. (2001). Coparenting: A link between marital conflict and parenting in two-parent families. *Journal of Family Psychology, 15*, 3–21.

Martin, J. A. (2000). Afterword: The changing nature of military service and military family life. In J. A. Martin, L. N. Rosen, & L. R. Sparacino (Eds.), *The military family: A practice guide for human service providers* (pp. 257–270). Westport, CN: Praeger.

Martin, J. A., Mancini, D. L., Bowen, G. L., Mancini, J. A., & Orthner, D. (2004). *Building strong communities for military families.* Minneapolis, MN: National Council on Family Relations.

McCubbin, H. I., Patterson, J., & Glynn, T. (1982). Social Support Index (SSI). In H. I. McCubbin, A. I. Thompson & M. A. McCubbin (Eds.), *Family assessment: Resiliency, coping and adaptation - inventories for research and practice* (pp. 357–389). Madison, WI: University of Wisconsin System.

McHale, J. P., & Rotman, T. (2007). Is seeing believing? Expectant parents' outlooks on coparenting and later coparenting solidarity. *Infant Behavior & Development, 30*, 63–81.

Mercer, R. T. (2004). Becoming a mother versus maternal role attainment. *Journal of Nursing Scholarship, 36*, 226–232.

Nelson, A. M. (2003). Transition to motherhood. *Journal of Obstetric, Gynecologic, & Neonatal Nursing, 32*, 465–477.

Norbeck, J. S. (1981). Social support: a model for clinical research and application. *ANS Advances in Nursing Science, 3*(4), 43–59.

Norbeck, J. S., & Anderson, N. J. (1989). Life stress, social support, and anxiety in mid- and late-pregnancy among low income women. *Research in Nursing & Health, 12*(5), 281–287.

Olson, D. H. (1995). Family systems: Understanding your roots. In R. D. Day, K. R. Gilbert, B. H. Settles & W. R. Burr (Eds.), *Research and theory in family science* (pp. 131–153). Pacific Grove, CA: Brooks/Cole Publishing Company.

Olson, D. H. (2000). Circumplex model of marital and family systems. *The Association for Family Therapy and Systemic Practice, 22*, 144–167.

Olson, D. H., Bell, R., & Portner, J. (1992). *FACES II.* Minneapolis, MN: Life Innovations.

Olson, D. H., Sprenkle, D. H., & Russell, C. S. (1979). Circumplex model of marital and family system: I. Cohesion and adaptability dimensions, family types, and clinical applications. *Family Process, 18*, 3–28.

Orr, S. T. (2004). Social support and pregnancy outcome: a review of the literature. *Clinical Obstetrics and Gynecology, 47*(4), 842–855; discussion 881–842.

Procidano, M. E., & Heller, K. (1983). Measures of perceived social support from friends and from family: three validation studies. *American Journal of Community Psychology, 11*(1), 1–24.

Pryor, J. E., Thompson, J. M., Robinson, E., Clark, P. M., Becroft, D. M., Pattison, N. S., et al. (2003). Stress and lack of social support as risk factors for small-for-gestational-age birth. *Acta Paediatrica, 92*(1), 62–64.

Ramsey, C. N., Jr., Abell, T. D., & Baker, L. C. (1986). The relationship between family functioning, life events, family structure, and the outcome of pregnancy. *Journal of Family Practice, 22*, 521–527.

Reeb, K. G., Graham, A. V., Zyzanski, S. J., & Kitson, G. C. (1987). Predicting low birthweight and complicated labor in urban black women: a biopsychosocial perspective. *Social Science and Medicine, 25*(12), 1321–1327.

Reece, S. M. (1995). Stress and maternal adaptation in first-time mothers more than 35 years old. *Applied Nursing Research, 8*, 61–66.

Rubin, R. (1984). *Maternal identity and the maternal experience*. New York: Springer.

Rubin, R. (1977). Binding-in in the postpartum period. *Maternal-Child Nursing Journal, 6,* 67–75.

Salmela-Aro, K., Aunola, K., Saisto, T., Halmesmaki, E., & Nurmi, J.E. (2006). Couples share similar changes in depressive symptoms and marital satisfaction anticipating the birth of a child. *Journal of Social and Personal Relationships, 23,* 781–803.

Schachman, K. A., Lee, R. K., & Lederman, R. P. (2004). Baby boot camp: Facilitating maternal role adaptation among military wives. *Nursing Research, 53,* 107–115.

Shereshefsky, P. M., & Yarrow, L. J. (1973). *Psychological aspects of a first pregnancy and early postnatal adaptation*. New York: Raven Press.

Sidani, S., & Braden, C. (1998). *Evaluating nursing interventions: a theory-driven approach*. Thousand Oaks, CA: Sage Publications.

Singer, J. D. (1998). Using SAS PROC MIXED to fit multilevel models, hierarchical models, and individual growth models. *Journal of Educational and Behavioral Statistics, 24,* 323–355.

Slade, A., Grienenberger, J., Bernback, E., Levy, D., & Locker, A. (2005). Maternal reflective functioning, attachment, and the transmission gap: A preliminary study. *Attachment and Human Development, 7,* 283–298.

Sleutel, M. R. (2003). Intrapartum nursing: integrating Rubin's framework with social support theory. *Journal of Obstetric, Gynecologic, and Neonatal Nursing, 32*(1), 76–82.

Smith, S. R., & Ingoldsby, B. B. (2009). *Exploring family theories* (2nd ed.). New York: Oxford University Press.

Splonskowski, J. M., & Twiss, J. J. (1995). Maternal coping adaptations, social support, and transition difficulties to parenthood of first-time civilian and military mothers. *Military Medicine, 160*(1), 28–32.

Swann, W. B., & Brown, J. D. (1990). From self to health: Self-verification and identity disruption. In B. R. Sarason, I. G. Sarason, & G. R. Pierce (Eds.), *Social support: An interactional view* (pp. 150–172). New York: Wiley.

Trad, P. V. (1991). Adaptation to developmental transformations during various phases of motherhood. *The Journal of the American Academy of Psychoanalysis, 19,* 403–421.

Vega, W. A., Patterson, T., Sallis, J., Nader, P., Atkins, C., & Abramson, I. (1986). Cohesion and adaptability in Mexican-American and Anglo families. *Journal of Marriage and the Family, 48,* 857–867.

Walker, L. O., & Montgomery, E. (1994). Maternal identity and role attainment: Long-term relations to child development. *Nursing Research, 43,* 105–110.

Weis, K. L. (2006). *Maternal identity formation in a military sample: A longitudinal perspective*. Unpublished Dissertation, University of North Carolina, Chapel Hill.

Weiss, R. S. (1974). The provisions of social relationships. In Z. Rubin (Ed.), *Doing unto others* (pp. 17–26). Englewood Cliffs, NJ: Prentice-Hall.

Weiss, S. J., & Chen, J. L. (2002). Factors influencing maternal mental health and family functioning during the low birthweight infant's first year of life. *Journal of Pediatric Nursing, 17*(2), 114–125.

Whitchurch, G., & Constantine, L. (1993). System theory. In P. G. Boss, W. J. Doherty, R. LaRossa, W. Schumm & S. Steinmetz (Eds.), *Sourcebook of family theories and methods: A contextual approach* (pp. 325–352). New York: Plenum.

Wood, D. (2004). Going it alone. *Air Force Times, 64,* 26.

Chapter 10
Prenatal Adaptation Among Multigravidas

In this chapter we present results of both quantitative analysis of prenatal psychosocial adaptation scale differences and differences based on content analyses of the primigravid and multigravid recorded interviews of primigravidas and multigravidas.

10.1 Quantitative Results: Statistical Analysis of Psychosocial Adaptation to Pregnancy Based on Parity

We have conducted research to compare psychosocial development, anxiety, and depression in primigravid and multigravid women across each trimester of pregnancy to determine mean level differences and pattern variations. The large study sample was comprised of 689 multicultural, low-income normal Caucasian (54.2%), African American (29%), and Hispanic English speaking (16.8%) gravidas, aged 18–44 years, attending a southwestern university hospital obstetric clinic (Lederman, Harrison, & Worsham, 1995). The majority of patients in the clinic were on Medicaid and had no health insurance. Most of the mothers were multigravidas (74.1%) with no history of premature delivery (87%). The Prenatal Self-Evaluation Questionnaire (PSEQ) was administered to the participants once in each trimester. Data were collected from cross-sectional sample populations with smaller sub-samples participating in at least two or all three trimesters of pregnancy.

Group comparisons on the PSEQ scales, the State-Trait Anxiety Inventory, and the Beck Depression Inventory were calculated using analysis of variance and post hoc Sheffé tests to identify significant group mean differences, shown in Table 10.1 Float. The Cronbach reliability coefficients for the seven PSEQ scales in all three trimesters ranged from 0.71 to 0.93.

The results show that multigravid women experience greater state anxiety and developmental conflict concerning Acceptance of Pregnancy and Relationship to (the gravida's) Mother in third trimester pregnancy. Primigravid women experience greater anxiety concerning their preparedness for labor in all trimesters of pregnancy, and fears concerning helplessness and loss of control in labor in the last two trimesters. These differences, particularly the number of differences in third trimester

R. Lederman and K. Weis, *Psychosocial Adaptation to Pregnancy*,
DOI 10.1007/978-1-4419-0288-7_10, © Springer Science+Business Media, LLC 2009

Table 10.1 Group Means ± Standard Deviation (*n*) of Primigravid and Multigravid Women

	Primigravidas	*Multigravidas*	t(*df*)
State anxiety, third trimester	39.2 ± 10 (141)	41.9 ± 10.6 (224)	−2.40 (363)*
Acceptance of pregnancy, third trimester	24.6 ± 7.6 (144)	28.1 ± 9.4 (235)	−3.75 (377)***
Relationship to mother, third trimester	15.9 ± 6.8 (143)	19.4 ± 7.9 (227)	−4.32 (368)***
Preparation for labor, first trimester	23.9 ± 5.4 (88)	18.2 ± 5.5 (118)	7.45 (204)***
Second trimester	22.5 ± 5.9 (132)	17.4 ± 5.3 (173)	7.94 (303)***
Third trimester	20.9 ± 5.5 (145)	17.6 ± 5.4 (235)	5.70 (378)***
Fear of pain, helplessness, and loss of control in labor, second trimester	22.2 ± 5.4 (132)	20.8 ± 5.6 (172)	2.24 (302)*
Third trimester	22.0 ± 5.0 (145)	20.1 ± 5.5 (235)	3.27 (378)**

Note. Significant differences in group mean pairs are identified with *$p< 0.05$, **$p< 0.01$, ***$p< 0.001$

of pregnancy, indicate that unresolved conflict is associated with greater anxiety as pregnancy advances to term. It is noteworthy that no parity differences were found in Identification with a Motherhood Role and Relationship with Husband, trait anxiety, or depression. These results indicate a need for a differential emphasis in education and counseling regarding the fears and concerns of primigravid and multigravid women. Green and Baston (2003) found similar results with regard to prenatal expectations and feelings of control in labor, with multigravidas reporting significantly greater control regarding the hospital staff, their own behavior, and control during contractions. They also recommended separate childbirth education for both primigravidas and multigravidas. While research reporting difference in parity is rare, our significant results may be a reflection of the large sample, and the diversity or uniqueness of sample characteristics.

10.2   Qualitative Analysis of Psychosocial Adaptation to Pregnancy Based on Parity

Another longitudinal study described in Chapter One was conducted with a sample comprised entirely of normal multigravid women (i.e., during a woman's second or subsequent pregnancies), age 20–42, in addition to a prior project with normal primigravid women. The 73 women participating in the project were followed from last trimester pregnancy, through labor and delivery, and up to 6 weeks postpartum. Data on psychosocial adaptation were collected in three prenatal interviews focusing on maternal adaptation concerning the seven prenatal personality dimensions, and two focusing on postnatal adaptation. Content analyses were conducted using the prenatal rating scales and scale definitions that were utilized with the sample of primigravidas. The responses of the multigravid women to the interview questions and scales are presented, and contrasted to primigravid responses.

As might be expected, the reactions and feelings expressed in interviews by women who have had a previous pregnancy, labor, and delivery, and who already were experiencing motherhood, differed from the reactions and feelings expressed by women experiencing pregnancy for the first time.

To the multigravidas, labor and delivery were more familiar events (Aaronson, Mural, & Pfoutz, 1988; Crowe, & von Baeyer, 1989; Morcos, Snart, & Harley, 1989). Their fears and anxieties were related to memories of their previous labor and delivery experiences, whereas primigravidas tended to experience more fears of the unknown (Kuczynski & Thompson, 1985; Moss, Bolland, Foxman, & Owen, 1987; Stolte, 1987). Primigravidas attempted to glean from the experiences of their own mothers or sisters an approximation of the events they would experience for themselves in labor, whereas multigravidas relied more heavily on their prior childbirth memories in formulating their images of childbirth and its challenges.

The multigravidas in this study, similar to earlier studies, differed from the primigravidas in the dimension of Identification with a Motherhood Role. Although this is generally a major adjustment, for primigravidas this dimension involved more encompassing changes in the perception of self (Brouse, 1988). That is, when a woman is pregnant with her first child, she takes the profound step from being a "woman without child to a woman with child," as noted in earlier chapters.

With the multigravidas, however, adaptation involved familiar as well as novel experiences. The women already were in a motherhood role, and the addition of another child spurred them to expand their identification with this role. The multigravidas' concerns involved coping with the many demands of another newborn, while continuing to provide care for their older child or children. Many women learn after having second and subsequent children that raising two children involves more than twice the work of raising one, and that the motherhood role is necessarily somewhat different with each child because of the unique personalities and varying needs and propensities of each child.

The women in this study reported a wide range of responses when questions were posed about the seven dimensions of prenatal adaptation. Many of these responses, and the ways in which they differed from the responses of primigravid women, are discussed throughout this chapter.

10.2.1 Acceptance of Pregnancy

There were no "typical" responses among the multigravidas on this dimension. The women tended to accept their pregnancies, and most were planned. Some of the pregnancies were unplanned and/or unwanted and the women had difficulty accepting them initially, but eventually either resigned themselves or learned to accept the pregnancy and the imminent labor and delivery. Condon and Esuvaranathan (1990) found that there were significantly more unplanned pregnancies among first-time expectant couples.

Ms. Roosevelt, a 32-year-old secretary who was pregnant with her second child, offered the following rationale for pregnancy.

Well, I describe pregnancy always as just a long ordeal, but I love children so it's a necessary ordeal.

This was a fairly common view among multigravidas. Only a few women actually stated that they enjoyed pregnancy, but, for the most part, they acknowledged pregnancy as a necessary "rite of passage" to having children.

Ms. Kennedy, a doctoral candidate, was shocked when she learned she was pregnant with her third child. "After we got over the initial shock, we decided that if we're ever going to have another child, this would be the best time to have one."

A 19-year-old participant in the study, Ms. Truman, accepted her pregnancy well although she said that it was not planned. She had two children already, and had a spontaneous abortion when she was 16 or 17. Ms. Truman exhibited very little noticeable pain or stress during labor, although she did lose her composure while pushing.

Ms. Truman relayed some conflictual responses to questions on acceptance of pregnancy. The fact that she was a mother at the young age of 19, and that none of her pregnancies was planned, contributed to the ambivalence she expressed regarding acceptance of pregnancy. For example, she said that she did not believe in abortion, but then remarked, "I, you know, I never wanted none [sic] of my kids, to tell you the truth." Admitting that she never wanted any of her children, but at the same time not considering abortion or more preventive planning any of the times she became pregnant revealed possibly opposing sentiments and may well have added to Ms. Truman's conflict regarding acceptance of pregnancy.

A 23-year-old woman, Ms. Johnson, did not plan her second pregnancy, but said she was happy about it. When comparing it to her first pregnancy, she said that she was "grouchy" and "hard to live with" the first time, but not the second time. Noticing an improvement in her attitude from the earlier pregnancy enabled Ms. Johnson to be more accepting of her current pregnancy.

Neither Ms. Johnson, nor Ms. Jackson, a 33-year-old full-time homemaker and mother of one child, indicated the reasons for their improved attitudes during interviews, although both said that they were more at ease with their second pregnancies because they knew what to expect. Ms. Jackson had planned her pregnancy and was pleased with it. She said that she felt "emotionally much better" than she did during her first pregnancy.

10.2.1.1 Body Image and Career Transitions during Pregnancy

Although she accepted the pregnancy and was familiar with the experience, Ms. Jackson had some problems accepting the appearance of her pregnant body and the limitations it placed on her activities. Her response was not infrequent among the women in this or in other projects (Lipps, 1985). "I like to be thin. I like to play tennis," she said.

Ms. Sharp, age 29, also had trouble accepting her pregnancy because she could not accept her pregnant body. In fact, she actually referred to her "inability to accept my body this way," and said, "I like being thin and I think that's more attractive than being pregnant, … a lot more attractive."

In contrast, body image had an unusual impact on Ms. O'Neill's acceptance of her pregnancy. She wrote in her dream diary that she enjoyed being pregnant because she already was overweight and that pregnancy gave her an excuse to wear loose-fitting clothing.

In addition to her body image difficulties, Ms. Sharp, who saw a therapist during the study, also seemed to be harboring some resentment concerning the pregnancy, which she said kept her from getting a promotion at work. She was a financial analyst with a master's degree in business, and it was clear that she felt the pregnancy interrupted her career plans.

> … once people at work knew I was pregnant, it really put a halt to any potential moves or promotions that could come up…. I know it will take the management a certain amount of time to adjust to the fact that I am still interested in a career and that I'm serious about working…

Yet another woman, Ms. Whitmire, aged 32 and the mother of one, was depressed because she found that she could no longer fit into her maternity clothes during the third trimester. However, this did not affect her acceptance of the pregnancy. She was excited about the pregnancy, but said she did not want to become pregnant again after the second child was born. In fact, she said she wished she could have twins because she would like to have three children, but did not want to be pregnant again.

Thus, a number of women had little appreciation for their expanding gestational girth and the detractions it imposed physically and in terms of self-image. Concern with interruption of a career compounded their sense of imposition.

10.2.1.2   The Impact of Experience and Family Planning on Acceptance of Pregnancy

Ms. Wilson, age 24, said that her second pregnancy was planned, and she appeared to have accepted it well for a number of reasons. She said she was happy about the pregnancy because her 3-year-old daughter needed a brother or sister. The second pregnancy also was better than her first because she did not cry as often. She added a comment that was by no means atypical among the multigravidas in the study. When queried about her acceptance of the pregnancy, she said that she knew this would be her last pregnancy. Some of the multigravidas experiencing what they hoped would be their last pregnancy expressed the feeling that they could accept the pregnancy and even enjoy it to an extent because they knew they were not planning to go through another pregnancy again.

In some cases, even though a pregnancy was unplanned, the women adapted to pregnancy fairly easily, expressing that their earlier childbirth experiences helped them with acceptance; this phenomenon was also noted by Shereshefsky and Yarrow (1973). Ms. Bradley said that she was comfortable with her third pregnancy "because I've been through it twice." Thus, the multigravid women in the study had a frame of reference from which to draw. They knew what to expect from pregnancy, and this seemed to make the transition easier to accept.

Ms. Carter, age 27, fully accepted her pregnancy because she had planned it for some time. She had been taking fertility drugs before she became pregnant. However, Ms. Carter said that early in the second trimester she began to feel that no one was paying attention to her or caring for her. Nevertheless, Ms. Carter expressed acceptance and happiness about her pregnancy.

Desire for another child did not always translate into overall acceptance of pregnancy among the multigravidas. Ms. Cleveland, an assistant librarian with a 2-year-old daughter, said that she had been trying for 3 years to become pregnant again. But she expressed some ambivalence saying that although she was "happy" about the pregnancy and that it was "mostly planned," she was worried about caring for another child. It is possible that her reticence was related in some way to her past mental health, and the challenge presented by caring for another child. She had attempted suicide several times, had been in a psychiatric hospital, and had been seeing a psychiatrist following her discharge.

10.2.1.3   Other Factors Bearing on Acceptance of Pregnancy

Several factors seemed to have influenced the multigravidas' acceptance of their pregnancies to some degree, such as spousal response, fear of abandonment, and fears concerning labor. In the case of Ms. Stevenson, her husband's extreme and outspoken lack of acceptance made it difficult for her to accept the pregnancy. Ms. Stevenson, a 33-year-old homemaker, was pregnant with her fourth child. She said that the pregnancy was unexpected and came as a shock to her and her husband, a minister. He rejected the pregnancy so totally that he refused to accompany Ms. Stevenson to the hospital and was not present during the labor or delivery. Her husband's attitude made Ms. Stevenson's pregnancy rather unpleasant for her, and the pregnancy had a profound impact on their marital relationship. This will be discussed in greater detail in the section on Relationship to Husband.

Another woman whose husband did not want a fourth child was Ms. Moyers, a 32-year-old homemaker, Ms. Moyers already had children aged 13, 6, and 3 years. Her husband was a yard worker and was concerned about the adequacy of his income. However, in Ms. Moyers' case, her husband's attitude did not seem to affect her acceptance of the pregnancy to a great degree. She said that she had been trying for 2 years to talk her husband into having a fourth child, and also talked at great length about how she felt it would not be more financially burdensome to have another child. This was a woman who loved newborns and infants, which eased her acceptance of another pregnancy.

One woman's comments gave the appearance that she had accepted her pregnancies so well that she did not experience the normal discomforts of pregnancy. Ms. Richards had two children, 2 and 4 years old, and had planned her third pregnancy. She said that she had experienced no pain and commented, "I haven't even really considered myself pregnant." However, in her dream diary, Ms. Richards said she had dreamed that she was in a cafeteria with an old boyfriend, and that her husband was with another girl who was "beautiful and thin." Ms. Richards frequently dreamed that her husband would leave her, and also dreamed that he compared her with more attractive women and found her lacking. Ms. Richards was a devoutly religious person, referring to herself as a "born again Christian." She also indicated that her beliefs had taught her to place a high premium on motherhood. It is possible that Ms. Richards felt a moral and spiritual obligation to accept and be happy about the pregnancy, while at the same time feeling ambivalence that manifested itself in her dreams of abandonment and rejection.

Ms. Patman, already the mother of a 15-month-old infant, expressed many conflicts about the acceptance of pregnancy. This was attributed, in part, to an admitted fear of death that seemed to permeate many of her responses. Although Ms. Patman said that she had planned her pregnancy, dreams and other statements indicated she experienced conflict. For example, she dreamed about having a baby without having to go through labor, and also dreamed about having general anesthesia during labor so that she would not remember the experience. Concerning her pregnancy, Ms. Patman said, "I've just been wanting to get it over with." She also said, "I still think it's too soon to have another one [child]." These statements, as well as her dreams, indicated she was experiencing some conflict in acceptance of the pregnancy, although the ratings on scales indicated moderate to low conflict in this area. Ms. Patman's responses did not indicate any cause for the difference between her answers to interview questions and her answers on the questionnaires.

10.2.1.4   Financial Considerations of a Larger Family

The very real concern of having an additional child to provide for can constitute a hindrance to acceptance of pregnancy, and one that is more pronounced than in a first pregnancy.

Multigravidas who worked outside the home, such as Ms. Pepper, had additional concerns with which to contend while trying to accept another pregnancy. Ms. Pepper, an editorial assistant and mother of one, said that her pregnancy was not planned, adding: "And it was a bad time for us because…our finances are in really bad shape." However, some of the women in this study were full-time home-makers and mothers, and did not work outside their homes. The majority of women, approximately 60%, had worked outside the home at some point prior to participat-ing in the study, while almost 10% had never worked outside the home. It is likely that pregnancy was easier to accept for those women who did not work outside the home after delivery, because they did not have to worry about finances, taking time off from work, finding child care in order to return to work, or other concerns facing working mothers. Condon and Esuvaranathan (1990) reported that multigravidas are employed significantly less than primigravidas.

Acceptance of pregnancy did not necessarily mean wholehearted enjoyment of pregnancy. Ms. Cisneros, age 36, said she had planned her pregnancy and, in fact, had made major plans to accommodate having and raising a second child. Nevertheless, she obviously was eager for pregnancy to end and stated, "We feel, both of us, I think, as if I'd been pregnant for a year and a half instead of eight months.…I think my body is just plain tired of being pregnant."

Ms. Cisneros, like several other women in the study, dreamed about being able to have a child without going through labor and delivery.

10.2.1.5 Summary: Acceptance of Pregnancy

It is clear that many factors enter into a multigravida's acceptance of pregnancy. Financial and career considerations, as well as the anticipated impact on the established family unit, play a role in how well a woman accepts being pregnant. Body image also affects a multigravida's acceptance, although perhaps not to the degree that it affects a woman who has never before been pregnant. Additionally, concerns over spousal acceptance of pregnancy are very real regardless of one's age, parity, or ethnicity (Nelson, 2003). Research shows that pregnancy is accepted with greater ease if it was planned (Condon & Corkindale, 1997; Finer & Henshaw, 2006), but the participants in this study all seemed to learn to accept or, at least, resign themselves to being pregnant. It is clear from many of the interview responses that the multigravidas found it easier to accept their pregnancies because they had undergone the experience before, found it familiar, and were not as dismayed by the changes in their bodies and emotions.

10.2.2 Identification with a Motherhood Role

As mentioned previously, and as documented elsewhere (Brouse, 1988; Hiser, 1987), the dimensions Acceptance of Pregnancy and Identification with a Motherhood Role were necessarily different for multigravidas and primigravidas because of the nature of the changes taking place, and because multigravidas had additional children.

The multigravidas in the study, particularly those pregnant with their second child, were concerned primarily with how their children were going to accept a sibling (Ching, 1986). Even though these women already had made the transition to the role of woman with child, they again had to form an identity with the role of "mother with a newborn" (Hiser, 1987). Other researchers (Condon & Esuvaranathan, 1990; Haedt & Keel, 2007) have noted that second-time expectant parents tended to be more stressed, but less attached to their unborn infants than first-time expectant parents. The authors reasoned that second-timers were more stressed as a result of environmental variables (financial problems, the demands of other children) and less attached because of a decreased novelty in experiencing the parental–fetal relationship in a subsequent pregnancy.

10.2.2.1 Anxiety About Anticipated Life Changes and the Unknown Child

Ms. Roosevelt compared the process of forming the identification of a motherhood role during her second pregnancy with that of her first.

> Looking back on the first pregnancy, the first delivery of a child, I didn't realize the extent to which it would change my life, and now I anticipate an equal extent, and the thing is you can't tell ahead of time exactly how that will affect you and what your life will be like afterward.

Ms. Roosevelt expressed a great deal of anxiety over the changes a second child would bring and said she had observed that having children "takes over" the lives of some of her friends. She also said that she could not visualize her baby as a person until it was born. A woman who seemed to be under a great deal of stress, Ms. Patman, also seemed to have difficulty expanding her identification of a motherhood role. She became upset and began crying during an interview while discussing how she would manage with two children to care for. After her second child was born, Ms. Patman continued to have trouble adjusting to her expanded motherhood role. When discussing the extra attention that her first child needed during this time, Ms. Patman said, "Sometimes I wish that the other one [child] wasn't around so much so I could spend more time with him [the newborn child]." It is clear that she found it difficult to fulfill the demands of both children.

Ms. Kennedy, on the other hand, seemed to more readily identify with an expanded motherhood role. When asked about what changes the new baby would bring, she said it would be more expensive, but that she anticipated no other major changes.

10.2.2.2   Preparing Children for a Sibling

Regarding material preparations for motherhood, Ms. Kennedy said during her third trimester that she was "ill-prepared" for the baby in terms of its room and belongings. However, she said that she had been discussing the baby with her children. In this way, Ms. Kennedy was taking care of the concern that was a priority for her – her children's reactions to the new baby.

Ms. Bradley also stated that she was concerned about her two other children feeling neglected after the new baby was born.

Ms. McGovern, a 32-year old with three children, said after her baby was born that one of the children kept calling him "ugly." Such reactions among older children were common. Women who had more than one child, such as Ms. McGovern, knew about and expected manifestations of sibling rivalry and were not surprised by it.

A 35-year-old pathologist and mother of one, Ms. Brooks, said that she was worried about the feelings of her older child. Before the new baby was born, her daughter kept going around the house, pointing at things and saying "mine." "I would say she's changing for the bad," Ms. Brooks said. Indeed, after the baby was born, Ms. Brooks said that the older child began showing jealous behavior. She said, "Whenever I was not with her [the new child], I had to be with the older one to make her feel better."

Ms. Bullock, a 30-year-old mother of one, said she was fairly sure that having another baby would change her life, but seemed unclear about exactly what aspects of her life would change. After the baby was born, she appeared worried that her older child was feeling neglected because of all the attention focused on the baby.

10.2.2.3   The Impact of Past Experience with Motherhood

Past experience with motherhood was an asset to most of the multigravidas during the process of identification with a motherhood role (Brouse, 1988; Hiser, 1987).

Ms. Wilson said that she envisioned becoming a better mother with her second child because she would know what to expect in terms of behavior and development.

> I can see a lot of improvement [in myself as a mother]....I could see where I would want to improve myself as a mother.... [I] have a little bit more patience, maybe. [I] know what to expect, when to expect it [children's misbehavior], and what to do when they do it.

This proved true as revealed in one of her postpartum interviews. Ms. Wilson said that the new baby held his breath when having temper tantrums, and that her family would get extremely concerned, but that she did not worry about it because she knew what was happening from experience with her first child. On the other hand, Ms. Wilson commented that she did not remember motherhood chores being so time consuming. Moreover, she said that she viewed the baby as a financial burden. Postpartally, she was rated as having high conflict on the dimension Satisfaction with Life Circumstances.

As can be seen from the previous examples, as well as subsequent anecdotes, maternal confidence regarding childcare tasks needs to be differentiated from satisfaction gained from the motherhood role and activities.

Feelings of security based on knowing how to care for their newborns were commonly expressed by the multigravidas (Hiser, 1987). Ms. Whitmire said,

> I probably had more doubts with the first one. I think I feel pretty secure right now because I think I feel I know how to do everything now since I've been through it once before.

Ms. Whitmire was the woman who stated that she would like to have twins, because she wanted to have three children without going through three pregnancies. In actuality, she seemed satisfied with and thus well adapted to her role, as evidenced by the following statement: "I just love my little girl – I wouldn't mind tripling the joy." Thus, Ms. Whitmire's negative statement about the chore of pregnancy did not have an ominous parallel in the development of a motherhood role.

Likewise, Ms. Cisneros said that having a second child would not cause a total upheaval in her life because she knew what to expect. However, just as having experience with mothering a newborn helped some of the multigravidas better identify with a motherhood role. This same experience caused anxiety in others (Brouse, 1988; Hiser, 1987). Ms. Humphrey, a 29-year-old registered nurse, said during her postpartum interview that she was not really excited about being a mother again. She said she thought this was because she knew what it was like to have a newborn – the colic, the 4 a.m. feedings, the crying, and other things.

One of the multigravidas, Ms. Cleveland, expressed some anxiety over identification with a motherhood role, even though she already had a 17-month-old child. "It's like having the first one. You can't imagine what having two is going to be like until it happens."

Nevertheless, Ms. Cleveland expected the new baby to be "more work, but more fun." She said that she wanted to be as effective a mother for her second child as she was for her first. She had experienced postpartum depression after her first delivery, and expected it again, but did not appear overly concerned about it.

Ms. Truman, who was only 19 years old and already had two children, was firmly established in a motherhood role. She said that she knew it would be harder to care and provide for a third child, but said she did not expect it to change her life in any major way.

Another mother of two, Ms. Rayburn, said she did not expect that having a third child would change her life. She identified with being a mother, although no one in her support network was happy about her having another child.

The number of children the women already had did not seem to have a substantial effect on their ability to expand their identification of a motherhood role (Hiser, 1987; Mercer, Ferketich, DeJoseph, May, & Sollid, 1988). For example, Ms. Hobby, who already had three children, said that she was not concerned about the changes another baby would bring about. She also said that she considered caring for an infant "fun." Her youngest child was 4 years old at the time of the study, so it had been some time since she had had an infant to care for.

Ms. King, a 28-year-old woman with one child, said that her pregnancy was not interrupting her plans to finish her master's degree. Indeed, she seemed quite well adapted to assuming a motherhood role, expressing that it turned out to be satisfying and healthy for herself and her family. After the baby was born, she reported that she and her husband were going out together more, "just the two of them," than they had gone out following the birth of their first baby.

Ms. Pepper also reported that her attitudes had changed since her first child was born. She had not started her first child on bottle feeding before returning to work and had had a great deal of trouble weaning him. Because of her prior experience, she decided that she would start her second baby on bottle feeding sooner, to make the transition easier for all concerned. After her second child was born, Ms. Pepper said that she was getting to know her second child better and sooner than her first. She said the fact that this was her second child enabled her to make many decisions.

Prior experience provided the mothers with a repertoire of resources in preparation for the care of a second child, and with an element of confidence regarding the nature of tasks to be performed.

10.2.2.4   Anticipation of Life Changes

The multigravidas who anticipated major life changes seemed, for the most part, to take the changes in stride. Ms. Carter said she realized that having a third child would tie her down a little more, but had no problems adjusting to the new baby. Postpartally, she also noted that she was not getting as angry about the new baby's crying and demands as she had with her first two children.

Ms. McGovern was optimistic about the changes a fourth baby would bring into her life. She wrote in her diary that she dreamed of having a new baby to care for. She said she liked the idea of having a new baby around. In a postpartum interview she said, "It's a big change in our family and in our life, but it's all been positive."

Ms. Bentsen, aged 39 and mother of one, said she expected that the new baby would change her life "a lot," but did not believe her life would be "completely consumed" by the new baby. She was working on her doctoral dissertation and was concerned with completing this endeavor in the pockets of time that would occur between the many childcare tasks she anticipated.

Ms. Brooks also reflected on the upcoming changes in her life.

> I know I'm not going to have time for myself in the sense of listening to records or reading a book or going to the pictures that I like, or to the symphony, or whatever.

Many of the women in the study were making different types of arrangements for their new babies from those they had made for their first baby. For example, Ms. Jackson said she had made plans to have a high school student stay with her older child and the new baby, so that she could have a day off each week. "I learned that the hard way last time. I was so protective. I was afraid to even leave him with a sitter."

This time, however, Ms. Jackson seemed to look forward to her new baby gaining a little independence. She dreamed that her newborn would be much more developed than normal at birth – that he would be talking, moving about, and other things. She also dreamed of being unmarried and "free" again. Although she had identified with a motherhood role, Ms. Jackson still had some conflict about how much care and attention the newborn would need.

It was not uncommon for the women in this study to have even higher conflict levels regarding their motherhood role following the birth of the baby. Ms. Moyers was one such woman. In her first prenatal interview, she said that she was eager to have another baby, but in her final postpartum interview she seemed distressed with the care of her other children.

Ms. Moyers said that she was depressed from being locked in the house with four kids day after day. This type of reaction could have been due to a transitory postpartum depression, a common and short-lived occurrence which she and other mothers experienced. Nevertheless, expressions such as being "locked in the house" also would seem to indicate a certain amount of resentment toward the extra work involved in having another child and the accompanying loss of personal freedom (Kennerly & Gath, 1989; Knight & Thirkettle, 1987).

10.2.2.5 Summary: Identification with a Motherhood Role

Women who have once before experienced a pregnancy, labor, delivery, and childrearing clearly have developed some sort of identification with a motherhood role. While it can be assumed that it would be easier for a multigravida to identify with this role than for a primigravida to do so, there still are certain hurdles in the identification process. The woman who already has one or more children must determine what her role will be in terms of having additional children. Also, she must prepare herself emotionally, physically, financially, and in other ways for the challenges that inevitably occur as the result of being the mother of more than one child. It appears that the participants in this study were pensive about the many meanings of motherhood role expansion to accommodate another child.

10.2.3 Relationship with Mother

Regardless of how many children the women had, each tended to think about their own mothers in relation to their pregnancy and their expanded motherhood role, although to a lesser extent than during a first pregnancy. Since these women had been previously pregnant and already had children, it was no longer as important as it once had been to reminisce with their mothers about pregnancy and childbirth experiences. It appears that a woman's natural mother is the motherhood prototype for a primigravid woman, while the standard for a multigravida is her own previous mothering experience (Belsky & Isabella, 1985).

10.2.3.1 Motherhood as a Maturational and Developmental Milestone

The most common expressions used by the gravidas to describe their feelings toward their mothers were "tolerance" and "understanding." These women felt that they could better understand their mothers' actions because they themselves were now mothers. This was true even in cases in which the woman did not have a good relationship with her mother. The excerpts that follow illustrate the dynamics of this developmental milestone.

Ms. Roosevelt said that both she and her mother were demanding, but that she tended to be less demanding than her mother. She also said her relationship with her mother had grown "more accepting." "I think that anyone who goes through the experience of bearing a child and trying to raise the child understands a lot more of what anyone who's done the same thing goes through."

Ms. Roosevelt experienced considerable conflict in the relationship with her mother and had some unresolved conflicts from her childhood. She began crying when discussing her family, remarking, "We were not affectionate. We were not warm and loving."

Ms. Wilson said that she became more tolerant of her mother since having her own children. She said that her parents had a "bad" divorce and that her mother handled it poorly. In fact, Ms. Wilson's mother had left her in her father's care when she was a child. However, some of her negative feelings toward her mother began to diminish as she started her own family.

> She left us kids with my father and so we stayed with my father, but at the time I didn't understand that she had no way of supporting us.... She had no job.... She just thought it was totally over for her. Kids were gone. Her husband is gone. Her whole life was gone.

Another woman who said that she was more tolerant of her mother after having a child of her own was Ms. Cleveland. She stated that she wanted to be the same kind of mother her own mother was, with "an infinite amount of patience and love." It was common for the women in this study to report that their feelings toward their mothers became more positive after having children of their own. This dynamic was greater among multigravidas than among primigravidas, perhaps because, in addition to bearing a child, they also were raising a child or children. Attitudes and perceptions of their mothers shifted, as they identified more fully with a mother-hood role themselves (Belsky & Isabella, 1985).

Ms. Jackson, when speaking about the changes in the relationship with her mother, said, "We have a lot more in common, obviously."

Ms. Brooks said, "… if anything, you tend to understand your mother more when you have children."

One possible explanation for the multigravidas' change of attitude is that they had come to realize that their mothers' advice on pregnancy and childrearing had some value in their lives. By experiencing the same things their mothers had experienced, the women were able to understand that their mothers did, indeed, know what they were talking about. Another possibility is that the women found their mothers' actions, beliefs, and behaviors more understandable after becoming mothers themselves.

Ms. Wright, a housewife and former art teacher with two children, said that she had gained respect for her mother through her own childrearing experiences. Ms. King also said she had more respect for her mother. This response was common among the gravidas.

10.2.3.2 The Impact of a Current Negative or Nonexistent Relationship with the Mother

There were some women who responded negatively to questions about the relationship with their mothers. Ms. Moyers, for example, said during a postpartum interview that she was frustrated with her mother because her mother thought she should stay home with the children all the time and never go out. Ms. O'Neill said her mother would not discuss labor and delivery with her at all, and seemed "squeamish" and disapproving of her plans to breastfeed. Most of the multigravidas seemed to have gained a measure of autonomy in their subsequent pregnancies, and their mothers' disapproval did not devastate them.

Ms. Humphrey said that she felt more in control of her temper and more under-standing of her own children than her mother was of her as a child. She said she resented some of the things that her mother did when she was a child. Sustained conflicts of this nature usually meant that the woman did not, or felt she could not, depend on her mother as a source of support during her pregnancy.

The only significant remark Ms. Cisneros made about her mother was that she seemed to care about her more when she was pregnant. It is common for family members to give more attention to a woman who is "heavy with child." This might lead some women to feel that their value as persons is not as high as their value as mothers, a deduction also evident in the testimony of other mothers' remarks.

As might be expected, women whose mothers were unavailable because of death, divorce, or other reasons experienced remorse with regard to the loss of their mothers (Belsky & Isabella, 1985). The women experienced this absence as a painful void that was particularly pronounced during pregnancy.

Ms. Hightower's parents were dead, and she said she missed her mother very much and wished that she were around to give her support and guidance during her pregnancies, as well as with bringing up her children.

Ms. McGovern said she got along much better with her stepmother than with her real mother, and counted on her stepmother for support and guidance. In fact, she said that she did not want her real mother to be with her after the baby was born. She also said she was like her real mother, although she did not want to be.

> ... I look like her [my mother]. I'm built like her, and I have a lot of her personality in me... And... when I get tired, I find myself sitting there yelling at the kids.... And of course, when I think back on it, my mother had lost her control very often.... So I can see a lot of her in me.

Nevertheless, Ms. McGovern's feelings toward her mother seemed to soften somewhat as her own identification with a motherhood role expanded.

> She is demanding and... critical ... Since I've had children. ... I do understand what she went through so I can understand why she is like she is, which does help.

Ms. Brooks was adamant about not wanting either of her parents around while she was in labor. She was not unique. In contrast to primigravid women, most of the multigravidas said that they did not think about their parents or in-laws when they envisioned the trial of labor for themselves. This was not necessarily indicative of the quality of relationships with the parents. Based on previous experience with childbirth and motherhood, the multigravidas had solidified an identification of themselves as wives and mothers, and their preference for support during labor was even more exclusively the husband.

10.2.3.3   Summary: Relationship with Mother

Pregnancy, labor, and delivery are times of great vulnerability in a woman's life and, as such, are times when a woman's thoughts and feelings are likely to turn toward her own mother. If the relationship between the gravid woman and her mother is a supportive one, then this will enhance the gravid woman's sense of self-esteem and, as a result, the perceptions she retains about her pregnancy experience. If, however, the relationship is unsupportive, it can negatively color the childbearing experience. Because of the novelty inherent in primigravid pregnancy and the parallel heightened sense of vulnerability, it follows that the relationship with the mother will have a somewhat lesser impact on the multigravid than on the primigravid woman. Overall, however, this is a time when women tend to reflect upon their relationships with their mothers while continuing to formulate an expanded motherhood role for themselves.

It appears that the significance of fostering mutual support and understanding of the mother and grandmother for each other is worthy of the continued attention of health care workers and should be addressed in prenatal care.

10.2.4 Relationship with Husband or Partner

The multigravidas and primigravidas in this study also differed in the ways that their relationships with their husbands changed during pregnancy, and in how these changes affected their coping responses in labor and delivery.

For the primigravida, pregnancy is a completely novel experience, and the attendant changes in the marriage often are startling (Bailey & Hailey, 1986–1987; Glazer, 1989; Saunders & Robins, 1987; Teichman & Lahav, 1987; Tomlinson, 1987). The multigravidas, however, seem to accept these changes, although they do not always like them (Glazer, 1989; Teichman & Lahav, 1987).

Ms. Bentsen said she and her husband were discovering that their lives were no longer centered on each other because they had a child, and were soon to have another to think about. Not only the woman, but also the couple were making the transition to being a family. Now that they were having more children, they found that they needed to expand their identification as a family (Broom, 1984; Glazer, 1989; Mercer & Ferketich, 1988).

The multigravidas indicated that they depended on their husbands for emotional support during pregnancy, and an overwhelming majority said they wanted their husbands with them during labor and delivery, a finding commonly observed (Brown, 1986a, b; Moss et al., 1987). The reasons that women gave for wanting their husbands with them during labor varied greatly. Some of their remarks were made in jest, with a bit of sarcasm, as were Ms. Kennedy's. "It's half his fault anyway, so he should be in on what's happening."

Another woman, Ms. Wilson, said she wanted her husband with her because "he is my strength." She said that he had been very helpful in caring for their first child. Ms. Wilson also stated that her husband was ignored by the hospital staff during her first labor and delivery, that none of the medical staff explained to her husband what was happening during labor, and that he did not know how to help her. She was sure he would be more helpful during the second labor, "if things were better explained to him," an expectation noted by other investigators (Berry, 1988; Glazer, 1989). Ms. Wilson's faith in her husband turned out to be justified, according to one of her postpartum interviews. She said that her husband provided moral support during labor, that he was better than he was with the first baby, and that he helped "take her mind off" contractions. Her husband did not, however, go into the delivery room with her.

In the case of Ms. Waxman, her husband empathized with her pain in labor and delivery. In fact, Ms. Waxman said that her husband became angry with their first child because of the pain that labor and delivery caused her, a response noted by others (Glazer, 1989).

A young wife and mother, Ms. Truman, said her husband was more interested in her current pregnancy than he had been in the first one. Perhaps this was due, in part, to the youth of the couple and the changes necessitated by an unexpected first pregnancy (Glazer, 1989). Her husband was just 22 years old.

Ms. Brooks indicated high satisfaction with her husband's support and help. She said that even though she felt bad about her appearance, her husband was supportive. She still was apprehensive that with another baby she and her husband would have even less time together than they had with only one child. Nevertheless, she felt that her husband might adjust more easily to having a second child.

> Well, the first baby, you make major adjustments. It's not all the other things, but I guess somebody coming along between you after being married for five years and being alone. And some new person comes and you have to adjust to spare some hours for that person ... and I think he [her husband] adjusted with greater difficulty [to the first baby] than I did. But I feel with this one, after having the first one, ... I don't think he's going to have any difficulty.

Ms. Carter considered herself fortunate, because her husband was a tremendous help at home during her pregnancy. Ms. McGovern said that although her husband was not always understanding about the pains and discomforts of pregnancy, he became more considerate as the pregnancy progressed.

Although pregnancy tended to enhance the marital bond in most cases, this was not always so. Ms. Roosevelt, who experienced moderate to high conflict in the relationship with her husband, said, "I'm more concerned with the pregnancy than with him."

After the baby was born, Ms. Roosevelt continued to feel conflict in her relationship with her husband and concern about her husband's response to the new baby. She said that he only held the baby when it was being "good" or "cute." Once, when she was planning to get out of the house by herself, her husband objected saying, "You're not going to do that, are you? Leave me with the two kids?" In making this remark, he seemed oblivious to the fact that Ms. Roosevelt spent most of her time alone with the two children.

One multigravida, Ms. Foley, said she had noticed changes in the relationship with her husband, but did not attribute these to her pregnancy.

> Our relationship has probably changed a fair amount in the last year, but it's more ... I wouldn't say it's due to being pregnant again, except that .... I'm probably more emotionally unstable now and ... more willing to let him take the brunt of it.

Because she had experienced the emotional lability of pregnancy before, Ms. Foley felt comfortable telling her husband about her feelings, thereby sharing some of the burden with him (Teichman & Lahav, 1987). She had learned from her previous experiences that she did not have to handle everything by herself.

Several of the women expressed the desire to have their husbands become more helpful with housework and childcare duties, and to become more sensitive to their moods and feelings during pregnancy; such wishes were reported in other studies as well (Brown, 1986a, b; Tomlinson, 1987). Among these women was Ms. Cleveland. She stated that she depended more on her husband for emotional support while pregnant than she did when she was not pregnant, but found him unavailable to give this support. She said she was not sure that her husband understood that she wanted him to help her more, and that he did not seem to accept the reality of her pregnancy or all the changes it would bring. Ms. Cleveland's husband was so preoccupied with his hobby of building model airplanes that he claimed to have no time to help with their child, to assist her with housework, or to lend emotional support. In fact, he became irate when Ms. Cleveland interrupted him at his hobby for any reason. This problem became more pronounced after the second baby was born.

In her dream diary, Ms. Cleveland recorded a dream in which her husband left her because she was being "bitchy." She discussed this with him, and he said that he did not want any more children because it placed too much of a strain on their marriage, emotionally and financially.

This lack of spousal support was compounded by what Ms. Cleveland perceived as a lack of acceptance by her husband's family. She said her husband's family did not wish to form a close relationship with her, and that they were adamant that her second child should be a boy. Ms. Cleveland remarked that she was afraid her in-laws would not want anything to do with the new baby if it was a girl. Fortunately, she had a son.

Ms. Kennedy said that her husband was "amenable," but not solicitous to her. Ms. Humphrey also said that her husband had very little sympathy for her changing moods and no sympathy at all for her tears.

One woman, Ms. Cisneros, said her husband liked her better as a mother than as a pregnant lady, indicating that while he may have accepted the change in status from couple to family, he still had problems in giving credence to the pregnancy and in lending support to his wife. In a later interview, Ms. Cisneros revealed that her husband was not accepting the pregnancy as well as she had hoped he would.

Several women were basing their expectations of their husbands' support and acceptance on their earlier pregnancies; if the husband had been supportive and sensitive during an earlier pregnancy, the multigravida assumed that she would receive similar support during subsequent pregnancies. When this was not the case, it resulted in disappointment and conflict (Glazer, 1989; Kemp & Hatmaker, 1989).

Some of the husbands said things which they may have considered innocent remarks, but which were perceived as insensitive and harsh by the multigravidas. For example, Ms. Hightower's husband told her that he was concerned that her legs would not be as attractive after having "all the babies." She was pregnant with her third child. Though the remark bothered Ms. Hightower, it did not precipitate an overt emotional response. Perhaps she was accustomed to such remarks by her third pregnancy and did not view them as a threat.

Ms. Humphrey said she feared that her husband might be sexually turned off by her large shape. She also feared he might be seeing another woman.

Ms. Wilson did not receive the support she needed from her husband because he had lost his job and "needs to be constantly entertained." She found this difficult to adjust to, because she was not as genial during her pregnancy as her husband wished. Because of this, Ms. Wilson said her husband had been "pretty grouchy." She reported during one interview that she had had a crying spell after a fight with her husband.

Ms. Whitmire said that her husband was trying to help more around the house, but that "he's kind of clumsy." She said she did not expect to get a great deal of assistance from him with the new baby. Generally, the multigravida is envisioned by others as experienced and capable, and additional support is not necessarily seen as needed.

10.2.4.1   Changes in the Sexual Relationship During Pregnancy

One substantial change that often occurs during pregnancy is the couple's sexual relations (Tomlinson, 1987). Once again, a wide range of responses occurred among the multigravidas regarding how pregnancy affected their sexual lives.

Ms. Kennedy, Ms. Carter, and Ms. Hobby said there was no real change in the frequency of sexual intercourse with their husbands. Ms. Foley said that she was more interested in continuing sexual relations with her husband during her current pregnancy than she had been during her two previous pregnancies.

However, Ms. Wilson and Ms. Cleveland said intercourse was less frequent. Ms. Truman said she did not enjoy intercourse during pregnancy. Ms. Wright said that she had lost all interest in sex. Ms. Moyers said during her second prenatal interview that her husband was disgusted with her because she did not feel like having sexual intercourse.

A few of the women expressed a reluctance to have sexual intercourse because of fear of harming the fetus. Ms. O'Neill said: "It's hard for me to really believe that it doesn't do some harm to the baby."

Ms. King said her desire for sexual intercourse, as well as her husband's desire, had decreased, adding: "I don't think I'm sexually appealing at this point, anyway."

Ms. Johnson also said she was "scared" of having sexual intercourse during pregnancy, but feared that if she did not have intercourse despite her apprehension, it would ruin her marriage.

In a few isolated instances, it was the man who was reluctant to continue sexual relations during the pregnancy. Ms. McGovern said that she had no objections to having sexual intercourse during pregnancy, but that her husband did not have the desire.

These responses approximated those of primigravidas, and it appears that responses do not change much in this regard compared to earlier pregnancies. However, sensitivity and adaptation to the changing needs of one or both partners may require further assessment and supportive, informative counseling if it is not accomplished independently by the marital partners.

10.2.4.2   Family and Social Support

The research literature has documented that family and social support are important contributors to a successful adaptation to and outcome of pregnancy and childbirth, and are significant determinants of individual reactions to the stress of parenthood (Cutrona, 1984; Oakley, 1985; Oakley, Rajan, & Grant, 1990).

For example, Oakley et al. (1990) recruited 509 women with histories of having low-birthweight babies in order to examine the effects of social support on infant birthweight. The women were recruited from the antenatal booking clinics for four hospitals and randomized to receive either a social intervention from midwives during pregnancy in addition to standard antenatal care, or to receive standard antenatal care only. At delivery, the mean birthweight of babies whose mothers had received the social intervention was 38 grams higher than babies whose mothers had received standard prenatal care only. Moreover, fewer women in the social intervention group were admitted to the hospital during pregnancy, and spontaneous onset of labor and vaginal delivery were more common, epidural anesthesia was used less, and the babies and mothers were significantly healthier in the following weeks.

During pregnancy, most partners have good intentions and want to support each other, but individuals may have different perceptions about what behaviors are supportive, especially during stressful changes such as the transition to parenthood (Brown, 1987). The husband may be trying to support his wife, but may find his efforts ineffective if he is giving the type of support he values rather than discovering the type of support his wife values. For this reason, it is important for couples to clearly state their specific needs for support (Brown, 1987).

Furthermore, there may be differences between expectant mothers and fathers in the perception of social support. In a study by Brown (1986a, b), partner support appeared to be the most important variable in understanding expectant fathers' health during pregnancy, but social support for expectant mothers included a larger domain, and social networks contributed to their health in much the same way as did partner support.

Jordan (1989) examined the types of social support and the specific behaviors identified as helpful by mothers and fathers having a second or subsequent child. During the prenatal period, both mothers and fathers thought that behaviors which provided tangible, material support were helpful, and they desired more of this type of support. In addition, emotional and informational support was perceived as helpful.

Social support sometimes diminishes during a second pregnancy, often because family and friends expect the mother to be more experienced and to require less assistance. However, the mother, who is normally fatigued, may need more rather than less assistance.

One of the women who was cited in an earlier section, Ms. Stevenson, received no support from her husband. He was so resentful and angry about her pregnancy (this was their fourth child) that he was physically, verbally, and emotionally abusive to Ms. Stevenson throughout and after the pregnancy. He did not accompany her to the hospital when labor began. As discussed in the literature, spousal involvement in pregnancy correlates with low anxiety in men (Teichman & Lahav, 1987). If the converse can be assumed to be true, Mr. Stevenson's refusal to become involved in the pregnancy may have been related to his high anxiety and resultant abusive behavior (Glazer, 1989). Ms. Stevenson tried to motivate her husband, a minister, to go to a marriage counselor with her and told him she would leave him if he did not. She said,

> I am a very sensitive person and my husband is a very critical person .... He also just cannot take children .... He has a very low frustration level .... Children frustrate him just too much because everything's not just perfect .... He almost went off the deep end when I became pregnant this time.

Throughout the prenatal interviews, Ms. Stevenson reported that her husband kept pressuring her to have an abortion, even though he was a fundamentalist minister. He told her that having so many children made them appear "low class," and he accused her of becoming pregnant deliberately. Mr. Stevenson was so full of rage at the idea of having another child that he would not touch Ms. Stevenson in any kind of affectionate or sexual way, and said that he would not pay any of her medical expenses. He also refused to help with the other children or the housework, saying that he was not going to "condone" his wife's "irresponsibility" in getting pregnant, or make anything easier on her. In other studies (Condon & Esuvaranathan, 1990) second-time fathers scored significantly lower on global fetal attachment than first-time fathers.

The situation did not improve after the baby was born. Ms. Stevenson went to the hospital and had the baby, not telling her husband until the delivery was over. Her husband called her a "baby factory" and said that she still looked pregnant after the baby was born.

Clearly, this is an extreme example of lack of support from a husband. However, the problem was only partly due to Ms. Stevenson's pregnancy; in great part it appeared due to her husband's insensitivity and general lack of maturity. Ms. Stevenson's pregnancy was the stimulus that brought these problems to light (Robson & Mandel, 1985). In any case, Mr. Stevenson's attitude did not dampen Ms. Stevenson's enthusiasm for having another child or cause her problems in labor and delivery, although it did appear to contribute to her severe postpartum depression. Marital disharmony has been associated with postpartum depression (blues) by other investigators (Cutrona, 1984, Kennerly & Gath, 1989). Researchers (Condon & Esuvaranathan, 1990) have noted that second-time fathers were significantly more stressed and depressed than first-time fathers, while mothers do not show such differences.

10.2.4.3   Summary: Relationship with Husband or Partner

One of the most significant relationships in a woman's life is her relationship with her husband. The importance of this relationship often is intensified during pregnancy, labor, and delivery. This is particularly true for a woman who has borne a child previously and has experienced the degree to which her relationship with her husband can help or hinder the childbirth experience. Krieg (2007) identified that both first- and second-time mothers experienced increased stress postnatally associated with their marital relationship. It is believed that mothers who have been married longer may have established a routine that reduces conflict in the relationship (Krieg). For multigravidas who had had a positive earlier birth experience together with their husbands, the relationship was something to be depended upon, something on which to rely. But for women whose husbands had not been supportive and helpful during earlier birth experiences, the relationship was another source of stress and tension, and one which was not generally broached in prenatal health care. Condon and Esuvaranathan (1990) noted that prenatal classes are structured primarily for first-time expectant parents than the needs of second-timers. First-time parents are focused on learning more about the labor and the birthing experience, whereas multiparous women are more interested in the particular institutions rules and the environment in which they will deliver.

10.2.5   Preparation for Labor

Multigravidas had a wide range of methods for preparing for the physical and emotional rigors of labor and delivery. Some attended expectant parent classes, others read literature, and still others depended on their memories of earlier pregnancy experiences (Aaronson et al., 1988; Crowe & von Baeyer, 1989; Reading & Cox, 1985; Stolte, 1987).

10.2.5.1 Childbirth Preparation Classes and Books

Ms. Roosevelt and her husband were enrolled in a refresher childbirth class, but she said, "We're not as enthusiastic as we were the first time, and we're not practicing like we should." She did not, however, anticipate any difficulties with labor. She said her first delivery was a wonderful experience and that she would like her second delivery to be like the first.

Ms. Roosevelt said she knew that she would be able to cope with the pain of labor and delivery. "So now I know…more what to expect in terms of actual labor and delivery." Ms. Roosevelt's response was a typical response among the multigravidas. In general, if a woman had a positive experience with previous deliveries, she expected the coming experience to be positive. Conversely, if a woman had experienced something frightening or unpleasant with a previous delivery, then anxiety and apprehension about labor and delivery were common (Crowe & von Baeyer, 1989; Lowe, 1989).

Ms. Foley, whose second baby was born with its head in a posterior position, was a bit worried throughout her third pregnancy that this might occur again. When discussing the value of childbirth classes during her deliveries, Ms. Foley said,

> Particularly, I think just knowing what to expect [in the second delivery] was a big help and breathing helped a lot, and I think it [the childbirth preparation method] was probably more helpful with the first baby than the second one.

Ms. O'Neill said that with her first pregnancy, she was not aware of the signals indicating that labor had begun, but that she knew what to look for with her current pregnancy because of the experience of her first pregnancy. Ms. O'Neill had been caught completely off guard with her first labor because the baby's birth was precipitous. As a result, she learned to pay more attention to Braxton-Hicks contractions during her second pregnancy so that she would not be totally surprised.

After her baby was born, Ms. Roosevelt said labor was exactly what she thought it would be and that she felt better prepared having experienced it before. Although she did not do so during her first pregnancy, Ms. Wilson was planning to go to "breathing classes" [childbirth classes] during the study. "I think I'm going into it a little bit different than last time." Ms. Wilson also had read a book on natural childbirth, but was doubtful that the techniques would prove helpful during labor. "It's got a lot of good pointers in it, but I don't think … it's for me. I don't think I could go totally natural." During Ms. Wilson's first delivery, the obstetrician used forceps as a "teaching tool" for other medical residents. This was not a pleasant experience for Ms. Wilson, and she carried the memory over into her second pregnancy. She did not understand how childbirth breathing techniques could possibly have helped in a situation such as a forceps delivery. The natural childbirth book did not succeed in helping Ms. Wilson prepare for labor, because she did not realize she was having contractions when labor began, even though it was her second childbirth experience.

Ms. Cisneros, who was pregnant with her second child, attended childbirth classes as she had done during her first pregnancy. She said she got a lot out of the classes with her first pregnancy, but that this pregnancy was different. "This time, I just didn't get into it as much as usual." This was a typical response for the multigravidas. The novelty of pregnancy, labor, and delivery was diminished, and the multigravidas were not as excited and intrigued because the things they were being taught were already well known to them (Moss et al., 1987). Ms. Cisneros said that she was not as worried about the delivery as she had been during her first pregnancy, and was not practicing her exercises as much.

Some women who used childbirth preparation methods with earlier pregnancies were disillusioned and skeptical about whether the techniques actually helped (Copstick, Taylor, Hayes, & Morris, 1986; Coussens & Coussens, 1984; Melzack, 1984). One such woman, Ms. Waxman, said,

> … I've been very aware of body changes, but I haven't looked at the material like I did the first time …. I took the classes before with my first child. At the time, changes seemed worthwhile, but when I actually got down to using what I had learned I was really disappointed.

Ms. Brooks said she had no time for expectant parent classes or for reading books on the subject, adding, "I guess it's kind of I'm familiar with it now from the first pregnancy." After her baby was born, Ms. Brooks said the labor experience was better the second time, and that it was important to her that the medical staff was "nice."

Ms. Cleveland was not attending childbirth classes. She said her husband was helping her practice breathing exercises, but that he was not very enthusiastic about it. She said she expected to be more prepared for her upcoming labor, and that she hoped labor and delivery would be shorter than it had been with her first child. This was a universal sentiment, especially among the multigravidas who were having their second baby. Because the first experience of labor generally is longer in duration, the gravidas were apprehensive about the advent of another lengthy labor. Almost all the women who were pregnant with their second baby said they wanted a shorter labor.

Ms. Truman, who was pregnant with her third child, had never been to childbirth classes, but it seemed that her previous childbirth experiences helped her through the third childbirth. She exhibited little noticeable pain or stress during labor.

Ms. Patman's husband did not wish to help her practice breathing exercises, and she was not attending childbirth classes during her pregnancy.

Ms. Whitmire said she had read books on preparation for labor, but that she still wished to have a child without going through labor. She had a moderate amount of conflict about labor.

Ms. Kennedy had not gone to expectant parent classes during any of her pregnancies. Her mother-in-law was an obstetrical nurse and had taught her the various exercises and breathing techniques. Like the vast majority of women, Ms. Kennedy said she wanted to be awake and aware during labor, and that she felt labor would not be too bad if it were short.

Ms. Cleveland said she wanted to be as aware as possible, but that if the pain got too bad, she wanted to retain the option of receiving pain medication. Because she had been through the experience before, Ms. Cleveland said she realized labor was "supposed to hurt some," but that she also had learned it would not last forever.

During the most difficult parts of labor, many primigravidas have doubts that labor will ever end, even though they know intellectually that it cannot last forever (Aaronson et al., 1988; Crowe & von Baeyer, 1989). Multigravidas, on the other hand, know for a fact that labor will end eventually.

10.2.5.2 Summary: Preparation for Labor

In general, the multigravidas in this study did not feel the same overwhelming need to seek outside preparation for labor and delivery as they had felt during their first pregnancies. Indeed, these women seemed to depend more on their own labor and delivery experiences, on shared conversations with their mothers, and on their own basic knowledge of labor and delivery than they had as primigravidas. It is likely that the novelty of being pregnant and preparing for labor and delivery was altered for the multigravidas. Therefore, it could be expected that these women were not as dependent upon childbirth preparation classes for second and subsequent pregnancies, though many found the childbirth refresher courses worthwhile.

10.2.6 Fear of Pain, Helplessness, and Loss of Control in Labor

The multigravidas seemed to know whether they might lose control during labor and delivery, based on their past experiences. The idea of losing control was upsetting to some, but was not mentioned as being the worst thing that could happen during labor and delivery.

Virtually all the women said the worst thing that could happen would be if the baby died, was injured, or was abnormal in some way, or if something (such as death or injury) happened to themselves. Primigravidas, compared to multigravidas, tend to have more concern about the well-being of themselves and their babies in labor, about being prepared for labor, and about loss of control, pain, and helplessness in labor (Beebe, Lee, Carrieri-Kohlman, & Humphreys, 2007).

One woman, Ms. Johnson, either did not experience any pain or fear of loss of self-control during her previous labor, or did not remember it if she did. She said, "I don't think about pain [regarding the upcoming labor and delivery] because I don't remember any pain."

Ms. Brooks also had few, if any, fears of losing control based on her past labor and delivery experience. In fact, she said that she would like labor and delivery to be the same as they were with her first pregnancy because, "It's a wonderful time." Ms. Foley said she did not think there was anything in labor or delivery that could make her lose her temper. However, she said she would be very distressed if she lost control, probably because it rarely happened to her. Ms. Foley said she could handle pain as long as there was a reason for it, such as being in labor. Moore (2004) observed that multigravidas', but not primigravidas', expectations of control of their behavior in labor and during contractions was a major predictor of their actual control. In general, multigravidas were more confident about coping with labor (Beebe et al., 2007).

Ms. Roosevelt was extremely forthright about the fact that she "goes to pieces" when she loses control, but said she realized that "nothing dire is going to happen" during labor and delivery, and that the baby eventually would be born.

It was apparent that Ms. Roosevelt's positive memories of her first labor and delivery framed her confidence (Crowe & von Baeyer, 1989; Lowe, 1989; Moss et al., 1987), and helped her realize that no matter how bad things got, it was unlikely that any harm would come to her or to the baby. Ms. Roosevelt had few conflicts concerning fear of loss of control, but had somewhat more conflict regarding concern for her well-being in labor.

Ms. Wilson said that she might lose her temper during labor, but did not think she would lose control completely. In fact, she thought she would be more in control than with her previous labor. This woman previously had a forceps delivery after having labor induced, and her memories of labor were not pleasant. She said she definitely did not want an induced labor the second time, because she felt that she could be more in control of her responses to contractions if they occurred naturally. She had moderately high anxiety concerning fear of pain, which likely was related to her traumatic first delivery.

Another woman, Ms. Patman also said she might scream during labor, but that it would not be a "big deal" if she did.

Ms. Cisneros, who said she was "nasty" and "ill-tempered" during her first delivery, said she might be "rude" to whoever happened to be around during the transition phase of labor, but that she was not worried about this because she felt it was a normal reaction to this phase of labor.

Ms. Cleveland lost her temper during her first labor and yelled at her husband. She realized that she might lose her temper again, but did not seem too concerned about it. She also said she was not worried about having a difficult delivery because she had been through a difficult delivery before. As it happened, labor events proceeded more smoothly than Ms. Cleveland felt they would. In a postpartum interview, Ms. Cleveland reported that she felt "under control" when labor began and that labor was "much easier" than she had expected.

Ms. Bentsen, who attended childbirth classes, did not indicate during her prenatal interviews that she had any particular fears of losing control. However, she did say she had a fear of death because of previous antepartum and labor and delivery complications. This fear was exacerbated by the fact that she reported being hypertensive even when she was not pregnant. In spite of Ms. Bentsen's stated fear of death, the observer who was with her during labor and delivery said she never lost control. It is probable that Ms. Bentsen felt that having had the experience once, she was prepared for anything that might occur in labor.

Ms. Jackson, who experienced a particularly painful delivery with her first child, had persistent fears of pain. She said, "the horror of that delivery stayed with me for at least a year." Ms. Jackson reported being in so much pain during her first delivery that she told her husband it would have to be their only child, because she did not want to risk having to go through the agony again. Ms. Jackson was emphatic about wanting epidural anesthesia so that she would not be so physically exhausted by pain that she could not participate in labor and delivery. She seemed convinced that her second labor and delivery would be painful and unpleasant, no matter what she did. She said, "It's not going to be a joy, and I'm not going to pretend it is."

Ms. Jackson, as might be expected, experienced considerable fear of pain in labor and conflict concerning gratification from childbirth. After the baby was born, she said she felt much better than she had after her first baby. Labor was shorter and the baby was not "posterior" this time. Nonetheless, Ms. Jackson's pervasive prenatal fears of pain, retained from her prior experience, appeared to contribute to her anxiety and stress level when labor began (Lowe, 1989).

Ms. Rayburn, whose ratings on all scales showed low conflict, also did not express any fears about pain or loss of control during labor in her prenatal interviews. However, after her baby was born she said the labor pains were severe, and that she had not known whether she was going to be able to cope with the pain. Evidently, Ms. Rayburn had relatively painless labor experiences before and was surprised by the intensity of her most recent childbirth experience.

For another gravida an early childhood experience with hospitalization and surgery also precipitated memories of uncontrollable fear and pain. Ms. Waxman had had an unpleasant experience having her tonsils removed when she was young, and her fears of pain and loss of control stemmed from that experience. She said she thought about pain a great deal, but that knowing labor would end would help her get through it.

In some cases, unpleasant past experiences with medical personnel were associated with fears of loss of control in labor (Moss et al., 1987). Ms. Patman was adamant about whom she would allow to give her anesthesia, if it became necessary. Only the highest-ranking medical physicians would be permitted to render medical care to her. She said, "I don't want any OB. resident touching me."

Labor and delivery can produce feelings of helplessness even in well-prepared women, and one of the contributing factors to this sense of helplessness may be the approach and management of care by the medical staff. If a woman felt that she was helpless in the care of doctors and nurses, she thought she had more reason to fear losing control. But if she could exercise some control over whom she allowed to treat her, it was likely to diminish the fear of helplessness (Crowe & von Baeyer, 1989; Mercer & Ferketich, 1988; Mercer et al., 1988; Slavazza, Mercer, Marut, & Shnider, 1985).

10.2.6.1   Summary: Fear of Pain, Helplessness, and Loss of Control in Labor

Regardless of a woman's level of experience in pregnancy, labor, and delivery, there always seems to be an underlying fear of pain, helplessness, and loss of control during labor. This is an area where, at times, experience in childbearing can be a detriment rather than an asset. For the multigravida, fears of this kind may be well grounded. A woman who has delivered a child knows that there is some pain involved, regardless of what is taught in prepared childbirth classes. To some degree a woman expects to feel helpless as well as some loss of control during such an experience. Memories of previous childbirths are almost certain to arouse some unpleasant thoughts about pain and fears of being alone and of having little control over some of the events. However, the advantage a multigravida has is that she knows childbirth will end eventually, and that, more likely than not, she and her new child will come through the experience safely.

10.2.7 Concerns for Well-Being of Self and Baby

Many primigravidas, and a number of multigravidas, worry throughout their pregnancies that their babies will be abnormal. This can add to the anxiety and stress a woman feels during labor and delivery. However, if a woman knows from experience that the likelihood of abnormalities is rather remote, she has less fear (Aaronson et al., 1988).

Ms. King said,

> I think having gone through a pregnancy and having a healthy baby, I'm not nearly as concerned [about possible abnormalities]. I work with the handicapped, and that was really a major concern the first time, and that really hasn't entered my head as much during this pregnancy.

It was uncommon for multigravidas to express fears that their babies would be too large to pass through their bodies, or that their babies would simply "fall out." Ms. Johnson said this was not a concern during her second pregnancy, but that she worried during her first pregnancy that her baby would be too large, which would have complicated her delivery.

The women had learned from their childbirth experiences that the human body is amazingly adaptable when it comes to giving birth (Aaronson et al., 1988; Crowe & von Baeyer, 1989). Women with a previous successful delivery were confident of successful outcomes in childbirth, while women with memories of unpleasant events and extraordinary pain were considerably more fearful (Lowe, 1989). Primigravidas more often had a greater concern for their well-being and that of their babies in labor than did multigravidas Van den Bussche, Crombex, Eccleston, and Sullivan (2007).

10.2.8 Fear of Loss of Self-Esteem in Labor

To the extent that a woman's sense of self is connected to her coping abilities in pregnancy, labor, and delivery, she is vulnerable to fears of losing self-esteem if a threatening event occurs (Bailey & Hailey, 1986–1987; Crowe & von Baeyer, 1989; Kemp & Page, 1987; Melzack, 1984; Mercer & Ferketich, 1988). Multigravidas usually have more realistic expectations of labor pain and feel more confident about coping with pain (McCrea, Wright, & Stringer, 2000).

For the most part, the multigravidas in this study, having been through the labor and delivery experience before, did not have the same basis for fears of loss of self-esteem in labor and delivery that the primigravidas had. However, this does not mean that the multigravidas experienced no fears of losing their self-esteem.

Instead, the multigravidas' fears along this dimension were related to how they envisioned they would be treated in labor and delivery by hospital staff, to their relationships with their husbands, and to how they imagined they would "perform" during labor and delivery (Melzack, 1984; Morcos et al., 1989). Pregnant women have high expectations for maintaining control during labor and delivery, particularly after attending childbirth preparation classes. Consequently, it is not uncommon for them to fear a loss of self-esteem during the labor and delivery process if they do not live up to their own expectations (Mercer et al., 1988).

Ms. Roosevelt retained an unpleasant memory from her first delivery, and it was associated with fears of loss of self-esteem. Her obstetrician at the time seemed to be in a hurry each time she saw him for a prenatal examination. The night she went into labor, the doctor had personal plans. Ms. Roosevelt said, "He stopped in his dress suit and said that he wouldn't be able to make it." This was degrading to Ms. Roosevelt's self-esteem; in her eyes, the obstetrician was saying that she was not important enough for him to deliver her baby on a night that he had a social engagement. She wanted to take steps to ensure that this situation did not happen with her second baby.

Another woman with a negative attitude toward medical professionals, Ms. Pepper, based her attitude on her belief that the doctors had not taken good care of her son when he was ill. While her son was sick, Ms. Pepper felt that doctors were discounting her opinion and not putting much credence in her insistence that something was wrong with her son. This was a blow to her credibility and sense of self at a sensitive moment, and this unpleasant memory was carried forward to her current pregnancy (Moss et al., 1987). Ms. Pepper projected her mistrust of medical personnel to the hospital staff long before she went into labor.

Ms. Hobby, who had had prior unsuccessful saddle blocks and had been administered anesthesia during her previous deliveries, was convinced early in her pregnancy that labor and delivery were going to hurt. Unpleasant experiences of this kind appear to have a long-lasting negative impact on a woman's self-esteem.

Painful memories of labor and delivery are not dissipated easily, as evidenced by Ms. Waxman. During her first delivery, she had had a fourth-degree episiotomy tear, which spread into her rectum. She was worried that this would happen again, referred to her first delivery as "awful," and seemed to harbor doubts about the competence of medical professionals. This experience was not only physically painful, but embarrassing as well. Ms. Waxman was frightened that she would have to go through another experience like the earlier one.

Ms. Wilson, whose contractions caught her unaware during her second labor, said in her postpartum interview that she had been extremely afraid she would tear herself while pushing. She admitted to being unprepared for labor and delivery, and this contributed somewhat to a loss of self-esteem.

Ms. Wilson was adamant about having a tubal ligation following the birth of her baby. Her sense of self-worth did not seem to be tied completely to motherhood, a relationship that varies among women (Kemp & Page, 1987). Ms. Wilson was aware she would always be a mother, but she was not "totally dependent on being a mommy." That sentiment, combined with her fears during labor and delivery, were significant contributing factors in her decision to be "sterilized" after delivery.

Ms. Cleveland, who had a history of suicide attempts and psychiatric counseling, had problems with self-esteem that were unrelated to her pregnancy. She had many dreams about death while she was pregnant, and also said that if the baby were not healthy, she would feel guilty because she smoked during pregnancy. In this case, apprehension over her baby's well-being and a disposition to self-blame may have been manifestations of Ms. Cleveland's low self-esteem (Kemp & Page, 1987). Low self-esteem has been associated with an expectation of poor delivery outcome and self-blame (Jones, 1986) and with a perception of inadequate motherhood role qualities (Curry, 1982; Kemp & Page, 1987).

A 19-year-old woman, Ms. Truman, had high ratings on fear of loss of self-esteem, but these fears likely were associated with her lack of education (Kemp & Page, 1987), and that she was about to have a third child while she was still a teenager. Authors have reported associations between self-esteem, birth order, and number of births (Brouse, 1985; Kemp & Page, 1987). However, Ms. Truman was tolerant, and her responses during interviews did not indicate that her sense of self was related to her coping skills in labor and delivery.

Ms. Carter reported after her baby was born that she had been very afraid about going into her third labor, in spite of the fact that she really wanted another baby and was well prepared for labor. She could not explain what caused this fear; it may have been caused, she opined, by fears of losing self-esteem.

In Ms. Stevenson's case, having an abusive husband lowered her self-esteem considerably, even before labor began. As mentioned earlier, Ms. Stevenson's husband did not accompany her to the hospital; she called him after the delivery to tell him his fourth child had been born. Even though her husband had made it clear he did not want the child, he relented somewhat toward the end of the pregnancy and said he would take her to the hospital. When she went into labor, Ms. Stevenson called her husband at a moment he considered an inconvenience, so she made other arrangements for getting to the hospital and did not contact her husband again until the baby was born.

The conscious decision to leave her husband out of the process at the last minute was perhaps the only way Ms. Stevenson could cope with labor and still retain some self-esteem. She did not explicitly state this in an interview, but it was clear that she knew she would not receive support from her husband, and that he would likely be a hindrance and a source of tension if he were with her during labor and delivery. The last straw seemed to be when Ms. Stevenson called her husband to tell him she was in labor, and he did not want to take her to the hospital. It appears that Ms. Stevenson decided she was going to take control of this significant event in her life.

10.2.8.1   Summary: Fear of Loss of Self-Esteem

A common observation regarding childbearing is that women somehow forget some of the unpleasantness involved with earlier trials of childbirth. This, however, may not be entirely true. For the women in this study, one of the events that repeatedly surfaced during interviews was the experiences each woman had had in her previous labor and delivery, and whether these experiences were beneficial or detrimental to her self-esteem. A negative physical experience in an earlier labor would likely contribute to a fear of loss of self-esteem (Crowe & von Baeyer, 1989; Kemp & Page, 1987; Melzack, 1984). In like manner, a negative experience with a member of the medical staff during a previous labor or delivery would be likely to render a pregnant woman wary of medical professionals during a subsequent pregnancy. Thus, prior experience often aided women in labor and delivery, but also had the potential of adding to their fears of losing self-esteem, depending upon the nature and memory of previous experiences.

10.3   Summary

Overall, multigravidas have the benefit of experience, a vantage point from which to envision the events that will happen to them during pregnancy as well as in labor, delivery, and childcare.

Although multigravidas still experience the wonder of such events as fetal movement, these events are familiar to them from their previous pregnancies. They also know more of what to expect in terms of pain during labor, postpartum depression, and the many added responsibilities of motherhood (Kennerly & Gath, 1989; Knight & Thirkettle, 1987).

On the other hand, multigravidas have adjustments to make that primigravidas do not. The multigravid woman is concerned with how to give adequate attention to all of her children and with keeping sibling jealousy to a minimum. She also has to consider the financial issues associated with feeding, clothing, and providing for another child, while at the same time maintaining a relationship with her husband and continuing her career, whether inside or outside the home. Certainly, the husband no longer ranks first in claims upon his wife but must accept the child's or children's right to priority (Russell, 1974). Interesting, Russell found that the first child was negatively related to crisis within the family and while the position of hierarchy was not a significant determining variable for women, the lower the role of the father within the "hierarchy of identities" the greater the level of crisis.

Thus, one can see that while multigravidas experience anxiety, fear, and apprehension concerning the approaching birth experience, by and large, these are not the same fears and anxieties experienced by women who have never confronted the challenge of labor and childbirth or dealt with the challenges of transitioning a couple of parenthood.

References

Aaronson, L., Mural, C., & Pfoutz, S. (1988). Seeking information: Where do pregnant women go? *Health Education Quarterly, 15*, 335–345.

Bailey, L., & Hailey, B. (1986–1987). The psychological experience of pregnancy. *International Journal of Psychiatry in Medicine, 16*, 263–274.

Beebe, K. R., Lee, K. A., Carrieri-Kohlman, V., & Humphreys, J. (2007). The effects of childbirth self-efficacy and anxiety during pregnancy on prehospitalization labor. *Journal of Obstetric, Gynecologic, and Neonatal Nursing, 35*, 410–418.

Belsky, J., & Isabella, R. (1985). Marital and parent-child relationships in family of origin and marital change following the birth of a baby: A retrospective analysis. *Child Development, 56*, 342–349.

Berry, L. (1988). Realistic expectations of the labor coach. *Journal of Obstetric, Gynecologic, and Neonatal Nursing, 17*, 354–355.

Broom, B. (1984). Consensus about the marital relationship during transition to parenthood. *Nursing Research, 33*, 223–228.

Brouse, S. (1985). Effect of gender role identity on patterns of feminine and self-concept scores from late pregnancy to early postpartum. *Advances in Nursing Science, 7*, 32–48.

Brouse, A. (1988). Easing the transition to the maternal role. *Journal of Advanced Nursing, 13*, 167–172.

Brown, M. A. (1986a). Marital support during pregnancy. *Journal of Obstetric, Gynecologic, and Neonatal Nursing, 15*, 475–483.

Brown, M. A. (1986b). Social support, stress, and health: A comparison of expectant mothers and fathers. *Nursing Research, 35*, 72–76.

Brown, M. A. (1987). How fathers and mothers perceive prenatal support. *Maternal Child Nursing 12*, 414–418.

Ching, G. T. (1986). The psychological effects of complicated pregnancy. *Xianggang Hu Li Za Zhi, 41*, 74–76.

Condon, J. T., & Corkindale, C. (1997). The correlates of antenatal attachment in pregnant women. *British Journal of Medical Psychology, 70*, 359–372.

Condon, J. T., & Esuvaranathan, V. (1990). The influence of parity on the experience of pregnancy: A comparison of first- and second-time expectant couples. *British Journal of Medical Psychology63*, 369–367.

Copstick, S., Taylor, K., Hayes, R., & Morris, N. (1986). Partner support and the use of coping techniques in labour. *Journal of Psychosomatic Research, 30*, 497–503.

Coussens, W. & Coussens, P. (1984). Maximizing preparation for childbirth. *Health Care for Women International, 5*, 335–353.

Curry, M. A. (1983) Variables related to adaptation to motherhood in "normal" primiparous women. *Journal of Obstetric, Gynecologic, and Neonatal Nursing, 12*(2):115–21.

Crowe, K., & von Baeyer, C. (1989). Predictors of a positive childbirth experience. *Birth, 16*, 59–63.

Cutrona, C. E. (1984). Social support and stress in the transition to parenthood. *Journal of Abnormal Psychology, 93*, 378–390.

Finer, L. B., & Henshaw, S. K. (2006). Disparities in rates of unintended pregnancy in the United States, 1994–2001. *Perspectives in Sexual and Reproductive Health, 38*, 90–96.

Glazer, G. (1989). Anxiety and stressors of expectant fathers. *Western Journal of Nursing Research, 11*, 47–59.

Green, J. M., & Baston, H. A. (2003). Feeling in control during labor: Concepts, correlates, and consequences. *Birth, 30*, 235–247.

Haedt, A., & Keel, P. (2007). Maternal attachment, depression, and body dissatisfaction in pregnant women. *Journal of Reproductive and Infant Psychology, 25*, 285–295.

Hiser, P. (1987). Concerns of multiparas during the second postpartum week. *Journal of Obstetric, Gynecologic, and Neonatal Nursing, 16*, 195–203.

Jones, E. E. (1986) Interpreting interpersonal behavior: The effects of expectancies. *Science, 234,* 41–46.

Jordan, P. L. (1989). Support behaviors identified as helpful and desired by second-time parents over the perinatal period. *Maternal-Child Nursing Journal, 18,* 133–145.

Kemp, V., & Page, C. (1987). Maternal self-esteem and prenatal attachment in high-risk pregnancy. *Maternal-Child Nursing Journal, 16,* 195–206.

Kemp, V. H., & Hatmaker, D. D. (1989). Stress and social support in high-risk pregnancy. *Research in Nursing and Health, 12,* 331–336

Kennerly, H., & Gath, D. (1989). Maternity blues, III: Associations with obstetric, psychological, and psychiatric factors. *British Journal of Psychiatry, 155,* 367–373.

Knight, R., & Thirkettle, J. (1987). The relationship between expectations of pregnancy and birth, and transient depression in the immediate postpartum period. *Journal of Psychosomatic Research, 31,* 351–357.

Krieg, D. B. (2007). Does motherhood get easier the second-time around? Examining parenting stress and marital quality among mothers having their first or second child. *Parenting Science and Practice, 7,* 149–175.

Kuczynski, J., & Thompson, L. (1985). Be prepared. *Nursing Mirror, 160,* 26–28.

Lederman, R., Harrison, J., & Worsham, S. (1995). *Differences in maternal development in primigravid and multigravid women.* San Diego, CA: The Society of Behavioral Medicine.

Lipps, H. (1985). A longitudinal study of the reporting of emotional and somatic symptoms during and after pregnancy. *Social Science and Medicine, 21,* 631–640.

Lowe, N. (1989). Explaining the pain of active labor: The importance of maternal confidence. *Research in Nursing & Health, 12,* 237–245.

McCrea, H., Wright, M. E., & Stringer, M. (2000). Psychosocial factors influencing personal control in pain relief. *International Journal of Nursing Studies, 37,* 493–503.

Melzack, R. (1984). The myth of painless childbirth (the John J. Bonica lecture). *Pain, 19,* 321–337.

Mercer, R., & Ferketich, S. (1988). Stress and social support as predictors of anxiety and depression during pregnancy. *Advances in Nursing Science, 10,* 26–39.

Mercer, R., Ferketich, S., DeJoseph, J., May, K., & Sollid, D. (1988). Effect of stress on family function during pregnancy. *Nursing Research, 37,* 268–275.

Moore, M. L. (2004) Perceptions of nurses and mothers in four studies of the peripartum period. *The Journal of Perinatal Education, 13*(3), 55–57.

Morcos, F. H., Snart, F. D., & Harley, D. D. (1989). Comparison of parents' expectations and importance ratings for specific aspects of childbirth. *Canadian Medical Association Journal, 141,* 909–914.

Moss, P., Bolland, G., Foxman, R., & Owen, C. (1987). The hospital inpatient stay: The experience of first-time parents. *Child: Care, Health, and Development, 13,* 153–167.

Nelson, A. M. (2003). Transition to motherhood. *Journal of Obstetrics, Gynecologic, and Neonatal Nursing, 32,* 465–477.

Oakley, A. (1985). Social support in pregnancy: The 'soft' way to increase birthweight? *Social Science and Medicine, 21,* 1259–1268.

Oakley, A., Rajan, L., & Grant, A. (1990). Social support and pregnancy outcome. *British Journal of Obstetrics and Gynaecology, 97,* 155–162.

Reading, A. E., & Cox, D. N. (1985). Psychosocial predictors of labor pain. *Pain, 22,* 309–315.

Robson, B., & Mandel, D. (1985). Marital adjustment and fatherhood. *Canadian Journal of Psychiatry, 30,* 169–172.

Russell, C. S. (1974). Transition to parenthood: Problems and gratifications. *Journal of Marriage and the Family, 36,* 294–301.

Saunders, R., & Robins, E. (1987). Changes in the marital relationship during the first pregnancy. *Health Care for Women International, 8,* 361–377.

Shereshefsky, P. M., & Yarrow, L. J. (Eds.). (1973). *Psychological aspects of a first pregnancy and early postpartum adaptation.* New York: Raven.

Slavazza, K., Mercer, R., Marut, J., & Shnider, S. (1985). Anesthesia, analgesia for vaginal childbirth: Differences in maternal perceptions. *Journal of Obstetric, Gynecologic, and Neonatal Nursing, 14*, 321–329.

Stolte, K. (1987). A comparison of women's expectations of labor with the actual event. *Birth, 14*, 99–103.

Teichman, Y., & Lahav, Y. (1987). Expectant fathers: Emotional reactions, physical symptoms and coping styles. *British Journal of Medical Psychology, 60*, 225–232.

Tomlinson, P. (1987). Spousal differences in marital satisfaction during transition to parenthood. *Nursing Research, 36*, 239–243.

Van den Bussche, E., Crombex, G., Eccleston, C., & Sullivan, M. J. L. (2007). Why women prefer epidural analgesia during childbirth: The role of beliefs about epidural analgesia and pain catastrophizing. *European Journal of Pain, 11*, 275–282.

Chapter 11
Methods of Assessment: Psychosocial Adaptation to Pregnancy Questionnaire Scales and Interview Schedules, and Review of Interventions to Enhance Adaptation

Preceding chapters describe seven psychosocial dimensions of maternal prenatal development for both primigravid and multigravid women. This chapter discusses methods of assessment for identifying gravid women who may be experiencing difficulties in one or more of the seven major psychosocial dimensions discussed. A self-report questionnaire (Lederman, 1996) developed for providing parallel measures of the major dimensions assessed in the clinical interviews is described, as well as the psychometric properties and validation results of its use to date. Suggestions are provided for conducting clinical interviews and for summarizing the information obtained in the form of quantitative ratings. Methods for learning and developing proficiency in assessment skills are also provided. Suggestions are made for clinical interventions and research applications of both interview and questionnaire assessment of maternal psychosocial development and adaptation to pregnancy.

In the last section of the chapter we present a brief review of potential therapeutic interventions to reduce anxiety and conflict, and to promote psychosocial adaptation to pregnancy.

11.1 Prenatal Self-Evaluation Questionnaire and Psychometric Data[1]

11.1.1 Description of the Seven Scales of the Prenatal Self-Evaluation Questionnaire and Sample Items

The questionnaire items for the Prenatal Self-Evaluation Questionnaire parallel the types of responses received in the prenatal interviews. The questionnaire contains 79 statements, each with four response categories. The expectant woman reads the

---

[1] Further information on the Prenatal Self-Evaluation Questionnaire and other research instruments cited in Chapter 11 can be obtained by contacting the first author at rlederma@utmb.edu, reginalederman@yahoo.com, 713 666 0172, 409 772 6570, or 832 228 1983.

R. Lederman and K. Weis, *Psychosocial Adaptation to Pregnancy*,
DOI 10.1007/978-1-4419-0288-7_11, © Springer Science+Business Media, LLC 2009

statements and indicates the extent to which they reflect her feelings by marking one of the four response categories. The objectively scored questionnaire takes approximately 10–20 min to complete and provides measures of seven personality dimensions.

The research results presented in Chapter 1 provided the basis for determining the scales to be constructed. A questionnaire composed of the initial statements was written to define the dimensions and then was administered to a group of 122 gravid women. The item analysis data obtained from this group were used to revise the questionnaire items. Our goal was to develop reliable and statistically independent scales. The final form of the questionnaire was administered to a second group of 119 primigravidas and multigravidas from two university hospitals. The data presented in this chapter were obtained from the second group of subjects.

The first five scales reflect the content presented in Chapters 2–6. The sixth scale reflects content found in Chapters 7 and 8. The rating scales measuring fears concerning, pain, helplessness, and loss of control, and loss of self-esteem were the core variables in the original eight-variable cluster with the highest intercorrelations. The statements written to reflect these concerns also were highly intercorrelated, and therefore were combined into a single scale, which is sufficient for the purpose of identifying gravid women with these related concerns. When counseling patients, however, a conceptual distinction among the concerns should be made. The seventh scale, Concern for Well-Being of Self and Baby, focuses on additional concerns of the gravida regarding her and her infant's overall well-being. These concerns, fear of reproductive adequacy and fear of injury and death, originally were represented by two rating scales in the interview data presented in Chapter 1. Descriptions and sample items for each of the scales are provided.

11.1.1.1 Acceptance of Pregnancy

The Acceptance of Pregnancy scale items specifically focus on the gravida's response to the pregnancy, rather than her response to the baby. The items pertain to her enjoyment of pregnancy, tolerance of discomforts, and the extent of ambivalence. Sample items include:

> This is a good time for me to be pregnant.
> I wish I wasn't having the baby now.
> This pregnancy has been a source of frustration to me.
> I am happy about this pregnancy.

11.1.1.2 Identification of a Motherhood Role

The second scale, Identification with a Motherhood Role, focuses on the extent to which the gravida looks forward to assuming a motherhood role, and anticipates the gratification that comes from caring for her baby. Our experience, based on the analysis of interview data presented in Chapters 2 and 3, suggests that it is important to conceptually distinguish between acceptance of pregnancy and identification of a motherhood role, although it is expected that the two will be related. For example, the older mother may feel a sense of immediacy about parenthood, expressing a "now or never" attitude, but she may not actually look forward to child care responsibilities inherent in a motherhood role. Sample items are:

I look forward to caring for the baby.
It will be difficult for me to give enough attention to a baby.
I think about the kind of mother I want to be.
I believe I can be a good mother.

11.1.1.3   Relationship with Mother

The Relationship with Mother scale measures the closeness, support, and empathy between the gravida and her mother. Some items in this scale include:

It's easy to talk to my mother about my problems.
I feel good when I'm with my mother.
When we get together my mother and I tend to argue.
My mother reassures me when I have doubts about myself.

11.1.1.4   Relationship with Husband/Partner

Items in the Relationship with Husband/Partner scale deal with mutuality, support, and communication patterns in the marital or partner relationship. Items included are:

My husband/partner is interested in discussing the pregnancy with me.
My husband/partner helps me at home when I need it.
I can count on my husband's/partner's support in labor.
I can count on my husband/partner to share in the care of the baby.

The questionnaire is available in two alternative forms, one which includes statements which refer to "husband," and one which includes items which refer to "partner/husband," as in the items cited earlier.

11.1.1.5   Preparation for Labor

The Preparation for Labor scale assesses the extent to which the gravida feels informed and prepared to cope with the events of labor. Sample items are:

I have a good idea of what to expect during labor and delivery.
I feel prepared for what happens in labor.
I know some things I can do to help myself in labor.
I look forward to childbirth.

11.1.1.6 Fear of Pain, Helplessness, and Loss of Control in Labor

Items in this scale deal with the stress and pain in labor, and the gravida's self-estimated ability to maintain control and cope with the events of labor. The scale includes items such as:

> I can cope well with pain.
> I feel that the stress of labor will be too much for me to handle.
> I think I can bear the discomfort of labor.

11.1.1.7 Concern for Well-being of Self and Baby in Labor

This final scale focuses on concerns the gravida may have regarding potential complications arising in labor, which could result in injury to herself or her baby. This scale provides a measure of specific concerns about labor, in terms commonly used by the gravidas, such as:

> I am worried that something will go wrong during labor.
> I am afraid that I will be harmed during delivery.
> I am anxious about complications occurring in labor.

11.1.2 Psychometric Data

11.1.2.1 Descriptive Data and Reliability Coefficients

Table 11.1 presents the number of items, the means, standard deviations, reliability coefficients, and the number of respondents for each scale. Reliability for the scales was determined by Cronbach's coefficient alpha, a measure of internal consistency of response.

11.1.2.2 Intercorrelations Among the Scales

Table 11.2 shows the intercorrelations among all the scales. The Cronbach alpha reliability coefficients are included at the bottom of the table for purposes of comparison with the correlations.

The scales were constructed so that each would provide some unique information. The Cronbach alpha reliability coefficients of the scales for the group of 119 primigravidas and multigravidas ranged from 0.75 to 0.92. The intercorrelation coefficients among the scales ranged from 0.06 to 0.54. These correlations are considerably lower than the reliabilities for the scales. It can be seen that the scales are relatively independent and that separate measures are justified for each of these constructs.

Table 11.1 Descriptive Data for Seven Scales of the Prenatal Self-Evaluation Questionnaire

				Scales			
Data	Acceptance of pregnancy	Identification with a motherhood role	Relationship with mother	Relationship with husband	Preparation for labor	Fear of pain, helplessness, and loss of control in labor	Concern for well-being of self and baby in labor
Number of items	14	15	10	10	10	10	10
Mean	22.3	20.2	17.3	16.2	15.9	18.2	16.5
Standard deviation	7.0	4.6	6.9	5.1	4.5	4.2	4.8
Alpha	0.90	0.79	0.92	0.82	0.80	0.75	0.83
n	119	119	115	115	119	118	119

Table 11.2 Intercorrelations Among the Seven Scales of the Prenatal Self-Evaluation Questionnaire (n = 115–119)

Scales	Acceptance of Pregnancy	Identification with a motherhood role	Relationship with mother	Relationship with husband	Preparation for labor	Fear of pain, helplessness, and loss of control in labor	Concern for well-being of self and baby in labor
Acceptance of pregnancy		0.54	0.27	0.25	0.33	0.36	0.31
Identification with a motherhood role		0.35	0.24	0.28	0.28	0.21	
Relationship with mother		0.30	0.25	0.18	0.11		
Relationship with husband		0.15	0.06	0.19			
Preparation for labor		0.47	0.35				
Fear of pain, helplessness, and loss of control in labor		0.52					
(Alpha)	0.90	0.79	0.92	0.82	0.80	0.75	0.83

Scales with Moderate Intercorrelations

The intercorrelation coefficient between acceptance of pregnancy and identification of a motherhood role is 0.54. This is not surprising since the extent to which a pregnancy is desired or accepted is closely related to the extent to which the gravida thinks about and identifies with a motherhood role. Identification with a Motherhood Role and Relationship with Mother have an intercorrelation coefficient of 0.35, indicating the developmental influence of the mother upon the gravida.

The intercorrelation coefficient between Preparation for Labor and the Fear of Pain, Helplessness, and Loss of Control in Labor is 0.47, suggesting that if the gravida feels uninformed and unprepared to cope with the events of labor, her fears of pain, helplessness, and loss of control in labor may increase. A lower but moderate intercorrelation of .35 was obtained between Preparation for Labor and concern for the Well-being of Self and Baby in Labor. Concern for the well-being of self and baby and the fear of pain, helplessness, and loss of control in labor have an intercorrelation coefficient of 0.52, indicating that the extent of the gravida's concern for her well-being and that of her baby is particularly related to the extent of her fears about pain, helplessness, and loss of control in labor. The three scales are interrelated possibly because they all deal with fears and concerns about labor. However, since the scales are only moderately correlated, it is useful to make a distinction among these different types of concerns.

Comparison of Scale Mean Levels Based on Parity

Mean differences between primigravidas and multigravidas on the seven scales are presented in Chapter 10 for a sample size of 689 gravidas. Lower mean conflict scores were obtained for primigravidas on acceptance of pregnancy, the relationship with mother, and state anxiety. These differences may possibly reflect increased stress between a couple that already has children, or it may be that multigravidas are more willing to acknowledge conflict in their marital relationships. Multigravidas, however, experienced lower conflict and anxiety concerning feelings of preparedness for labor, and fears concerning pain, helplessness, and loss of control in labor.

Also of interest are the remaining scales in which no differences were found based on parity. There were no significant differences between primigravidas and multigravidas on the following scales:

Identification with a motherhood role.
Relationship with husband/partner
Concerns about well-being of self and baby in labor.

One might expect that the experienced multigravida would have fewer fears and conflicts about motherhood and about having a normal childbirth. The data, however, suggest that this is not the case.

Congruence Between the Interview and Self-Report Questionnaire Responses

The subjects for this study (Lederman, Lederman, & Haller, 1981) were 73
married multigravidas, 20–42 years old, with no complicating medical or
obstetrical conditions. Clinical interviews were conducted with each patient at
32, 35, and 37 weeks of gestation. After reviewing tapes and transcripts, the
first author (R. Lederman) and a graduate nurse independently made ratings of
the maternal adjustment dimensions. At the completion of the final interview
the patient also responded to the 79-item Prenatal Self-Evaluation
Questionnaire.

Table 11.3 shows the reliability data for the questionnaire scales and the interview rating scales. The internal consistency coefficients for the questionnaire
scales range from 0.74 to 0.92. The correlations between the sets of interview
ratings range from 0.58 to 0.88. In some respects, the magnitude of the coefficients for the questionnaire parallels those for the interview ratings. For example, relatively high internal consistency in self-report and in rater agreement is
shown for the relationship with husband/partner dimension. The two lowest
coefficients for the questionnaire scales are those for fear of pain, helplessness,
and loss of control and for identification of a motherhood role. These dimensions also show lower correlations between the sets of independent interview
ratings.

Table 11.3 also shows the correlations (congruence) between the questionnaire
scale scores and scores from the sets of interview ratings. They show a wide range.
There are consistently higher correlations with the scores for relationship with
husband and for concern for well-being of self and baby in labor, and lower correlations for identification with a motherhood role and preparation for labor. It can also
be observed that despite the relatively high rater agreement on the preparation for
labor dimension, there are only moderate to low correlations with the corresponding
questionnaire scale. The data suggest that the degree of congruence between the questionnaire scales and the interview ratings is both a function of the reliability of the
measurements and the nature of the dimensions being assessed. The last column in
Table 11.3 shows that averaging the independent sets of interview ratings in order
to increase the reliability of the ratings results in somewhat higher congruence
between the questionnaire scales and ratings.

The next to the last (fifth) column in Table 11.3 shows the correlations of
the questionnaire scale scores with the scores of Rater 1 which were adjusted
after a discussion of score discrepancies with Rater 2. It can be seen that discussion of patients' adaptation by two raters enhances the reliability of the
interviewer's ratings and also results in higher congruence between the questionnaire and interview scales. In summary, utilization of discussion among
raters or of combined (averaged) rating scores enhances the reliability of
assessments. Further, the two methods of measurement – interview ratings and
questionnaire scale scores – should be used in tandem, since some differences
could result from the two methods in identifying patients who experience
greater conflict.

Table 11.3 Reliability and Congruence of the Questionnaire Scales and Prenatal Maternal Adaptation Ratings

| Prenatal variable | Reliability | | Questionnaire Scale congruence with ratings of same dimensions | | | |
	Questionnaire[a]	Ratings[b]	1[c]	2	1 Adjusted[d]	Average[e]
Acceptance of pregnancy	0.92	0.59	0.57	0.74	0.69	0.75
Identification of a motherhood role	0.75	0.62	0.32	0.44	0.35	0.45
Relationship with mother	0.87	0.75	0.64	0.58	0.65	0.63
Relationship with husband	0.85	0.88	0.77	0.76	0.78	0.78
Preparation for labor	0.77	0.72	0.54	0.37	0.54	0.47
Fear of pain, helplessness, and loss of control in labor	0.74	0.58	0.58	0.53	0.59	0.61
Concern for well-being of self and baby in labor	0.85	0.73	0.76	0.77	0.84	0.80

[a] Cronbach's alpha coefficients
[b] Determined by product–moment correlations between the independent ratings
[c] Determined by product–moment correlations for Rater 1 and for Rater 2 with the Questionnaire Scale scores
[d] Determined by product–moment correlations between the Questionnaire Scale scores and independent ratings of Rater-1 adjusted after discussion with Rater 2
[e] Determined by product–moment correlations between the Questionnaire Scale scores and an average of the independent, unadjusted ratings of Rater 1 and Rater 2

Prediction of Anxiety and Stress in Active Labor Using the Prenatal Self-Evaluation Questionnaire

In order to determine the predictive validity of the Prenatal Self-Evaluation Questionnaire to behavior in labor, Lederman, Lederman, and Kutzner (1983a, 1983b) undertook a study to examine the effects of prenatal developmental conflict on maternal anxiety in labor.

The research literature provides evidence for the deleterious effects of anxiety and stress on labor (Buchan, 1980; Lowe, 1987; Facchinetti, Ottolini, Fazzio, Rigatelli, & Volpe, 2007; Lobel, Hamilton, & Cannella, 2008; Wadhwa, 2005; Wuitchik, Bakal, & Lipshitz, 1989). Anxiety associated with unattended labor (Sosa, Kennell, Klaus, Robertson, & Urrutia, 1980; Kennell, Klaus, McGrath, Robertson, & Hinkley, 1991; Pascoe, 1993), and with prenatal conflicts about marriage, pregnancy, and motherhood (Lederman, Lederman, Work, & McCann, 1979; Terhi, 2001) has been correlated with prolonged labor (Sosa et al. 1980; Kennell et al. 1991; Pascoe, 1993). Lack of attendance and support of the laboring women, and the anxiety that may ensue, has also been associated with the rate of cesarean section deliveries, forceps deliveries, epidural anesthesia use, oxytocin administration, prolonged infant hospitalization, and maternal fever (Hodnett & Fredericks, 2003; Hodnett, Gates, Hofmeyr, & Sakala, 2007; Kennell et al. 1991; McGrath & Kennell, 2008). Lederman and colleagues (Lederman et al. 1979; Lederman, Lederman, Work, &

McCann 1981; Lederman, Lederman, Work, & McCann, 1985) have demonstrated that maternal anxiety during labor is associated with elevated stress-related hormones that can inhibit uterine contractions and cause placental vasoconstriction, which may lead to protracted labor and fetal anoxia.

The participants for this study were 53 of the 73 married multigravidas, 20–42 years old, with no complicating medical and obstetrical conditions, and who completed both the pregnancy and the childbirth anxiety questionnaires. As noted earlier, the seven prenatal dimensions of pregnancy adaptation were measured both in interviews at 32, 35, and 37 weeks of gestation and with the Prenatal Self-Evaluation Questionnaire which was completed by subjects at the end of the last interview. At 3-, 7-, and 10-cm. cervical dilation the women were asked to verbally respond to a self-report labor anxiety inventory which was read to them. Only the results for active phase labor at 3-cm. cervical dilatation are reported here.

Through the use of cluster analysis, three scales were derived from the 15 self-report items developed for the Labor Anxiety Inventory. Anxiety Scale 1 measures coping with contractions, Scale 2 measures concern about the safety of mother and baby, and Scale 3 measures fear of pain in labor. The reliability coefficients for Scales 1, 2, and 3 are 0.82, 0.72, and 0.82, respectively; the intercorrelations among the three scales are $r = 0.24$–0.39. Thus, there are three reliable independent measures relating to anxiety in active labor: Scale 1:Coping, Scale 2: Safety, and Scale 3: Pain. The instrument and the factor analysis of the scales are described in a paper (Lederman et al., 1983a), which is available on request.

Table 11.4 shows the correlations of the Prenatal Self-Evaluation Questionnaire scales and the prenatal interview ratings with the Labor Anxiety Scales of Coping, Safety, and Pain. The Pregnancy Factor is composed of four separate scales from the Prenatal Self-Evaluation Questionnaire and the prenatal interviews, including Acceptance of Pregnancy, Identification of a Motherhood Role, Relationship with Mother, and Relationship with Husband. The correlations among these four scales were consistently higher, with the highest relationship between Identification of a Motherhood Role and Acceptance of Pregnancy ($r = 0.64$, not shown in table). Based on the consistent pattern of relationships among the four scales, they were combined to form the Pregnancy Factor (Lederman et al., 1983a).

Table 11.4 shows that the interview ratings generally have higher and more significant correlations with the Labor Anxiety Scales than do the questionnaire scales. As expected, Table 11.4 reveals that on both the questionnaire and the interview ratings, prenatal Preparation for Labor has a significant relationship with Coping during Labor. Also as expected, prenatal Concerns for Well-Being of Self and Baby in Labor on both the questionnaire and interview ratings correlate significantly with concerns about Safety in Labor. Prenatal Concerns for Well-Being of Self and Baby also correlate significantly with Fear of Pain during Labor. Prenatal Fear of Pain during Labor, as measured in interviews, has a strong correlation with the subsequent Pain scale administered during labor, but the correla-

Table 11.4 Correlations of the Prenatal Self-Evaluation Questionnaire and Interview Scales with the Labor Anxiety Scales

Variables	Labor anxiety scales		
	1 – Coping	2 – Safety	3 – Pain
Questionnaire			
Pregnancy factor (ACCPR, IMORO, RHU, RMO)	0.13	0.07	0.15
Fear of pain, helplessness, loss of control	0.27	0.13	0.15
Concern for well-being of self and baby in labor	0.21	0.44*	0.38**
Preparation for labor	0.34**	0.16	0.05
Interview rating scales			
Pregnancy factor (ACCPR, IMORO, RHU, RMO)	0.17	−0.05	0.08
Fear of pain, helplessness, loss of control in labor	0.23	0.33**	0.52**
Concern for well-being of self and baby in labor	0.23*	0.57**	0.43**
Preparation for labor	0.49**	0.17	0.23*

ACCPR: acceptance of pregnancy *IMORO*: identification with a motherhood role; *RHU*: relationship with husband; *RMO*: relationship with mother
*$p < 0.05$
**$p < 0.01$

tion is not significant for the prenatal questionnaire scale for these data. Multiple regression analyses confirmed the findings of the correlational analyses (Lederman et al., 1983b).

The results support the predictive validity of the prenatal dimensions to anxiety in labor. Higher anxiety in labor also showed significant relationships to lower uterine activity, a longer duration of labor, and fetal heart rate deceleration (Lederman et al., 1985).

Prediction of Maternal Postpartum Adaptation Using the Prenatal Self-Evaluation Questionnaire

To further evaluate the criterion validity of the Prenatal Self-Evaluation Questionnaire, the predictive correlations of the Prenatal Self-Evaluation Questionnaire to measures of maternal postpartum adaptation were determined (Lederman, Lederman, Kutzner, & Haller, 1982a, 1982b; Lederman, 1989).

The participants were the same normal, married multigravidas, 20–42 years old (Lederman et al., 1982a, 1982b; Lederman, 1989) who completed the Prenatal Self-Evaluation Questionnaire and the prenatal interview schedules in last trimester pregnancy. Following labor and delivery, at 6–8 weeks postpartum, the Postpartum Self-Evaluation Questionnaire (Lederman, Weingarten, & Lederman, 1981) was administered. The scales of the Postpartum Self-Evaluation Questionnaire include Relationship with Husband, Perception of the Father's Participation in Child Care, Gratification from Labor and Delivery, Satisfaction with Life Circumstances, Confidence in Motherhood Role/Tasks, Satisfaction with Motherhood (with the Infant and Infant Care), and Support for Maternal Role from Family, Friends, and Others. Of the seven scales, two were utilized in the data analysis to specifically determine maternal role adaptation: Confidence in Maternal Role/Tasks and Satisfaction with Motherhood. The Cronbach alpha reliability coefficients for these two scales in the current sample are 0.84 and 0.66, respectively, and for an earlier sample ($n = 58$) are 0.74 and 0.78, respectively (Lederman et al. 1981). These results were replicated in a more recent study also examining relationships between prenatal and postnatal adaptation in a sample of gravidas (Lederman, 2008b).

Table 11.5 shows the Prenatal Self-Evaluation Questionnaire scales that were significantly related to the two measures of maternal postpartum adaptation. All scales were scored, as before, so that high scores reflect higher conflict, anxiety, and dissatisfaction. The four prenatal measures pertain to psychological development for motherhood and to adjustment in important interpersonal relationships, and they correlate in a consistent direction postpartally with Satisfaction with Motherhood and Confidence in a Motherhood Role. The highest correlations with the two postpartum adaptation scales are with the prenatal scales of Identification with a Motherhood Role and with Relationship to Husband. In addition, the prenatal measure of Relationship to Husband correlated significantly and highly with two related postpartum measures on Relationship to Husband ($r = 0.83$, $p = < 0.01$) and maternal perception of and satisfaction with Husband Participation in Childcare ($r = 0.79$, $p = 0.01$). These results, reported for the sample of 53 subjects, were supported for the total sample of 73 subjects (Lederman, 1989). Thus, attitudinal and value statements during pregnancy about a motherhood role appear to provide reliable long-term prediction of maternal confidence and satisfaction with motherhood.

The results of the study were replicated and extended in another study of the predictiveness of prenatal to postnatal maternal adaptation (Lederman, 2008b). Several prenatal measures had significant predictive correlations with the postpartum scale on Relationship with Husband, including Acceptance of Pregnancy ($r = 0.56$, $p = 0.02$), Identification of a Motherhood Role ($r = 0.59$, $p = 0.008$), Preparation of

Table 11.5 Correlations of Prenatal Personality Dimensions to Maternal Postpartum Adaptation

	Satisfaction with motherhood	Confidence in motherhood role
Acceptance of pregnancy	0.22	0.25
Identification with a motherhood role	0.39*	0.34*
Relationship with mother	0.21	0.29**
Relationship with husband	0.26**	0.36**

*$p < 0.05$, one-tailed
**$p < 0.01$, one-tailed

Labor, ($r = 0.48$, $p = 0.04$), Fears of Labor ($r = 0.51$, $p = 0.03$), as well as the Prenatal Relationship with Husband ($r = 0.45$, $p = 0.05$). Prenatal Acceptance of Pregnancy correlated significantly with all the Dyadic Adjustment and Maternal–Fetal Attachment scales.

The stability of maternal response is also supported in another longitudinal study conducted by Kutzner (1984), who used the same multigravid subjects and assessments obtained at 6 weeks, and obtained an additional measure of maternal adaptation at 2–3 years after birth. The results showed that the 6-week assessments were highly correlated and predictive of interview and questionnaire responses obtained at the 2–3-year measure, and indicates that maternal response to a motherhood role is relatively constant, and is not likely to vary without planned intervention.

The results of the studies further demonstrated the longitudinal significance of maternal role formulation in pregnancy, and the predictive validity of the Prenatal Self-Evaluation Questionnaire for identifying women with unusual difficulty in prenatal and postnatal adaptation so that early, preventive intervention approaches can be initiated. Other reports in the literature also support the significance of prenatal maternal adaptation to postpartum adaptation (Sieber, Germann, Barbir, & Ehlert, 2006). In a review of the literature on maternal role adaptation, Koniak-Griffin (1993) reported that significant correlations existed between prenatal and postnatal maternal self-confidence, and feelings toward the neonate and the mother herself, indicating stability over time.

Comparisons of Reliability Coefficients in Three Trimesters of Pregnancy and in Three Ethnic Groups: Mean Level Differences in the Total Group

We have conducted studies to examine the pattern of relationships across each trimester of pregnancy to determine mean level differences and pattern variations. If maladaptive patterns of maternal behavior can be identified early in pregnancy, then preventive counseling could be instituted earlier. The study sample was a multicultural, lower socioeconomic population of gravid women, enabling a simultaneous determination of scale reliabilities in three different ethnic groups (Lederman, Harrison, & Worsham, 1992).

The subjects were 689 normal Caucasian (54.2%), African American (29%), and Hispanic-English speaking (16.8%) gravidas attending a university hospital clinic for obstetric care. The majority of patients in the clinic are Medicaid recipients and have no health insurance. Most of the mothers were multigravidas (74.1%), and had no history of premature delivery (87%). The Prenatal Self-Evaluation Questionnaire was administered to the women once in each trimester. Data were collected from cross-sectional sample populations with smaller subsamples participating in two or all three trimesters of pregnancy.

Table 11.6 shows the Cronbach alpha reliability coefficients for the seven scales in each trimester. The alpha coefficients range from 0.71 to 0.93, with all scales at 0.80 or above, except Identification of a Motherhood Role and Fear of Pain, Helplessness, and Loss of Control in Labor.

Table 11.6 Reliability Coefficients (Cronbach's Alpha) of the Prenatal Self-Evaluation Questionnaire Sales in three Trimesters of Pregnancy

Scale	1st trimester	2nd trimester	3rd trimester
Concern for well-being of self and baby in labor	0.87	0.85	0.86
Acceptance of pregnancy	0.88	0.88	0.91
Identification with a motherhood role	0.76	0.71	0.73
Preparation for labor	0.87	0.80	0.79
Fear of pain, helplessness, and loss of control in labor	0.74	0.76	0.78
Relationship with mother	0.91	0.93	0.92
Relationship with husband	0.83	0.84	0.84

Note: $N = 196-203$ in first trimester, $N = 297-302$ in second trimester, and $N = 367-377$ in third trimester

Table 11.7 provides the Cronbach alphas by ethnic group for the seven prenatal dimensions in first trimester pregnancy. The reliability coefficients range from 0.75 to 0.91 for Caucasians, from 0.76 to 0.92 for African Americans, and from 0.72 to 0.88 for Hispanics. The magnitude of the reliability coefficients is similar for each ethnic group in trimesters 2 and 3 of pregnancy and are not presented here.

Table 11.7 Reliability Coefficients (Cronbach's Alpha) of the Prenatal Self-Evaluation Questionnaire Scales in Third trimester of Pregnancy for three Ethnic Groups

Scale	Caucasian	African American	Hispanic
Concern for well-being of self and baby in labor	0.88 (192)	0.86 (98)	0.79 (66)
Acceptance of pregnancy	0.91 (189)	0.90 (99)	0.88 (88)
Identification with a motherhood role	0.75 (187)	0.77 (94)	0.76 (67)
Preparation for labor	0.79 (189)	0.80 (94)	0.82 (64)
Fear of pain, helplessness, and loss of control in labor	0.77 (191)	0.76 (98)	0.72 (68)
Relationship with mother	0.93 (186)	0.92 (96)	0.84 (68)
Relationship with husband	0.87 (190)	0.79 (93)	0.79 (64)

Note: Numbers in parentheses are sample sizes. The total sample size includes the category "Other"

Tables 11.8–11.10 present the scale intercorrelations within each trimester of pregnancy for the total sample. The reliability coefficients are presented at the bottom of each table. A comparison of the results shows that the scale intercorrelations in all three tables are less than the reliability coefficients, providing support for the independence of the scales and the unique information embodied in each scale.

In summary, Tables 11.6–11.10 support the reliability of the instruments in each trimester of pregnancy and in three different ethnic groups of low socioeconomic origin.

Table 11.11 illustrates the mean score changes between trimesters. Maternal conflict concerning acceptance of the pregnancy decreased significantly between the first and third trimesters. Maternal concerns about labor regarding the Well-Being of Self and Baby and Preparation for Labor demonstrated significant

Table 11.8 Prenatal Self-Evaluation Questionnaire Scales: Intercorrelations in 1st Trimester of Pregnancy

Variable	WELLBE	ACCPREG	IDMORO	PREPLAB	HELPL	RELMOTH	RELHUS
Concern for well-being of self and baby in labor (WELLBE)	—	0.23	0.20	0.18	0.41	−0.01	0.10
Acceptance of pregnancy (ACCPREG)	—	—	0.63	0.34	0.39	0.32	0.37
Identification with a motherhood role (IDMORO)	—	—	—	0.41	0.38	0.32	0.43
Preparation for labor (PREPLAB)	—	—	—	—	0.52	0.14	0.20
Fear of pain, helplessness, and loss of control in labor (HELPL)	—	—	—	—	—	0.05	0.34
Relationship with mother (RELMOTH)	—	—	—	—	—	—	0.23

decreases from the first to the third trimester, while fears of Pain, Helplessness, and Loss of Control of Labor showed significant decreases from the second to the third trimester. These decreases demonstrate maternal changes in expected directions. That is, they may be interpreted as reflecting developmental maturity and adaptation of the mother as pregnancy progresses, or the acquisition of knowledge about the processes of labor and self-help skills for coping with labor (Crowe & von Baeyer, 1989).

Table 11.12 provides the prenatal scale correlations between the three trimesters of pregnancy. The moderate to high correlations across trimesters, together with the data presented in Table 11.11, suggest consistency in maternal developmental and adaptive status throughout pregnancy. Tables 11.11 and 11.12 provide additional support for the construct validity of the Prenatal Self-Evaluation Questionnaire scales.

Comparisons of Reliability Coefficients Obtained by Different Investigators in Administration to U.S. and non-U.S. Populations

The scale reliability coefficients reported by the investigators and cited in Table 11.13 show a similar magnitude of internal consistency and they are all ≥0.7. The study by Crook, with a smaller sample size, contained some alpha coefficients with

Table 11.9 Prenatal Self-Evaluation Questionnaire Scales: Intercorrelations in 2nd Trimester of Pregnancy

Variable	WELLBE[a]	ACCPREG	IDMORO	PREPLAB	HELPL	RELMOTH	RELHUS
Concern for well-being of self and baby in labor	—	0.37	0.33	0.18	0.51	0.07	0.22
Acceptance of pregnancy	—	—	0.61	0.36	0.41	0.33	0.44
Identification with a motherhood role	—	—	—	0.29	0.26	0.20	0.31
Preparation for labor	—	—	—	—	0.57	0.17	0.19
Fear of pain, helplessness, and loss of control in labor	—	—	—	—	—	0.18	0.21
Relationship with mother	—	—	—	—	—	—	0.18

[a] See Table 11.8 for identification of column headings

Table 11.10 Prenatal Self-Evaluation Questionnaire Scales: Intercorrelations in 3rd Trimester of Pregnancy

Variable	WELLBE[a]	ACCPREG	IDMORO	PREPLAB	HELPL	RELMOTH	RELHUS
Concern for well-being of self and baby in labor	—	0.30	0.38	0.37	0.57	0.04	0.17
Acceptance of pregnancy	—	—	0.63	0.41	0.39	0.44	0.51
Identification with a motherhood role	—	—	—	0.43	0.42	0.34	0.31
Preparation for labor	—	—	—	—	0.61	0.22	0.26
Fear of pain, helplessness, and loss of control in labor	—	—	—	—	—	0.13	0.28
Relationship with mother	—	—	—	—	—	—	0.34

[a] See 11.8 for identification of column heads

Table 11.11 Mean (SD) Differences of the Prenatal Self-Evaluation Scales over Three Trimesters of Pregnancy (Paired *t* tests)

Scales	1st-trimester	2nd trimester	3rd trimester	Mean difference
Concern for well-being of self and baby in labor	19.0 (6.3)	—	17.8 (5.8)	1.2*
Concern for well-being of self and baby in labor	—	20.0 (6.7)	18.2 (6.5)	18**
Acceptance of pregnancy	27.4 (9.0)	—	25.4 (8.8)	2.0*
Preparation for labor	20.6 (6.2)	—	18.8 (5.7)	1.8**
Fear of pain, helplessness, and loss of control in labor	—	22.0 (5.9)	20.9 (5.8)	1.1**

* $p < 0.05$
** $p < 0.01$

Table 11.12 Prenatal Self Evaluation Questionaire Scales: Correlations between Trimesters of Pregnancy

Scales		2nd trimester	3rd Trimester
Concern for well-being of self and baby in-labor	1st tri	0.69	0.74
	2nd tri	–	0.81
Acceptance of pregnancy	1st tri	0.89	0.71
	2nd tri	–	0.72
Identification with a motherhood role	1st tri	0.71	0.82
	2nd tri	–	0.73
Preparation for labor	1st tri	0.81	0.71
	2nd tri	–	0.71
Fear of pain, helplessness, and loss of control in, labor	1st tri	0.86	0.79
	2nd tri	–	0.78
Relationship with mother	1st tri	0.80	0.79
	2nd tri	–	0.79
Relationship with husband	1st tri	0.64	0.67
	2nd tri	–	0.7

moderately lower or higher values than the other study samples cited in Table 11.13 with larger sample sizes. While most investigators utilized middle-class, normal subject samples, Lederman's 1992 study incorporated a high-risk, lower socioeconomic triethnic sample of Caucasian, African American, and English-speaking Hispanic subjects. The results reported by Lederman (1984, 1990) in Table 11.3 for third trimester pregnancy are upheld for all trimesters and all ethnic populations when the alpha coefficients are calculated for first and second trimester and for the separate ethnic groups (Lederman et al. 1992). These results support the robustness of the instrument and its utility with diverse populations of varying ethnicity and in different geographic locations, including Western, Southwestern, and Midwestern regions of the United States, as well as populations from Canada. Overall, the highest reliability coefficients are obtained for Acceptance of Pregnancy and Relationship with Mother.

Table 11.13 Cronbach's Coefficient Alpha (n) for the Prenatal Self-Evaluation Questionnaire Scales

Scales	Lederman (1996)	Lederman (1990)	Lederman et al. (1992)	Zachariah (Canadian) (1984)	Schachman et al. (2001)	Kiehl & White (2003)	Curry (1987)	Stark (1997)	Crook (1986)	Hyle (1993)	Weis 2006
WELLBE[a]	0.83(119)	0.85(73)	0.85(361)	0.83(115)	0.84(91)	0.87(40)	0.82(90)	0.84(103)	0.69(42)	0.84(241)	0.84(421)
ACCPREG	0.90(119)	0.92(73)	0.90(357)	0.82(115)	0.94(91)	0.91(40)	0.86(95)	0.89(107)	0.84(42)	0.86(241)	0.89(421)
IDMORO	0.79(119)	0.75(73)	0.76(352)	0.67(115)	0.90(91)	0.79(40)	0.70(95)	0.81(107)	0.88(42)	0.76(241)	0.78(421)
PREPLAB	0.80(119)	0.77(73)	0.80(352)	0.82(115)	0.89(91)	0.89(40)	0.74(87)	0.85(106)	0.76(42)	0.77(241)	0.86(420)
HELPL	0.75(118)	0.74(73)	0.75(361)	0.70(115)	0.83(91)	0.81(40)	0.75(84)	0.77(107)	0.89(42)	0.70(241)	0.78(420)
RELMOTH	0.92(115)	0.87(73)	0.91(355)	0.85(115)	0.86(91)	0.89(40)	0.89(89)	0.92(101)	0.74(42)	0.94(241)	0.93(408)
RELHUS	0.82(115)	0.85(73)	0.83(351)	0.76(115)	0.91(91)	0.79(40)	0.79(89)	0.84(102)	0.81(42)	0.89(241)	0.85(417)

[a] See Table 11.8 for identification of scales

The Prenatal Self-Evaluation Questionnaire has been translated into several languages, including Spanish, Italian, German, Greek, Chinese, Swedish, and Norwegian, and it has been administered by researchers to pregnant women from these populations, as well as to populations from New Zealand and Australia.

11.2   Prenatal Clinical Interview Schedules and Rating Scales

The clinical interview serves a number of purposes. During the interview, opportunities exist for educating and counseling patients. A major purpose of our research interviews, however, was to obtain quantitative ratings of the status of the gravidas in relation to the pregnancy variables listed in the Chapter 1 tables. In order to systematically obtain the information needed to make the necessary assessments, an interview schedule containing specific questions was developed (see Appendix A). The questions from the interview schedule were presented in three sessions, with each session requiring 40 min to 1 hour. Spontaneous comments from the subjects were encouraged, and they also were asked to keep a diary and dream record which was discussed during the sessions. These sessions were tape recorded to facilitate later review of the content.

11.2.1   Clinical Practice Recommendations for Conducting Interviews

Preparation for parenthood involves contemplation about the new role to be assumed and about the relationship to be developed with the child. Pregnancy has long been viewed merely as the incubation period for the infant, but it also should be seen as the process necessary for the evolution of a parent. Researchers frequently describe processes of role development which are applicable only to the postnatal period, while prenatal processes in pregnancy are not thoroughly and systematically researched. Utilizing questions from the Interview Schedule in Appendix A, provides an avenue of inquiry that can be directed toward the gravida's motivation and specific preparation for motherhood, and her adaptation to anticipated changes in lifestyle. Our studies have provided considerable insight in to the status and importance accorded motherhood by the women in our studies, many of whom did not anticipate a traditional sex role for themselves. The intensity of motherhood-career conflicts appeared to support, rather than refute, the significance accorded motherhood by the subjects.

The interview provides an opportunity for the gravida to speak openly about thoughts or concerns she may have regarding her unborn child. The mother's description of her anticipated relationship with the child will necessarily be abstract to a certain extent, especially for the primigravida, and could represent an element of wish fulfillment of the mother's need for intimacy or a "warm, loving relationship." The interviewer therefore should seek to augment the mother's response with inquiry into her goals for the child's development, and how those goals might be achieved. Although this was not a specific aim of the interview, such inquiry served to set the mother, and often the father as well, on a course of contemplation that would otherwise not have been as well focused. Overall, the process of inquiry tends to stimulate and channel the gravida's thoughts toward productive reflection – alone and with others – and to integrate challenges which arise and the behaviors necessary to meet them. Pregnancy is widely acknowledged to be a time of openness and receptiveness, and a prime time for self-examination and eagerness to learn. Conflicts are more readily disclosed and options for resolution considered.

Several studies focusing on the gravida's relationship with her mother have emphasized the need for mother-daughter reconciliation, in order for the gravida to comfortably and independently evolve a workable motherhood identity for herself. When reported, however, the magnitude of correlations between relationship to mother and pregnancy adaptation generally was only low to moderate. This result indicates the significance of the factor, but also shows that several other factors affect pregnancy adaptation and motherhood identification (Shereshefsky & Yarrow, 1973; Leifer, 1977; Ballou, 1978; Lederman et al., 1979).

Chapter 4 on relationship with the mother identifies conditions and behaviors which support or obstruct the gravida's relationship with her mother. In a study of the influence of this relationship on reproductive adjustment, Uddenberg (1974) obtained more significant results when he evaluated closeness and power in the relationship. Therefore, it is important in evaluating the quality of the relationship to consider the influence the maternal grandmother exercises in the relationship, and how much the gravida seeks and values this relationship.

The relationship with the husband needs to be assessed with care. Grossman, Eichler, and Winickoff (1980) have noted that gravidas near term may be "unwilling or unable to acknowledge any difficulties in their marriages, sensing the extreme importance of a good relationship to the successful outcome of their undertaking." A number of studies failed to find significant correlations between the marital rela-tionship and pregnancy adaptation variables (Shereshefsky & Yarrow, 1973; Grossman, Eichler, & Winickoff, 1980), but others cite the marital relationship as the most significant influence on pregnancy adaptation (Wenner, Cohen, Wiegert, Kvarnes, Ohaneson, & Fearing, 1969). The work of Weis et al. (2008) with military families and the impact of the husband's deployment on acceptance of pregnancy and later postpartum adjustments (Weis, 2006) reinforce the significance of this relationship to maternal prenatal adaptation.

Based on an examination of data collection methods used by other investigators, as well as on the author's experience, several suggestions for increasing assessment accuracy are offered. Two very useful areas for inquiry deal with changes in *the couple's relationship*, and *how the partners resolve differences in their needs for sexual intercourse*. Responses to questions in both these areas did not appear to be influenced by social desirability; the questions called for statements of behavior which revealed sensitivity and responsiveness in the relationship. Questions about changes in the husband's behavior – increased concern, willingness to listen, assistance with household chores, attention to mutual preparation for childbirth and parent-hood, providing emotional reassurance and physical support – provided a better (that is, more revealing) indicator of the quality of the relationship than inquiry about the mother's feelings of increased closeness. Some gravidas responded that they always had a very close relationship with their husbands and that the closeness did not change with the pregnancy.

Husband–wife differences in sex drive throughout pregnancy have been noted by researchers (Condon, 2006; Masters, Johnson, & Kolodny, 1988; Solberg, Butler, & Wagner, 1973) who have measured frequency of sexual activity and reasons for its cessation or prohibition. Differences in sex drive were evaluated in our research as well. In addition, the gravida was asked to explain how differences were reconciled when they occurred.

Frequently, the gravida's interest in sex diminished while the husband's remained unchanged. Did the couple discuss differences in need and arrive at a mutually satisfying agreement? Or, did the gravida ignore her husband's approaches or respond with silent reproof? Did the husband respect his wife's feelings? Did the couple attempt to utilize alternative methods of gratification (which may be prohibited by some religions)? Did they eventually find a solution which was satisfying and acceptable to both, at least for the remainder of the gestation? The answers to these questions provided a basis for judging the marital relationship and the expectant couple's pattern of support and problem solving. It also was important to consider mutuality in the relationship, as well as dependence and interdependence of the partners as demonstrated in other areas of functioning.

The area of preparation for labor is one in which the health care worker, particularly the nurse, can readily assess knowledge and the appropriateness of anticipated coping behaviors. Usually, it is necessary for the interviewer to clarify some misunderstandings about labor processes and the emotional and physical sensations that will be experienced. For the woman who is preoccupied with other concerns, this may be the only opportunity for her to learn about labor from a reliable source and to reflect on how she will cope. This is an area in which nurses and childbirth educators can be particularly helpful.

One should inquire about the gravida's history of dealing with pain and with crises in general. Patterns of reaction to pain such as stoicism or endurance without pharmacological aids, and means for pain alleviation, tend to be predictive of similar behaviors in labor. In addition, one should discuss preferred comfort measures with the gravida before the onset of labor. Assessment of pain tolerance, relief measures, preferred physical support measures, and how the staff and the husband can be helpful will all reveal a great deal about personal coping mechanisms that are useful to be aware of, but difficult to discern at a later period in labor.

11.2.2 Summary Ratings

Quantitative ratings of the gravida's status on specific dimensions provided a useful summary of the information obtained in the interviews. The process of making ratings focuses attention on specific aspects of behavior that are useful in describing present adaptation or in making predictions for the future. Ratings also enable follow-up studies to be conducted. The ratings may be supplemented with narrative comments that will facilitate communication of the material among professional personnel. Additional suggestions for increasing accuracy using validating procedures are presented in the last section of this chapter.

Rating scales with which to summarize the interview responses are provided in Appendix B. These 5-point scales provide five categories, or levels, for describing patients; "1" indicates low conflict or fear and "5" indicates high conflict or fear. With experience, interviewers may wish to make finer distinctions regarding the adaptation of the gravid women. Additional levels of discrimination can be obtained by using half-point intervals or by adding more points to the scale.

The ratings are likely to be most useful when they reflect relative comparisons among patients. Relative comparisons provide a frame of reference which gives meaning to the ratings in a particular clinical setting, and are more likely to ensure congruence among different raters who might otherwise use varying subjective standards. For this reason, interviews with a number of patients should be conducted before ratings are made in order to make the rating standards as uniform and objective as possible.

The overall rating for a scale should be based on an integration of the material gathered from all the gravida's interviews. Several methods of integrating the relevant responses are possible in order to obtain a single rating. We recommend a global rather than an analytic method. An analytic method is used in inventories, where the single-scale score is based on the sum of responses to statements. The global method relies on a subjective synthesis of the responses obtained in the interviews. Since the principles of measurement for scales obtained by ratings are the same as those obtained from inventories, some factors determining the validity of inventory scales should be kept in mind when making ratings. Global synthesis of interview responses is an analogous process.

In an inventory, a range of statements are included to adequately define the dimension. Breadth of coverage increases the potential validity of the scale for predictive purposes, but it may lower the internal consistency of the responses to the statements. Reliability, however, can be increased by including more statements. The status of subjects on the scale is determined by their consistency of response; that is, the highest and lowest scoring subjects are those who respond consistently high or low on a scale. Interview responses differ in some ways from statements on inventories, and this should be taken into consideration when subjectively processing the information. Some of the subject's responses may be more detailed and revealing than others. These types of responses should be given more weight or influence in determining the rating, but not to the exclusion of other responses. Generalizability for the rating is best obtained by incorporating several of the patient's responses into the rating, and by considering the consistency of the responses before making a judgment.

Some additional cautions are worth noting. The rater should ensure that responses used to infer the patient's status for one scale do not infringe upon the definition of another scale or influence its rating, for this would obscure the unique information conveyed by each scale. Similarly, raters should guard against allowing a general impression of the patient to influence their judgments of her adaptations. The dimensions should each be viewed as relatively independent aspects of behavior.

11.3   Recommendations for Clinical Care and Research

11.3.1   Clinical Assessment: Continuity of Care and Assessment of Maternal Developmental Adaptation

In order to be clinically effective over the course of the maternity cycle, it is important that a pattern of continuity in follow-up and assessment be maintained. Ideally, the same person caring for the gravida in pregnancy should be with her during labor and delivery, and continue the assessment of mother, father, and infant during the period of postpartum adjustment. This process would require a reorganization in the delivery of clinical health care services, which currently divides and separates staff in obstetric/maternity units. Instead, a provision is needed that is more consonant with the case management approach to health care delivery, and is founded on consistency and continuity in patient care by a health care provider.

Continuity in obstetric case care would serve three important purposes. First, patients would receive the benefit of consistent provider support throughout the maternity cycle, a form of support very likely to be more informed, and offered with a greater interest in and commitment to the family's growth, development, and welfare. Second, it is principally through continuity in follow-up care and evaluation that developmental theory, embodying the entire maternity cycle, will evolve. And, very importantly, the prenatal identification of significant predictors of behavior in labor and postpartum adjustment will be facilitated by continuity of care. The discernment and discussion of longitudinal patterns of relationships can serve as the test ground and basis for the design of future research in this area. Through research, the identification of crucial predictive factors also will provide an important foundation and guide to methods of intervention. Utilization of a method of caretaker assessment based on continuity in assessment can be very well applied to learning exercises in the classroom, in workshops, and in the clinical environment.

A third, and often overlooked, advantage to continuity of care is that it is gratifying and rewarding work for the clinical practitioner. This aspect will foster continued attention to theory development – to the generation of assessment and evaluation instruments, and methods of intervention.

11.3.2   Suggestions for Clinical Research Studies

11.3.2.1   Assessment of Prenatal Adaptation and Determination of Labor and Delivery Outcomes

For obstetric clinics providing integrated maternal care services, a clinically beneficial research project would be to assess the prenatal adaptation of different groups of patients during pregnancy using the Prenatal Self-Evaluation Questionnaire, followed by an analysis and determination of the questionnaire's predictability of maternal anxiety and stress during labor, maternal/infant health outcomes of labor and delivery, and maternal postpartum adaptation. The research results presented in Chapters 1 and 11, as well as in the other chapters, provide support for the criterion validity of the interview and questionnaire assessment of the prenatal personality dimensions. Criterion or predictive validity is provided in the correlations of the prenatal dimensions with subsequent maternal and fetal labor events and delivery outcomes, as well as with maternal and child adaptation and development in the years after birth. A design which incorporates both interview and questionnaire assessment enables the researcher to also test the effectiveness of each instrument as a screening measure to identify subjects who may be at risk for adaptational problems and labor complications, as well as to determine the additional knowledge and predictive power provided by interview assessments and ratings.

The specific design for projects will depend on the research questions of interest in a particular patient population and the social, psychological, cultural, economic, and medical and reproductive characteristics of the population to be studied. Based on the research questions and population characteristics, additional instruments can be added to the prenatal assessment project in order to test related questions and to provide concurrent and construct validity for the instruments and the research results obtained with them.

The results obtained through research projects could then be analyzed to determine significant correlates of prenatal adaptation and predictors of maternal and fetal delivery outcomes, and could form the basis for designing intervention protocols. Since it is possible and likely that similar research methods used with different populations will yield varied results, it would be prudent for clinicians to conduct assessments with targeted populations before introducing and testing novel intervention protocols with a given population.

As noted, questionnaire assessment can be performed in conjunction with interview assessment and rating scale scoring on each of the seven dimensions. The schedules of interview assessment and the rating scales are provided in Appendices A and B. Skill in conducting interviews, and in assessment and rating scale score determination can be achieved through planned experiences in interviewing and in evaluation, which can be provided through workshops.[2]

Further information on assessment workshops can be obtained by contacting the first author at sites noted.

Prenatal Assessment for Screening, Identification, and Planned Intervention

A number of the prenatal dimensions correlated significantly with maternal anxiety in labor (see Table 11.4) and with measures of maternal postpartum adaptation (see Table 11.5). For example, prenatal Preparation for Labor correlated with maternal Coping during Labor. And prenatal Fear of Pain, Helplessness, and Loss of Control during Labor correlated with the actual Fear of Pain during Labor. Thus, it is possible to design studies for assessment of prenatal Preparation for Labor and for counseling and education intervention for women who are assessed to have low levels of knowledge or readiness for labor. Likewise, for women with a high prenatal Fear of Pain during

Labor, preventive intervention measures can be introduced during pregnancy to allay some degree of fear and anxiety, and to better assess individual maternal responses to pain and preferred measures for the alleviation of pain. The author has discerned during prenatal interviews that women can provide upon inquiry the details of ways in which they perceive and interpret pain, respond to different kinds of pain, and preferred methods for alleviating pain for themselves as well as through the provision of assistance activities from others. Some of these activities may not be included in the current prenatal classes which prepare women to cope with labor. Such detailed prenatal assessment, especially as can occur in interviews, can provide a rich foundation upon which to plan and develop protocols for the management of pain together with the gravid women during pregnancy and the provider of care during labor. The success of these individual protocols of care can be assessed in studies measuring the effectiveness of intervention and the gratification of the labor and delivery experience for women who receive and do not receive such customized plans of care.

Postpartally, measures of Satisfaction with Motherhood and Confidence in a Motherhood Role are correlated with prenatal measures of Identification of a Motherhood Role and with Relationship to Husband. These results should be further tested in replication studies by other investigators, as well as in intervention studies to strengthen the marital relationship when excessive conflict is assessed prenatally and to assist the expectant mother in making plans for childcare that are accordance with her motherhood role preferences. Prenatal assessment and intervention of this kind may be especially valuable not only in promoting adaptation to pregnancy and motherhood, but to preservation of the marriage and the family, and development of a sensitive, responsive mother-child relationship.

11.4 Research Intervention Trials for General and Pregnancy-Specific Anxiety Reduction

11.4.1 Assessment of the Seven PSEQ Dimensions as a Basis for Intervention

The studies, descriptions, and interpretations presented in this book provide detailed information about the type and timing of anxiety the gravida experiences prenatally as she progresses in maternal adaptation. Each dimension of psychosocial adaptation has been studied across trimesters and in different ethnic populations to describe the origin of individual differences in prenatal maternal adaptation, and the scientific basis and descriptions of low, moderate, and high psychosocial adaptation, which serve as a guide to interpretation of maternal behavior, and as the basis for the formulation of intervention therapies. This section on prenatal interventions is included to permit the reader to consider methods for addressing maternal maladaptive problems, as well as enhancement of psychosocial adaptation for all expectant women and families. It is prepared to familiarize the reader with available therapeutic interventions, rather than provide an exhaustive literature review of such interventions.

Intervention research requires an understanding of variables for which change can reasonably be expected as a result of therapeutic intervention. The dependent variables and the related constructs must be carefully specified and designed so that they can be anticipated and measured (Lipsey, 1993). Sensitive and accurate measures of dependent variables are vital to detect changes in predicted outcomes (Stewart & Archbold, 1993). The seven dimensions described for maternal prenatal psychosocial adaptation provide the systematic steps through which a gravida becomes a mother. Both the Prenatal Self-Evaluation Questionnaire (PSEQ) and the interview schedules provide a means of measuring pregnancy-specific anxiety and isolating the specific types of anxiety so that focused intervention can take place. Additionally, the PSEQ and interview schedules are designed to be administered at any point during pregnancy. They can then be used for pre- and post-test measurement.

11.4.1.1 Characteristics of Effective Interventions

Effective interventions require clear conceptual frameworks, systematic development, and rigorous testing (Olds, Sadler, & Kitzman, 2007; Scott & Sechrest, 1989). Theory guides the design and delivery of the intervention, which promotes a causal relationship to exist between the intervention and the intended outcomes. This relationship guides the interpretation of research findings whether significant or nonsignificant (Sidani & Braden, 1998). Future research should also adhere to high standards of randomization (Olds et al. 2007) to avoid selection bias and enhance generalization. Ideally, intervention therapies should be initiated before parenting and parent-child problems occur, and they are most effective with psychologically vulnerable, challenged populations, which may include most expectant mothers and fathers, but particularly those with a history of intimate partner violence, depression, psychosocial stress, economic disadvantage, limited sense of mastery, lower self-esteem, and greater ambivalence about pregnancy (Bloom, Curry, Durham, 2007; Olds et al., 2007). Both efficacy and effectiveness trials are needed, as well as cost analyses (Flay et al., 2004; Olds et al.). In the Bloom et al. study, such vulnerable subjects tended toward high utilization of prenatal medical services, clearly a factor in cost of care.

Prenatal prevention and treatment programs need to target improvement of maternal psychosocial health, including anxiety, depression, self-esteem, and close kin relationship problems as preventive interventions, just as parenting intervention programs have evolved for these purposes (Barlow, Coren, & Stewart-Brown, 2003).

11.5 The Panoply of Therapeutic Prenatal Interventions to Promote Maternal Psychosocial Adaptation to Pregnancy

Lederman (1995a) has conducted extensive reviews of literature (Lederman 1995a) on anxiety in pregnancy and therapies (Lederman 1995b) to ameliorate maternal anxiety and reduce adverse outcomes. Recent literature has documented the long-term and far-reaching effects of maternal anxiety associated with low birth weight for the mother and the fetus, newborn, infant, child, and adult continuum of psychosocial and physical health status. Relationships are reported for maternal prenatal depression and newborn biochemical/physiological profiles that mimic their mothers' prenatal biochemical/physiological depression profile (Field, Diego, & Hernandez-Reif, 2006). Maternal prenatal depression is also associated with newborn depressive brain organization. This same research group (Field, Diego, & Hernandez-Reif, 2008) further reported counterintuitive results regarding prenatal dysthymia versus major depression. The newborns of dysthymic versus major depression disorder mothers had a significantly shorter gestational age, a lower birthweight, shorter birth length, and less optimal obstetric complications scores. The neonates of dysthymic mothers also had lower orientation and motor scores and more depressive symptoms on the Brazelton Neonatal Behavioral Assessment Scale. Prenatal maternal anxiety and depression also predict negative behavioral reactivity in infancy (Davis, Snidman, Wadhwa, Dunkel-Schetter, Glynn, & Sandman, 2004). Given the well-known high correlation of depression and anxiety, one can tentatively extrapolate the effects of maternal prenatal anxiety to neonatal neurologic and behavioral responses. These recent data offer compelling evidence for the earliest assessment and intervention possible of maternal prenatal-specific psychosocial dimensions, assessment which to date is most inclusively accomplished with the seven dimensions of maternal psychosocial adaptation, measured with the Prenatal Self-Evaluation Questionnaire and/or the Interview Schedules and Rating Scales of the seven dimensions.

11.5.1   Intervention Research Demonstrating Effectiveness in High-Risk Prenatal Populations

Studies on socially supportive community intervention during pregnancy, though sparse, suggest that social support may have significant short- and long-term maternal–child benefits. When social support was provided by paraprofessional women to expectant teens at home, the teens were less likely to have a preterm birth (Rogers, Peoples-Sheps, & Suchrindran, 1996). A program based on four nurse home-visits to high-risk African-American pregnant women to assist with relationship problems with the gravida's mother and husband and to enhance self-esteem proved to be very effective in reducing low birth weight (LBW) to 9% in the experimental group, compared to 22% in a control group (Norbeck et al., 1996). Edwards et al. (1994) replicated these results by providing consistent supportive services to high-risk women by professional clinic staff. Another impressive personal intervention consisting of an average of 54–72 min of psychosocial services over the entire course of pregnancy to low-income women yielded significant differences in LBW outcomes in all ethnic groups, including Caucasian (Zimmer-Gembeck & Helfand, 1996). In Britain (Oakley, Hickey, Rajan, & Rigby, 1996), pregnant women who received social support from midwives likewise had fewer low birth weight infants and benefited from additional favorable maternal–child health outcomes. At a 7-year follow-up, significant health and development benefits for the children were sustained; the mothers' physical and psychosocial health also was preserved. Other supportive nurse home visitation program (Olds, Henderson, Kitzman, Eckenrode, Cole, & Tatelbaum, 1998; Olds, 2002) yielded maternal–child benefits over a period of 15 years, including an improvement in the mothers' health behaviors and the quality of infant/child caregiving. These effects were still observed at a 20-year follow-up and were strongest for mothers who were single and of lower socioeconomic backgrounds (Kitzman et al., 2000). The very enduring effects of supportive interventions on the reduction of adverse birth outcomes and maternal–child life course provide compelling evidence for greater supportive psychosocial interventions.

11.5.2   Intervention Research Demonstrating Effectiveness in Low-Risk Prenatal Populations

Most prenatal supportive interventions focus on health education (e.g., diet, exercise, maternal and newborn care, symptom relief, preparation for labor and childbirth, and recognition of complications). Few programs have a primary focus on maternal/paternal/family mental health and psychosocial well-being, or any foundations in scientific research if counseling is offered. From research literature reported throughout this book, it seems clear that intervention programs that would assist and support the mother and family in crystallizing parenthood roles, in preparing for the parenting challenges that lie ahead, in counseling to improve marital/partner communication and support, as well as other significant kin relationships, and in enhancing self-esteem, and coping and mastery skills with daily hassles and stressful life events would be highly warranted. As an example, a pilot study of 5-week maternal prenatal support groups (of 4–6 participants each) using a psychoeducational intervention based on the seven pregnancy-specific personality dimensions developed by Lederman, and additional measures of dyadic relationship and maternal–fetal attachment was implemented with a low-income multiethnic population in second-trimester pregnancy. All instruments had adequate Cronbach alpha reliability coefficients. The results, reported in professional scientific presentations (Lederman, 2008a), showed significant differences in pre-post group measures of Well-Being of Self and Baby in Labor across time and between groups. The Intervention group ($n = 21$) showed significantly decreased anxiety over time while the Control group ($n = 18$) reported increased anxiety. For Concerns about Preparation of Labor both Intervention and Control groups reported decreased anxiety, but the Intervention group reported greater decreases. On the abridged Dyadic Adjustment Scale (DAS) 3 on togetherness or altruism, both groups increased, but the Intervention group increased more. On DAS Scale 4 on time spent in outside interests by the couple the Intervention

Group increased and the control Group decreased significantly ($F = 8.229$, $p = 0.007$). These results show that the Psychosocial Support Group Intervention decreased maternal anxiety about well-being of herself and baby and about feelings of preparedness for labor compared to the Control Group. The Intervention Group also showed greater Dyadic Adjustment Scale benefits than the control group. It is also noteworthy that we again replicated findings wherein prenatal psychosocial adaptation was predictive of postnatal maternal psychosocial adaptation. Several prenatal measures had significant predictive correlations with the postpartum scale on Relationship with Husband, including Acceptance of Pregnancy ($r = 0.56$, $p = 0.02$), Identification with a Motherhood Role ($r = 0.59$, $p = 0.008$), Preparation of Labor ($r = 0.48$, $p = 0.04$), Fears of Labor ($r = 0.51$, $p = 0.03$), and Prenatal Relationship with Husband ($r = 0.45$, $p = 0.05$). These results provide support for the early prenatal implementation of psychosocial support groups to decrease anxiety and increase adaptation to pregnancy, which may have short-term benefits for improving birth outcomes, as well as long-term benefits for maternal and child mental health and development. A goal of this research is to contribute to positive intergenerational psychosocial relationships and health.

11.5.3 Marital/Partner Relationships as Factors Influencing Maternal Stress/Anxiety Responses, with Implications for Therapeutic Intervention

Marital and partner relationships are the most frequent and cogent factors cited in the transition to parenthood (Perren, Von Wyl, Burgin, Simoni, & von Klitzing, 2005). The significance of marital quality is underscored by recent reports of its association with the later marital quality of the parents' offspring (Amato & Booth, 2001), hence the origin of the notion of intergenerational transmission of marital quality across the transition to parenthood (Perren et al.). Several social factors pertaining to partner relationships have been identified as influencing paternal transition to parenthood, including partner communication, extended family involvement, relationship with partner, peer attitudes and expectations, uncertain normative expectations, intensity of emotions, feelings of isolation, inability to engage in the pregnancy, and lack of medical knowledge – factors which clearly present the multitude of and complexity surrounding paternal and parental adaptation in the transition to parenthood (Leite, 2007).

Significant differences in pregnancy adaptation have been found in relation to marital status disparities, without any further measurement of marital/partner relationship quality. Kiernan and Pickett (2006) found that cohabiting mothers (vs. married mothers) had a greater risk of adverse outcomes pertaining to smoking, while nonmarried women lacking an intimate relationship were more likely to smoke throughout the pregnancy than those more involved with the fathers. In contrast, stronger parental bonds were associated with the initiation of breast feeding and a decreased risk of maternal depression. Women who perceived barriers to communication about their emotions with their health providers or their family had significantly higher depression scores than those who did not (Sleath et al. 2005). Additionally, researchers (Talge, Neal, Glover, and the Early Stress Transitional Research and Prevention Science Network, 2007) have suggested that extra maternal vigilance and anxiety, readily distracted attention, or a hyperresponsive HPA axis may contribute to the vulnerability of childhood neurodevelopmental disorders.

11.5.4   Maternal and Paternal Coping Strategies and Birth Outcomes

A number of studies reveal poor maternal psychosocial coping skills and mastery in the appraisal of stress and in stress management. Anxiety has been found to be higher in women who are lower in mastery, have less positive attitudes about their pregnancy, and experience a larger number of stressful life events during pregnancy; such women also report increases in anxiety (vs. adaptation) from early to late pregnancy (Gorung, Dunkell-Schetter, Collins, Rini, & Hobel, 2005). Poor coping skills have been associated with preterm birth (Dole et al., 2004) and significantly low birthweight deliveries (Borders, Grobman, Amsden, & Holl, 2007). These results suggest that coping and mastery skills be incorporated into individual and group psychoeducational support interventions.

11.5.5   Complementary and Alternative Medical (CAM) Therapies

Numerous mind-body stress reduction interventions during pregnancy have been noted for their effects on perceived stress, mood, and perinatal outcomes (Guerreiro da Silva 2007, Beddoe & Lee, 2008). These interventions have included acupuncture, exercise, hypnosis, massage, psychoeducation, qi gong, progressive muscle relaxation, tai chi, yoga and meditation, other CAM therapies, and individual therapies. In the review of literature conducted by Beddoe and Lee, there were numerous methodological problems identified (absence of randomization or control of confounding variables). However, they still noted evidence of efficacy of mind-body modalities that included higher birthweight, shorter length of labor, fewer instrument-assisted births, and reduced perceived stress and anxiety. The authors aptly recommended that further research is necessary to predict characteristics of subgroups that might be most likely to benefit from different mind-body practices, and the examination of the cost effectiveness of these interventions on perinatal outcomes.

In the following paragraphs we briefly review some of the studies and major findings included in articles in the Beddoe and Lee review of literature, and others not included that have pertinent recommendations. In a study on active or passive (sitting) relaxation, both methods significantly reduced state anxiety and maternal heart rate, but active relaxation had a significantly greater effect (Teixeira, Martin, Prendiville, & Glover 2005). Another trial of stress reduction demonstrated significantly lower levels of stress, lower symptoms of depression, and negative affect, and lower cortisol levels under the stress reduction condition (Urizar et al., 2004). Bastani, Hidarnia, Kazemnejad, Vafaei, and Kashanian (2005) reported reduced measures of state anxiety and perceived stress, compared to a control group, for a randomized control trial of applied relaxation training. This same group of researchers (Bastani, Hidarnia, Montgomery, Aguilar-Vafaei, & Kazemnejad, 2006) showed that low-risk primigravid women with measurement of high anxiety levels who received applied relaxation training showed significant reductions in low birth weight, cesarean section, and/or instrumental delivery. One further study (Guerreiro da Silva, 2007) measuring emotional complaints in pregnancy regarding mood, sleep, relationships, social activities, sexual life, and joy of living showed that the intensity of distress decreased by at least half (60%) in patients participating in the experimental condition, compared to 26% of those in the control group ($p = 0.013$). While very few studies consider fetal effects of maternal anxiety, DiPietro and colleagues (DiPietro, Costigan, Nelson, & Gurewitsch, 2008) evaluated fetal responses to induced maternal relaxation in 100 maternal–fetal pairs using guided imagery relaxation. The results showed significant changes in maternal heart rate, skin conductance, respiration period, and respiratory sinus arrhythmia, and significant changes in fetal neurobehavior, including decreased fetal heart rate (FHR), increased FHR variability, suppression of fetal motor (FM) activity, and increased FM-FHR coupling. There were significant associations between maternal autonomic measures and fetal cardiac patterns, lower umbilical and uterine resistance, and declining salivary cortisol levels.

The aggregate of these studies strongly suggests that expectant women living under high anxiety and stressful conditions benefit from anxiety and stress reduction interventions, and that further studies are warranted and should include fetal response measures in relation to maternal anxiety responses.

The foregoing research results on intervention protocols strongly suggest that screening measures for maternal anxiety, stressful life events, supportive family and community systems, and coping skills be instituted as part of routine antenatal health screening for adaptation to pregnancy (Bentley, Melville, Berry, & Katon, 2007; Leigh & Milgrom, 2007). These recommendations are very much in agreement with the judicious Surgeon General's recent conclusions and recommendations for prenatal and perinatal maternal and family care (Office of the Surgeon General and the Eunice Kennedy Shriver National Institute of Child Health and Human Development, 2008).

Clinicians and researcher need to evaluate and discern the interventions appropriate for the populations to whom they offer health care and therapeutic interventions. It seems reasonable for health care providers to consider both pregnancy-specific psychosocial individual and group interventions, as well as complementary and alternative medical interventions for stress reduction, and combinations of these therapies in future randomized clinical intervention trials.

References

Amato, P. R., & Booth, A. (2001). *The legacy of parents' marital discord and divorce across generations: Results for a 20-year longitudinal study of two generations.* Paper presented at the European Conference of Developmental Psychology, Milano, Italy, August 27–31.

Ballou, J. (1978). *The psychology of pregnancy.* Lexington, MA: Lexington Books.

Bastani, F., Hidarnia, A., Kazemnejad, A., Vafaei, M., & Kashanian, M. (2005). A randomized controlled trial of the effects of applied relaxation training on reducing anxiety and perceived stress in pregnant women. *Journal of Midwifery and Women's Health.* 50(4):e36–e40.

Bastani F, Hidarnia A, Montgomery KS, Aguilar-Vafaei ME, & Kazemnejad A. (2006). Does relaxation education in anxious primigravid Iranian women influence adverse Pregnancy Outcomes? A randomized control trial. *Journal of Perinatal and Neonatal Nursing,* 20(2):138–46.

Barlow, J., Coren, E., & Stewart-Brown, S. S. B. (2003). Parent-training programs for improving maternal psychosocial health (Review). *Cochrane Database and Systematic Reviews,* 4, Art. No.: CD002020. DOI: 10.1002/14651858.CD002020.pub2.

Beddoe, A. E., & Lee, K. A. (2008). Mind–body interventions during pregnancy. *Journal of Obstetric, Gynecologic, and Neonatal Nursing, 37,* 165–175.

Bentley S. M., Melville J. L., Berry, B. D., & Katon, W. J. (2007). Implementing a clinical and research registry in obstetrics: overcoming the barriers. *General Hospital Psychiatry, 29,* 192–198

Bloom, T., Curry, M. A., & Durham, L. (2007). Abuse and Psychosocial stress as factors in high utilization of medical services during pregnancy. *Issues in Mental Health Nursing, 28,* 849–865.

Borders, A. E. B., Grobman, A. A., Amsden, L. B., & Holl, J. L. (2007). Chronic stress and low birth weight in a low-income population of women. *Obstetrics and Gynecology, 109*(2), 331–338.

Buchan, P. C. (1980). Emotional stress in childbirth and its modification by variations in obstetric management: Epidural analgesia and stress in labor. *Acta Obstetrica & Gynecologica Scandanavica, 59*(4) 319–321.

Condon, J. (2006). What about Dad? Psychosocial and mental health issues for new fathers. *Australian Family Physician, 35*(9), 690–692.

Crook, L. D. (1986). *The relationship of prenatal and postpartum dimensions to women's satisfaction with their childbirth experience.* Unpublished master's thesis, The University of Wisconsin-Madison, Madison, WI.

Crowe, K., & von Baeyer, C. (1989). Predictors of a positive childbirth experience. *Birth, 16*(2), 59–63.

Curry, M. A. (1987). Maternal behavior of hospitalized pregnant women. *Journal of Psychosomatic Obstetrics and Gynecology, 7*(3), 165–182.

Davis, E. P., Snidman, N., Wadhwa, P. D., Dunkel Schetter, C., Glynn, L. M., & Sandman, C. A. (2004). Prenatal Maternal anxiety and depression predict negative behavioral reactivity in infancy. *Infancy, 6*(3), 319–331.

DiPietro, J. A., Costigan, K. A., Nelson, P., Gurewitsch, E. (2008). Fetal response to induced maternal relaxation during pregnancy. *Biological Psychology, 77,* 11–19.

Dole, N., Savitz, D. A., Siega-Riz, A. M., Herta-Picciotto, I., McMahon, M. J., & Buekens, P. (2004). Psychosocial factors and preterm birth among African American and White women in central North Carolina. *American Journal of Public Health, 94*(8), 1358–1365.

Edwards, C. H., Knight, E. M., Johnson, A. A., Oyemade, U. J., Cole, O. J., Laryea, H., et al. (1994). Multiple factors as mediators of the reduced incidence of low birth weight in an urban clinic population. *Journal of Nutrition, 124,* 927S–935S.

Facchinetti, F., Ottolini, F., Fazzio, M., Rigatelli, M., & Volpe, A. (2007). Psychosocial factors associated with preterm uterine contractions. *Psychotherapy and Psychosomatics, 76,* 391–394.

Field, T., Diego, M., Hernandez-Reif, M. (2006). Prenatal depression effects on the fetus and newborn. *Infant Behavior & Development, 31*(2), 190–193

Field, T. Diego, M., Hernandez-Reif, M. (2008). Prenatal dysthymia versus major depression effects on the neonate. *Infant Behavior & Development, 29*(3), 445–455.

Flay, B. R., Biglan, A., Boruch, R. F., Castro, F. G., Gottfredson, D., Kellam, S. G., et al. (2004). Standards of evidence: Criteria for efficacy, effectiveness, and dissemination. Falls Church, VA: Society for prevention research.org/Standardsofevidencebook.pdf.

Fearing, J. M. (1969). Emotional problems in pregnancy. *Psychiatry, 32,* 389–410.

Gorung, R. A. R., Dunkell-Schetter, C., Collins, N., Rini, C., & Hobel, C. J. (2005). Psychosocial predictors of prenatal anxiety. *Journal of Social and Clinical Psychology, 24*(4), 497–519.

Grossman, F. K., Eichler, L. S., & Winickoff, S. A. (1980). *Pregnancy, birth, and parenthood.* San Francisco, CA: Jossey-Bass.

Guerreiro da Silva, J. B. (2007). Acupuncture for mild and moderate emotional complaints in pregnancy – A prospective, quasi-randomized, controlled study. *Acupuncture in Medicine, 25*(3), 65–71.

Hall, S. L. (1991). The development of self-concept during the three trimesters of pregnancy. (Doctoral dissertation, The University of Texas at Austin,). *Dissertation Abstracts International, 52*(4), 1953B.

Hodnett, E. D., Fredericks, S. (2003). Support during pregnancy for women at increased risk of low birthweight babies (Cochrane Review). *Cochrane Database of Systematic Reviews, 3,* Art. No.: CD000198. DOI: 10.1002/14651858.

Hodnett, E. D., Gates, S., Hofmeyr, G. J., & Sakala, C. (2007). Continuous support for women during childbirth. *Cochrane Database of Systematic Reviews, 3.* Art. No.: CD003766. DOI: 10.1002/14651858.CD003766.pub2.

Hyle, L. W. (1993) The relationship of sexual abuse to the birthweight of infants born to low income women. (Doctoral dissertation, The University of Maryland)

Kennell, M. D., Klaus, M., McGrath, S., Robertson, S., & Hinkley, C. (1991). Continuous Emotional Support During Labor in a U.S. Hospital. *Journal of the American Medical Association, 17,* 2197–2201.

Kiehl. E. M., & White, M. (2003) Maternal adaptation during childbearing in Norway, Sweden, and the United States. *Scandinavian Journal of Caring Sciences, 17,* 96–103

Kiernan, K., & Pickett, K. E. (2006). Marital status disparities in maternal smoking during pregnancy, breastfeeding, and maternal depression. *Social Science & Medicine, 63,* 335–346.

Kitzman, H., Olds, D., Sidora, K., Henderson, C. R., Hanks, C., Cole, R., et al. (2000). Enduring effects of nurse home visitation on maternal life course. *Journal of the American Medical Association, 282,* 1983–1989.

Koniak-Griffin, D. (1993). Maternal role attainment. *Image, 25,* 257–262.

Kutzner, S. K. (1984). *Adaptation to motherhood from postpartum to early childhood.* Unpublished doctoral dissertation, University of Michigan, Ann Arbor, MI.

Lederman, R. (1989, June). *Prediction of postpartum adaptation from maternal prenatal adaptation scales.* Paper presentation at the second International Nursing Research Conference on Social Support, Seoul, Korea.

Lederman, R. (1990, August). *Predicting anxiety at the onset of active labor for three prenatal instruments.* Presentation at the Ninety-Eighth Annual Convention of the American Psychological Association, Boston, MA.

Lederman, R. P. (Fall, 1995a). Relationship of anxiety, stress, and psychosocial development to reproductive health. *Behavioral Medicine, 21,* 101–112.

Lederman, R. P. (Fall, 1995b). Treatment strategies for anxiety, stress, and developmental conflict during reproduction. *Behavioral Medicine*, *21*, 113–122.

Lederman, R. P. (March 1996). *Psychosocial adaptation in pregnancy: Assessment of seven dimensions of maternal development* (2nd ed.). New York: Springer.

Lederman, R. P. (2008a) *Effectiveness of maternal prenatal psychosocial support for decreasing anxiety in experimental and control groups*. 28th Annual Meeting of the Society of Behavioral Medicine, San Diego, CA, March 22–25, 2008.

Lederman, R. P. (2008b) *Predictiveness of postpartum maternal psychosocial adaptation from prenatal scales of adaptation, dyadic adjustment, and maternal attachment*. 28th Annual Meeting of the Society of Behavioral Medicine, San Diego, CA, March 22–25, 2008

Lederman, R., Harrison, J. A., & Worsham, S. (1992). Psychosocial factors of low birthweight in a multicultural, high-risk population. In K. Wijma & B. von Schoultz (Eds.), *Reproductive life: Advances in research in psychosomatic obstetrics and gynaecology* (pp. 69–74). Casterton Hall, The United Kingdom: Parthenon.

Lederman, E., Lederman, R., & Haller, K. (1981, September). *Dimensions of prenatal maternal adjustment: Congruence between interview and self-report questionnaire responses*. Poster presentation at the Council of Nurse Researchers Annual Meeting, Washington, DC.

Lederman, R., Lederman, E., & Kutzner, S. (1983a, April). *Predicting anxiety at the onset of active labor, part I: Factor structure of pregnancy and labor instruments*. Paper presentation at the 7th Midwest Nursing Research Society Conference, Iowa City, Iowa.

Lederman, R., Lederman, E., & Kutzner, S. (1983b, April). *Predicting anxiety at the onset of active labor, part II: Multiple regression analysis to determine the predictability of three prenatal instruments to stress and anxiety in labor*. Paper presentation at the 7th Midwest Nursing Research Society Conference, Iowa City, IA.

Lederman, E., Lederman, R., Kutzner, S., & Haller, K. (1982a). *Prediction of multiparous mothers' satisfaction with infant care*. Paper presented at the 19th Annual Convention of the American Psychological Association, Washington, DC.

Lederman, E., Lederman, R., Kutzner, S., & Haller, K. (1982b). *Prenatal predictors of multigravid anxiety in labor*. Paper presented at the Tenth Annual Conference of Psychosomatic Obstetrics and Gynecology, San Francisco, CA.

Lederman, R., Lederman, E., Work, B. A., Jr., & McCann, D. S. (1979). Relationship of psychological factors in pregnancy to progress in labor. *Nursing Research*, *28*(2), 94–97.

Lederman, R., Lederman, E., Work, B. A., Jr., & McCann, D. S. (1981). Maternal psychological and physiologic correlates of fetal-newborn health status. *American Journal of Obstetrics and Gynecology*, *139*, 956–958.

Lederman, R., Lederman, E., Work, B. A., Jr., & McCann, D. S. (1985). Anxiety and epinephrine in multiparous labor: Relationship to duration of labor and fetal heart rate pattern. *American Journal of Obstetrics and Gynecology*, *153*(8), 870–877.

Lederman, R., Weingarten, C., & Lederman, E. (1981). Postpartum self-evaluation questionnaire: Measures of maternal adaptation. In R. Lederman & B. Raff (Eds.), *Perinatal parental behavior*. New York, NY: Liss-March of Dimes Birth Defects Foundation: Original Article Series, *17*(6), 201–231.

Leifer, M. (1977). Psychological changes accompanying pregnancy and motherhood. *Genetic Psychology Monographs*, *95*, 55–96.

Leigh, B. & Milgrom, J. (2007). Acceptability of antenatal screening for depression in routine antenatal care. *Austrian Journal of Advanced Nursing*, *24*(3), 14–18

Leite, R. (2007). An exploration of aspects of boundary ambiguity among young, unmarried fathers during the prenatal period. *Family Relations*, *56*, 162–167

Lipsey, M. W. (1993). Theories as methods. Small theories of treatments. *NewDirections of Program Evaluation*. *57*, 5–38.

Lobel, M., Hamilton, J. G., & Cannella, D. T. (2008). Psychosocial perspectives on pregnancy: Prenatal maternal stress and coping. *Social and Personality Psychology Compass*, *2*(4), 1600–1623.

Lowe, N. K. (1987). Individual variation in childbirth pain. *Journal of Psychosomatic Obstetrics and Gynaecology*, *7*, 183–192.

Masters, W. H., Johnson, V. E., & Kolodny, R. C. (1988). *Human Sexuality* (3rd ed.). Boston, MA: Scott, Foresman, and Co.

McGrath, S. K. & Kennell, J. H. (2008). A randomized controlled trial of continuous labor support for middle-class couples: Effect on cesarean delivery rates. Birth, *35*(2), 92–97.

Norbeck, J. S., DeJoseph, J. F., & Smith, R. T. (1996). A randomized trial of an empirically-derived social support intervention to prevent low birth weight among African-American women. *Social Science and Medicine*, *43*(6), 947–954.

Oakley, A., Hickey, D., Rajan, L., & Rigby, A. S. (1996). Social support in pregnancy: Does it have long-term effects? *Journal of Reproductive and Infant Psychology*, *14*, 7–22.

Olds, D. L. (2002). Prenatal and infancy home visiting by Nurses: From Randomized Trials to Community Replication. *Prevention Science, 3*(3), 153–172.

Olds, D., Henderson, C. Jr., Kitzman, H., Eckenrode, J., Cole, R., & Tatelbaum, R. (1998). The promise of home visitation: Results of two randomized trials. *Journal of Community Psychology*, *26*(1), 5–21.

Olds, D. L., Sadler, L., & Kitzman, H. (2007). Programs for parents and infants and toddlers: recent evidence from randomized trials. *Journal of Child Psychology and Psychiatry, 48*(3/4), 355–391.

Pascoe, J. M. (1993). Social support during labor and duration of labor: A community-based study. *Public Health Nursing, 10*, 97–99.

Perren, S., Von Wyl, A., Burgin, D., Simoni, H., & Von Klitzing, K. (2005). Intergenerational transmission of marital quality across the transition to parenthood. *Family Process, 44*(4), 441–459.

Rogers, M. M., Peoples-Sheps, M. D., & Suchrindran, C. (1996). Impact of a social support program and teenage prenatal care use and pregnancy outcomes. *Journal of Adolescent Health, 19*(12):132–140.

Saisto, T. (2001). *Prenatal conflicts about marriage, pregnancy, and motherhood.* Unpublished academic disserction, Univeristy of Helsinki, Helsinki.

Scott, A. G. & Sechrest, L. (1989). Strength of theory and theory of strength. *Evaluation and Program Planning, 12*, 329–336.

Shereshefsky, P. M., & Yarrow, L. J. (Eds.). (1973). *Psychological aspects of a first pregnancy and early postnatal adaptation.* New York, NY: Raven Press.

Sidani, S. & Braden, C. J. (1998). *Evaluating nursing interventions: A theory-driven approach.* Thousand Oaks, CA, Sage.

Sieber, S., Germann, N., Barbir, A., & Ehlert, U. (2006). Emotional well-being and predictors of birth-anxiety, self-efficacy, and psychosocial adaptation in healthy pregnant women. *Acta obstetricia et gynecologica Scandinavica, 85*(10), 1200–1207.

Sleath, B., West, S., Tudor, G., Perreira, K., King, V., & Morrisey, J. (2005). Ethnicity and prenatal depression: Women's experiences and perspectives on communicating about their emotions and feelings during pregnancy. *Patient Education and Counseling, 58*, 35–40.

Solberg, D. A., Butler, J., & Wagner, N. N. (1973). Sexual behavior in pregnancy. *New England Journal of Medicine, 288*, 1098–1103.

Sosa, R., Kennell, J., Klaus, M., Robertson, S., & Urrutia, J. (1980). The effect of a supportive companion or perinatal problems, length of labor, and mother–infant interaction. *The New England Journal of Medicine, 303*, 597–600.

Stark, M. A. (1997). Psychosocial adjustment during pregnancy: The experience of mature gravidas. *Journal of Obstetric, Gynecologic and Neonatal Nursing, 26*(2), 206–211.

Stewart, B. J. & Archbold, P. G. (1993). Nursing intervention studies require outcome measures that are sensitive to change: Part One. *Research in nursing & health. 15*(6):477–81.

Office of the Surgeon General and the Eunice Kennedy Shriver National Institute of Child Health and Human Development (NICHD) (2008). *The Surgeon General's Conference on the Prevention of Preterm Birth,* webcast on June 16 and June 17, 2008.

Talge, N. M., Neal, C., Glover, V., and the Early Stress Transitional Research and Prevention Science Network: Fetal and Neonatal Experience on Child and Adolescent Mental Health, (2007). Antenatal maternal stress and long-term development effects on child neurodevelopment: how and why? *Journal of Child Psychiatry and Psychology*, 48(3/4), 245–261.

Teixeira, J., Martin, D., Prendiville, O., & Glover, V. (2005). The effects of acute relaxation on indices of anxiety during pregnancy. *Journal of Psychosomatic Obstetrics & Gynecology*, 26(4) 271–276.

Terhi, S. (2001). Obstetric, psychological, and pain-related background and treatment of pain-related childbirth. Academic Dissertation. Department of Obstetrics and Gynecology, University of Helsinki, Finland.

Uddenberg, N. (1974). Reproductive adaptation in mother and daughter: A study of personality development and adaptation to motherhood. *Acta Psychiatrica Scandinavica*, 254, 1–115.

Urizar, G. G., Milazzo, M., Le, H. N., Delucchi, K., Sotelo, R., & Munoz, R. F. (2004). Impact of stress reduction instructions on stress and cortisol levels during pregnancy. *Biological Psychology*, 67, 275–282.

Wadhwa, P. D. (2005). Psychneuroendocrine processes in human pregnancy influence fetal development and health. *Psychneuroendocrinology*, 30, 724–723.

Wenner, N. K., Cohen, M. B., Wiegert, E. V., Kvarnes, R. G., Ohaneson, E. M., & Fearing, J. M. (1969). Emotional problems in pregnancy. *Psychiatry*, 32, 389–410.

Weis, K. L. (2006). Maternal identity formation in a military sample: A longitudinal perspective. *Dissertation Abstracts International*. University of North Carolina, Chapel Hill. *Dissertation Abstracts International*, 67, no. 02B p. 812. (UMI No. 3207315)

Weis, K. L., Lederman, R. P., Lilly, A. E., & Schaffer, J. (2008). The relationship of military imposed marital separations on maternal acceptance of pregnancy. *Research in Nursing and Health*, 31, 196–207.

Wuitchik, M., Bakal, D., & Lipshitz, J. (1989). The clinical significance of pain and cognitive activity in latent labor. *Obstetrics & Gynecology*, 73(1), 35–42.

Zachariah, R. C. (1984). Intergeneration attachment and psychological well-being during pregnancy. (Doctoral dissertation, The University of California, 1984). *Dissertation Abstracts International*, 46(5), 1515B.

Zimmer-Gembeck, M. J., & Helfand, M. (1996). Low birthweight in a public prenatal care program: Behavioral and psychosocial intervention. Social Science and Medicine, 43, 187–197.

Appendix A.
Interview Schedules for the Seven Dimensions of Maternal Adaptation to Pregnancy

Interview Schedules[1]

First Interview Session

1. If there are any concerns I don't mention, bring them up as they occur to you.
2. What are you doing now and before your pregnancy? Working? In school?
3. Do you think a mother should continue work or her education after the baby is born? If so, how soon after? Do you plan to return? If so, how soon after? What kinds of arrangements have you made for the care of the baby?
4. To what extent was this pregnancy planned? Initially wanted? How does this compare to your feelings now?
5. What has your pregnancy been like? How are you feeling? Are there any concerns about this pregnancy?
6. How will having a baby change your life? How will you manage at home? Who will help?
7. What do you think about most often when you think about the baby?
8. Do you have any concerns about the sex of the baby?
9. How do you think you will feel about the baby when you are at home with him?
10. Do you think about what kind of mother you want to be? In what ways do you want to be like your mother? In what ways different? Has your relationship to your mother changed since you've been pregnant?
11. How strong or serious are your doubts about being a mother and caring for the baby?
12. Whom did you turn to most often when you had problems as a child? As a teenager? Your mother? Father? Siblings? Friends? A favorite relative?
13. What kinds of reactions have your parents had to your pregnancy?
14. Have your parents helped you make any decisions about caring for the baby? What and how?

---

[1] Please note that the interview schedule is modified when used with multigravidas

15. Since you've been pregnant, have you recalled and discussed with your parents any events from your own childhood? What were they? What were your feelings? What were your parents' reactions? Do you wish it had been different? How would you like to handle this?

16. Have you ever wished you weren't having the baby at this time? If yes, why? What are the details? Does this bother you? How much? Why?

17. Are there any differences in your relationship to your husband1 partner now that you are pregnant? If so, how? Do you feel he understands you?

18. How does your husband/partner feel about this pregnancy? How does he react to you? How much does he help with the household chores? With care of the children?

19. How has your husband's/partner's family reacted to you? To this pregnancy?

20. What are your husband's/partner's primary concerns, if any about this pregnancy? How are they like or different from your own?

21. To what extent do you expect your relationship to your husband/partner to change after the birth of this baby?

22. Is there anything you would like to mention or ask?

Second Interview Session

23. Are there any aspects of the previous interview you would like to discuss?

24. How have you been feeling since I last saw you?

25. Has anything occurred since our last meeting that you would like to discuss now?

26. Do you intend to go or are you presently going to expectant parenthood or labor preparation classes? What do you hope to get out of these classes? Did they help? How do you feel as a result of attending classes? What have you read or discussed with others? Does your husband go to childbirth classes with you? How does he feel about this? Does he help you practice the exercises?

27. What have you heard or read about what labor is like? Do you think it will be like that for you?

28. What do you think about most often in relation to labor? Do you ever dream or daydream about being in labor? Do any dreams or thoughts occur more than once?

29. Do you ever wish you weren't pregnant and didn't have to go through labor? What are the details, circumstances?

30. What were your first thoughts about being in labor?

31. What do you imagine labor and delivery rooms are like?

32. What do you think contractions are like? Are they different in the beginning and the end of labor?

33. What aspect of labor do you think will be most difficult for you? How do you think you will cope with this?

34. Have you ever been in the hospital before? Had surgery? What were your thoughts about the medical and nursing care? About attention given to your

medical, physical, and emotional needs? Did you feel the staff understood you? Do you feel the doctors and nurses caring for you understand you now-your physical needs and feelings?

35. How bothered are you by the doctor's physical exam? By the gynecological exam? What about it seems to bother you?
36. Do you think about your parents and parents-in-law in relation to your labor?
37. Whom do you really want to be with you during labor? Your husband? Your mother? Someone else? What about this person makes him or her desirable at this time?
38. How does your husband/partner seem to react when you try to discuss labor? How are his feelings like and different from your own? Is the adjustment to this pregnancy easier for your husband than for you?
39. Will your husband/partner be with you during labor? During delivery? Do you anticipate he will help you? How much? How does he feel about it?
40. What sorts of things would you be uncomfortable discussing in your husband's/ partner's presence? How freely can you speak with him?
41. Is there anything you would like to ask me about the childbirth experience? Anything else you would like to mention or ask?

Third Interview Session

42. Is there anything from the previous session or anything that has occurred since then that you would like to mention?
43. How are you feeling now?
44. Have you made any recordings in your diary since last time? (Briefly discuss entries made.)
45. Have you made any preparations for the baby? What have you done? (If not, why not?)
46. How aware would you like to be during labor? During delivery? Can you say why you feel this way?
47. What is your reaction to pain in general? To abdominal cramps? Headaches? Minor injuries? How do you manage at these times?
48. How did you react to your first menstrual period?
49. How did you feel about menstruation in the years before you became pregnant?
50. How bothered are you by menstrual pain?
51. Did you ever think that you might be hurt during intercourse? Have you become upset about this? How do you feel about intercourse during pregnancy?
52. Since you became pregnant, is intercourse more or less frequent or the same? How does your husband/partner respond to the differences? Have you found alternative ways for satisfying each other?
53. Do you have any thoughts about what kind of anesthesia, if any, you would like during delivery?
54. Will you accept medication during labor? What are your thoughts about this?

55. Have you anticipated the possibility of losing your temper or of losing control in labor? In what way? How would you feel about it?

56. In second-stage labor you will have the urge to bear down, and you will be asked to push with contractions to assist in delivering your baby. This is the last stage, just before delivery. Is there anything, any feeling or doubt, that would prevent you from bearing down or pushing?

57. Do you sometimes think your body will be inadequate for the baby to pass through? What thoughts do you have about this?

58. What is the worst thing that could happen to you in labor? What will you do if this happens? How would you handle this? How would you feel?

59. What about you as a person will make it easier or more difficult for you to cope with labor and delivery?

60. Did your mother discuss your own delivery with you? When? What things did she mention? How did she feel about it? How did you feel about it?

61. Do you feel everything will turn out well with your delivery? Do you have any doubts about this? How often?

62. If you had to guess, do you think you would do the same, better, or worse than other women in labor?

63. Is there anything you would like to discuss further? This is our last meeting before labor. If any questions arise, you may reach me by phone if you wish to.

Appendix B
Rating Scales For Prenatal Interview

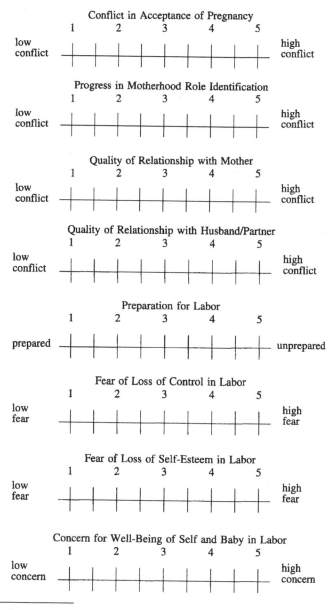

Note. Concern for Well-Being of Self and Baby in Labor is an additional dimension assessed in the Prenatal Self-Evaluation Questionnaire. These are additional concerns that may need to be addressed in interviews as well.

Index